TUBERCULOSIS

TUBERCULOSIS

A foundation for nursing and healthcare practice

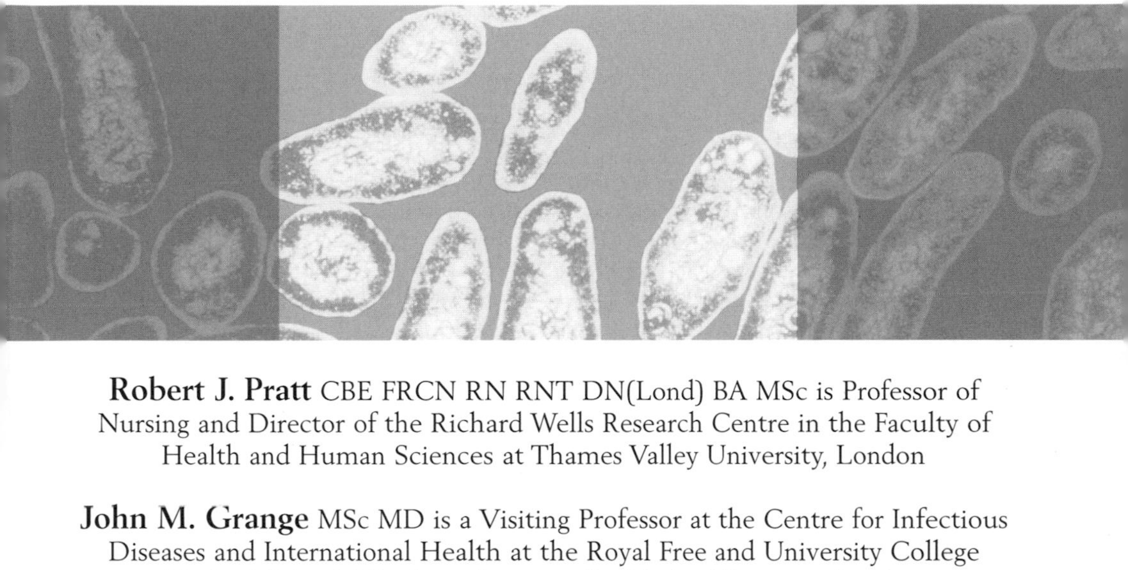

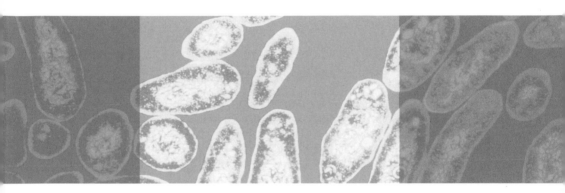

Robert J. Pratt CBE FRCN RN RNT DN(Lond) BA MSc is Professor of Nursing and Director of the Richard Wells Research Centre in the Faculty of Health and Human Sciences at Thames Valley University, London

John M. Grange MSc MD is a Visiting Professor at the Centre for Infectious Diseases and International Health at the Royal Free and University College Medical School, Windeyer Institute for Medical Sciences, London

Virginia G. Williams RN HV BNurs MSc is Head of the Nursing Division for the International Union Against Tuberculosis and Lung Disease (UNION), and Lecturer in the Public Health and Primary Care Unit at the St Bartholomew's School of Nursing and Midwifery, City University, London

Hodder Arnold

A MEMBER OF THE HODDER HEADLINE GROUP

First published in Great Britain in 2005 by
Hodder Education, a member of the Hodder Headline Group,
338 Euston Road, London NW1 3BH

http://www.hoddereducation.co.uk

Distributed in the United States of America by
Oxford University Press Inc.,
198 Madison Avenue, New York, NY10016
Oxford is a registered trademark of Oxford University Press

British Library Cataloguing in Publication Data
A catalogue record for this book is available from the British Library

Library of Congress Cataloging-in-Publication Data
A catalog record for this book is available from the Library of Congress

ISBN-10: 0 340 64568 7
ISBN-13: 978 0 340 64568 0

1 2 3 4 5 6 7 8 9 10

Commissioning Editor: Clare Christian
Development Editor: Heather Smith
Project Editor: Wendy Rooke
Production Controller: Jane Lawrence
Cover Design: Amina Dudhia
Indexer: Dr Laurence Errington

Typeset in 9 on 12pt Berling Roman by Phoenix Photosetting, Chatham, Kent
Printed and bound in Malta

Cover image © Kwangshin Kim/Science Photo Library

Contents

Contributors

Foreword
Professor Sir John Crofton
Emeritus Professor of Respiratory Diseases and Tuberculosis, University of Edinburgh
Honorary President of *TB Alert*

Chapter Authors

Chapter 14 – Adherence to Antituberculosis Therapy
Heather Loveday RN, RNT, MA
Principal Lecturer (Research), Richard Wells Research Centre, Thames Valley University, London
and
Caroline Smales RN, RNT, BSc
Senior Lecturer, Richard Wells Research Centre, Thames Valley University, London

Chapter 18 – Case Management
Joe Rowan RN, BA (Hons), MA
Lecturer Practitioner in Public Health and Tuberculosis, Public Health and Primary Care Unit, City University, London

Chapter Contributors and Advisors

Chapter 17 – The Individualized Care of Patients with Tuberculosis
Tim Stephens RN, BA (Hons) Nursing
Practice Facilitator, Critical Care Outreach Team, Barts and the London NHS Trust
and
Karen Gibson RN, BSc, MSc
Senior Lecturer, Faculty of Health and Human Sciences, Thames Valley University, London

Chapters 19 & 20 – The Tuberculosis Infection Control Plan: Risk Assessment and Risk Management
Evonne Curran RN, MPH
Lead Nurse Infection Control, North Glasgow University Hospitals NHS Trust (Glasgow Royal Infirmary), Honorary Lecturer, Glasgow University
and
Deborah Weston RN, BSc
Infection Control Advisor, East Kent Hospitals NHS Trust

Foreword

This is a most comprehensive book on all aspects of nursing and tuberculosis. It will be of great value as a reference book, particularly for teachers of nursing. Indeed it would be a valuable reference book for many doctors, not only for its extensively referenced medical chapters but also for study of the very practical chapters on nursing details. All too many doctors are less than knowledgeable about the capacities and skills of other health professionals.

Nurses are a vital component in the control, treatment and cure of tuberculosis. Most treatment nowadays is carried out in the community. There treatment is best supervised by nurses in regular contact with the patient. Patients find it much easier to talk to nurses about their anxieties, concern about treatment, problems with family, work etc. Consequently it is the nurses who can best assure that each patient successfully completes treatment. It is they who will most readily learn of the patient's social problems. If they cannot deal with them themselves, they will know where to seek help.

The book also covers in detail the precautions about spread of tuberculous infection to staff and other patients in hospital. These precautions are of supreme importance with patients who harbour, or may harbour, tubercle bacilli with multiple resistance to the standard drugs, especially if there are other patients with HIV infection. Such patients are exquisitely sensitive, both to infection and subsequent disease, even after the most transient exposure.

Readers, of course, may have to adapt the book's extensive recommendations to conditions in their own country or region. This will not be too difficult in most industrialised countries. It may be much more difficult with the often grossly inadequate resources in poor countries. In such countries, senior nurses, or international advisors, could use the book to extract or adapt, and express in simple language comprehensible locally, the book's wide sweep of knowledge and advice.

Professor Sir John Crofton
Emeritus Professor of Respiratory Diseases and Tuberculosis
University of Edinburgh
Honorary President, *TB Alert* (United Kingdom)

Preface

Tuberculosis is one of the most frequent causes of ill health throughout the world and, although in most cases completely curable, it continues to cause 2 million deaths each year and a further million deaths in HIV-infected people.

Nurses need to acquire a general understanding of the underlying science driving the global pandemic of tuberculosis. They need an opportunity to explore the clinical consequences of infection and to increase their skills in using a needs-based model of nursing to assess, plan, implement and evaluate appropriate nursing care and case management for those with active disease. Nurses also need insights into how to support patients in adhering to antituberculosis therapy and to help them confront the stigma that is frequently associated with this disease. Preventing the nosocomial transmission of tubercle bacilli in healthcare settings is a high priority for caregivers and an extensive discussion of the assessment and management of this risk, within the context of clinical governance, facilitates nurses in developing effective infection prevention and control strategies.

This book has been written to provide nurses and other healthcare practitioners with authoritative information that they can use to develop evidence-based prevention and care strategies. Each chapter is introduced with clear and pertinent learning outcomes that can be used as self-assessment tools. Relevant website resources and recommendations for further reading are given at the end of each chapter and a comprehensive glossary of technical terms is provided.

Although generally focused on the nursing management of patients with tuberculosis in the United Kingdom, the general principles described in this text can be adapted and applied in healthcare setting in most countries.

Tuberculosis continues to present an unparalleled threat to the public health of people throughout the world. We hope this book will help nurses and other healthcare practitioners to develop a confident and competent approach to caring for patients with tuberculosis and make the defining difference to the quality of care these patients receive.

RJP, JMG, VGW
London January 2005

Acknowledgements

The authors are indebted to those who have contributed to this text, especially our co-authors, **Joe Rowan**, at City University, London, **Heather Loveday**, **Caroline Smales** and **Karen Gibson** at Thames Valley University, London, and **Tim Stephens** at Barts and the London NHS Trust. **Dr Roger Woodruff** at the Austin and Repatriation Medical Centre in Melbourne, Australia, provided invaluable insights into palliative care for which we're grateful. We also wish to acknowledge the invaluable input of our infection control nurse advisors, **Evonne Curran** at the Glasgow Royal Infirmary and **Deborah Weston** at the East Kent Hospitals NHS Trust.

We are grateful to **Professor Sir John Crofton,** Emeritus Professor of Respiratory Disease and Tuberculosis at the University of Edinburgh, and Honorary President of *TB Alert*, for his critical comment and for providing the Foreword to this text.

We would like to also thank the staff at Hodder Arnold (Hodder Headline Group) in London, our publisher. We are particularly indebted to our editors, **Clare Christian** (commissioning editor)**, Heather Smith** (development editor), **Wendy Rooke**, (project editor) and **Jane Smith** (copy editor) and to **Harriet Stewart-Jones** (proof-reader) and **Dr Laurence Errington** (indexer).

Dedication

This text is dedicated to all of our friends and colleagues at ***TB Alert***, the premier UK tuberculosis charity which is devoted to increasing the awareness in Great Britain of the threat of this disease, both at home and abroad, and to raise funds to support prevention and care efforts in those countries most affected by it. We also dedicate this text to all of our friends, colleagues, students and patients whose lives have been affected by tuberculosis. http://www.tbalert.org

CHAPTER 1

The story of an evolving pandemic

> The captain of all these men of death that came against him to take him away, was the Consumption, for it was that that brought him down to the grave.
>
> *John Bunyan* – The life and death of Mr. Badman *(1680)*.

Introduction

Tuberculosis has been a scourge of mankind since the beginning of recorded human history. It is a disease that should have been reduced to a mere shadow of its former self by judicious use of the powerful control tools now available. Yet, today, there are more cases of tuberculosis in the world than at any period of previous human history. So serious is the threat of this disease that, in 1993, the World Health Organization took the unprecedented step of declaring it a global emergency. To understand why this preventable and treatable disease is now so prevalent, and to know what could be and is being done to conquer it, we must first trace its course through the millennia and see how this course has set the scene for tuberculosis today. In turn, by gaining an understanding of the particular problems that beset us today, we can rationally consider what we need to do in the future to conquer this, the 'white plague', which has taken such a grim toll of human lives for far too long.

Learning outcomes

After studying and reflecting on the material in this chapter, you will be able to:

- give a brief account of the history of tuberculosis,
- describe what is meant by epidemiology and the terms used,
- discuss the factors affecting the spread of tuberculosis in a community,
- describe the present-day extent of tuberculosis in the world,
- explain why tuberculosis today is so different from the disease in the past,
- outline and discuss the major factors – human immunodeficiency virus infection, drug resistance, poverty, inequity and conflict – that pose particular challenges to tuberculosis control.

HISTORY OF TUBERCULOSIS

There is skeletal evidence of tuberculosis in what is now south-west Germany as far back as 5000 BC and in Egyptian mummies dating back to 4000 BC. By around 2500 BC to 1500 BC, tuberculosis was well established in Europe and probably came to Britain 1000 or more years later during the Roman occupation.

Tuberculosis (or a tuberculosis-like disease) is now known to have been endemic in American Indians living in some regions of North and South America long before their first contact with Europeans and probably since pre-historic times.

The earliest written descriptions of a disease that was almost certainly tuberculosis are found in the *Rig Veda*, dating back to between 2000 and 1500 BC. In this and other early Indian literature, the disease was called *Rogaraj* – the king of diseases – and *Rajayakshma* – the disease of kings.

Various manifestations of tuberculosis have been recorded throughout the ages. In ancient Greece, Hippocrates (c. 460–c. 370 BC), the physician who is recognized as the father of medicine, described pulmonary tuberculosis and called it **phthisis**, a Greek word meaning 'to waste away'. Other early physicians referred to pulmonary tuberculosis as **consumption** and described extrapulmonary forms of tuberculosis, including spinal tuberculosis (also known as **Pott's disease**, named after Sir Percival Pott, an eighteenth-century surgeon at St Bartholomew's Hospital, London) and **scrofula** (enlarged, sometimes discharging, tuberculous lymph glands in the neck). Physicians continued to use the terms 'consumption' and 'phthisis' to describe pulmonary tuberculosis well into the first decades of the twentieth century. The term **tuberculosis** is in allusion to the pulmonary lesions first observed by Hippocrates and termed **tubercles** because they looked like small potato tubers. The term tubercle appears in the writings of the French pathologist Franciscus Sylvius (1614–1672) and the English physician Richard Morton (1637–1698). The first use of the word tuberculosis as the name of the disease is accredited to the German physician Johann Schönlein (1793–1864), who also described purpura and introduced the term haemophilia. Probably first used around 1840, the name tuberculosis came into more general use during the early part of the twentieth century.

The natural history of tuberculosis was described in the early nineteenth century by the French physicians Gaspard Laurent Bayle (1774–1816) and René Laënnec (1781–1826), both of whom died from the disease. Bayle, by his detailed pathological studies, put the investigation of tuberculosis on a firm scientific basis, while the invention of the stethoscope by his close friend Laënnec in 1816 facilitated detailed descriptions of the clinical signs of the disease in the human lung.

The bacterial cause of tuberculosis, initially simply termed the tubercle bacillus but later formally named *Mycobacterium tuberculosis*, was identified in 1882 by the German microbiologist Robert Koch. Following this important discovery, Koch was appointed a 'civil servant' and came under great pressure from the German government to discover a cure for the disease. In 1890, he attempted to use injections of a heat-concentrated filtrate of the medium in which tubercle bacilli had been grown (a preparation known as Old Tuberculin) as a therapeutic agent for tuberculosis, but with very variable results. Although Old Tuberculin was not a reliable treatment for active tuberculosis, in 1907 the Austrian physician Clemens von Pirquet used it as a skin test reagent to indicate previous infection by *M. tuberculosis*. This laid the foundations for the use of tuberculin in **Mantoux** and **Heaf** tests, which continue to be used today as important diagnostic and epidemiological tools.

In 1898, at Harvard University, the American bacteriologist Theobald Smith described the bovine tubercle bacillus *Mycobacterium bovis*, a variant of *M. tuberculosis* that infects and causes disease in cattle. Although there was some initial confusion and controversy over the role of *M. bovis* as a cause of tuberculosis in human beings (due to an error by none less than Robert Koch), a growing awareness of its importance in causing human tuberculosis led to the commencement of animal tuberculosis control programmes in several industrialized countries during the early decades of the twentieth century. These programmes were based on the identification (by tuberculin testing) and slaughter of infected cattle, meat inspection and the widespread heat-treatment (pasteurization) of cows' milk. In several of the industrially developed nations, including the UK, Canada and the USA, this had a dramatic effect on reducing the number of new cases of human tuberculosis, especially amongst farm workers and children.

During the time that the serious public health threat of bovine tuberculosis was being brought under control, the causative bacillus, *M. bovis*, was being harnessed into the service of humankind as a vaccine to prevent tuberculosis. A strain of this bacillus was gradually weakened (attenuated) by repeated subculturing by the French bacteriologists Albert Léon Calmette and Camille Guérin. Eventually the vaccine, termed **Bacille Calmette–Guérin** (BCG), was produced and first used in 1921 and continues to be used throughout the world today.

In 1944, *streptomycin*, the first antibiotic that was truly effective in treating tuberculosis, was discovered by the soil microbiologists Selman Waksman and Albert Schatz, working at Rutgers Agricultural College in New Brunswick, New Jersey. This was quickly followed by the discovery of other drugs, notably *isoniazid* and *para-aminosalicylic acid* (PAS), which, together with streptomycin, would prove to be almost miraculous in the treatment of tuberculosis. Since then, an impressive repertoire of drugs has been developed to treat tuberculosis, including *rifampicin*, *ethambutol* and *pyrazinamide*.

Even a brief study of the history of tuberculosis reveals the major impact made by the disease throughout human history and its challenge to the efforts of countless medical scientists. More extensive historical reviews are to be found in several excellent books and chapters.[1–5]

INTRODUCING EPIDEMIOLOGY

Epidemiology is the study of the causes, distribution, frequency and control of disease in populations. It is characterized by having a 'population perspective', that is, it attempts to relate disease events or individuals with disease to the population from which they derive. The word **epidemic** comes from the Greek word *epidêmos*, meaning 'on, or upon, the people', and was originally used to describe sudden outbreaks of disease such as plague or cholera. It has the same meaning today and is used to describe an outbreak of a contagious disease that spreads rapidly and widely. The term **pandemic** refers to an epidemic that occurs over a wide geographical area, such as the current global pandemic of human immunodeficiency virus (HIV) disease. By contrast, the term **endemic** refers to an infection or disease that is present, and usually prevalent, in a population or geographical area at all times. It can, for example, be stated that some level of active tuberculosis is endemic in many countries. Endemic disease may, at times, become epidemic, and epidemics may, of course, become pandemics.

Defining the terms used in epidemiology

The epidemiological terms commonly used to describe the rate or 'disease frequency' in the community are prevalence, incidence, the attack rate, the annual infection rate or annual risk of infection, the contagion (or transmission) parameter and the disease ratio (Box 1.1).

BOX 1.1 Definition of some terms used in the science of epidemiology

Prevalence	The total number of cases of a disease present in a defined population at or over a given time
Annual prevalence	The total number of cases of a disease present in a defined population over a period of 1 year
Point prevalence	The total number of cases of a disease present in a defined population at a precise time, such as a given date
Incidence rate	The number of *new* cases of a disease notified in a defined population over a specified period of time, usually 1 year
Annual infection rate or annual risk of infection	The number of people in a defined population who are infected with a given microbial pathogen over a period of 1 year
Attack rate	The incidence rate in a specific episode of risk
Contagion or transmission parameter	The average number of people infected by a single infectious source case
Disease ratio	The risk of a person infected by an infectious agent developing clinically evident active disease

Prevalence refers to the actual number of cases of an infectious disease at or over a given time in a specified population and is usually given as the number of cases over a year – **annual prevalence** – or over a much shorter period of time – **point prevalence**. The latter is important in monitoring an acute illness such as influenza, whereas the former is appropriate for a much more chronic disease such as tuberculosis. For example, we could count the number of all people who were living in London during 2003 and those who had active tuberculosis, irrespective of when they were diagnosed. The total number of people with the disease would be the prevalence rate of tuberculosis in London in that year. It is conventional to express the prevalence, and the incidence as defined below, as the number of those with the disease in every 100 000 of the population.

The **incidence rate** is the number of *new* cases of a disease which are notified over a specified period of time, usually a year, in either the total population or in a specified unit of population at risk. For example, counting the number of new cases of tuberculosis that occurred in people known to be infected with HIV in London during 1996 would give us the incidence rate of tuberculosis in this population for that year. The **attack rate** is a special form of incidence rate that is used in situations in which there is a specific episode of risk. An example might be a group of nurses who were exposed to a patient with infectious tuberculosis for a short period of time before that patient was diagnosed and rendered non-infectious by therapy. The attack rate would be the proportion of those nurses who became infected with *M. tuberculosis* following this brief period of exposure. In calculating attack rates, it is not necessary to specify a time period because it is assumed that the group (population) has been observed for the period in which it was at risk following the episode of infection.

The **contagion** (or **transmission**) **parameter** is the average number of people infected by a single infectious source case and is affected by overcrowding and other living and working conditions such as ventilation and exposure to sunlight. The **annual infection rate** or **annual risk of infection** is the number of people infected with a microbial pathogen in the course of a year. This may be considerably higher than the actual incidence of the disease, as not all those infected with the tubercle bacillus actually develop active and clinically evident disease as a result.

The ratio of infection to overt disease is termed the **disease ratio** and is affected by the age and immune status of the infected people and the virulence of the infecting organism. Thus, Louis Pasteur remarked that the outcome of an infection depends on the state of the 'seed' (the infecting organism) and the 'soil' (the infected person). As a general rule, the disease ratio in neonates and infants following infection with *M. tuberculosis* is relatively high, being over 30 per cent. Later in life, around 5 per cent of those infected develop so-called primary tuberculosis within 5 years of infection, and a further 5 per cent develop post-primary disease at some future period in their lives. This disease ratio varies from region to region, being affected by various factors, including genetic and nutritional ones and causes of immune suppression, but there are very few data concerning the exact disease ratio in any given region. Not all forms of tuberculosis are infectious – about half of those with overt disease, or 1 in 20 of those infected, are able to transmit the disease to other people.

The contagion parameter and the disease ratio determine the epidemiological trend of an infectious disease over time in a community. Thus, for example, if 1 in 20 infected people developed the infectious form of tuberculosis and each of these infected 20 other people, the incidence of the disease in a relatively stable community would remain constant. If the contagion parameter was lowered by reducing crowding in living and working conditions, however, the incidence would decline, but, conversely, if the risk of developing overt disease after infection was increased in a community by, for example, widespread HIV infection, the incidence would increase.

Epidemics of infectious diseases often wax and wane throughout the course of time, alternating between periods of high and increasing incidence and low and decreasing incidence, much like a roller coaster ride. This has been the pattern of tuberculosis in many countries over the last 500 years.[5]

Ideally, the recorded prevalence and incidence of tuberculosis are determined by notification of all diagnosed cases. In practice, epidemiology based on notification gives a gross underestimate of the actual numbers of cases of the disease. In many regions only a proportion of patients are diagnosed, primarily those with open pulmonary tuberculosis detected by microscopical examination of sputum smears. Cases of sputum smear-negative pulmonary, extrapulmonary and childhood tuberculosis are often underdiagnosed. Also, even in those countries where notification is a statutory requirement, physicians not infrequently forget or neglect to notify cases to the appropriate authorities.

Estimates of prevalence are thus often made indirectly by means of the tuberculin test, which, subject to various factors considered in Chapter 7, detects those infected by the tubercle bacillus.[6,7] This estimation may best be done by tuberculin testing a group of people annually and noting the number that have converted to tuberculin reactivity (i.e. development of a positive tuberculin test) over the previous 12 months. This gives a direct indication of the annual infection rate but is often impracticable. Alternatively, therefore, people of a given age, such as a group of military recruits, may be tested on just one occasion and the number of reactors compared with the number in the analogous groups tested in previous years. Although only giving an indirect estimate of the annual infection rate, it allows increases or decreases in the transmissibility of the disease in the community to be determined. From this information the total number of cases of active tuberculosis and the number of infectious cases in a community may be extrapolated, although various confounding factors render the calculated numbers no more than a rough estimate.[8]

The epidemiology of tuberculosis in former days

After becoming established in Europe approximately 2000 years before the birth of Christ, both the prevalence and incidence of tuberculosis continued to increase in each following century. The reasons for this continuing increase, which would ultimately lead to a global tuberculosis pandemic stemming from Europe by the beginning of the eighteenth century, included the following.

Population growth

For most of human existence, the world population has increased slowly, by about 0.002 per cent per year, or 20 per million inhabitants. From the end of the Middle Ages, populations increased in all European countries and this increase accelerated dramatically during the seventeenth and eighteenth centuries, principally due to advances in sanitation, technology and food distribution which had brought about a declining death rate. At the beginning of the eighteenth century, the population of England and Wales was about 5.5 million and had increased to 9 million by the beginning of the nineteenth century.

Urbanization, poverty and malnutrition

Poverty, starvation, overcrowding and poor housing were all factors associated with disease and deaths from tuberculosis long before Koch identified the tubercle bacillus. From the end of the seventeenth century onwards, urbanization increased and European cities became overcrowded with impoverished and malnourished citizens. As more and more people in England moved into the cities and became infected (and infectious), the number of new cases of tuberculosis started to increase dramatically. This process of urbanization, with increased exposure and infection, accelerated during the Industrial Revolution in the late eighteenth and early nineteenth centuries in Great Britain. Tuberculosis had gone from being endemic to becoming epidemic during the mid-sixteenth century, and the seeds were planted for one of the great European plagues, which would, for hundreds of years to come, change the course of history throughout the world.

The European epidemic

The incidence of tuberculosis was extremely high in London during the middle of the seventeenth century and the disease accounted for approximately 20 per cent of all deaths in the period 1656–1700. From the middle of the seventeenth to the beginning of the eighteenth century, deaths from tuberculosis decreased somewhat, falling to just 12 per cent in 1700. The worst was yet to come, however, and tuberculosis would come to dominate the eighteenth century in Great Britain. From 1730 onwards, the percentage of deaths in the general population caused by tuberculosis relentlessly increased, rising to 26 per cent by the end of the eighteenth century. In addition to pulmonary tuberculosis, many people, particularly young people, in England suffered from scrofula (enlarged, sometimes discharging, tuberculous lymph glands in the neck) during the nineteenth century, principally as a result of drinking milk containing *M. bovis*. Migration of Europeans to America, South Africa and Australia in the eighteenth, but more significantly in the nineteenth, century facilitated the spread of tuberculosis out of Europe (as colonization had done in earlier centuries). In both Europe and America, tuberculosis raged with the fervour of a medieval plague, reaching its zenith between the end of the eighteenth and the first half of the nineteenth centuries.

The white plague

As pulmonary tuberculosis gained in epidemic force throughout most of Europe and North America during the eighteenth and nineteenth centuries, becoming known as the **white plague of Europe**, it swept through most major cities, especially London, Paris, Berlin and New York City, infecting half the world's population and killing millions of people every year. By the end of the nineteenth century, tuberculosis was responsible for one in seven deaths among adults, principally young adults, and it would continue into the twenty-first century to cause more deaths throughout the world than any other infectious disease known to humankind.

The decline of tuberculosis in Europe and America during the nineteenth century

In some cities in the USA, and in some countries in Europe, the number of people with tuberculosis started to decline slowly from the middle of the nineteenth century. In England and Wales, this decline started around 1838 and would continue, if somewhat unevenly, well into the next century. In Germany, a significant decline in mortality from tuberculosis commenced only after Robert Koch had discovered the bacterial cause of the disease, while in Ireland and Norway, tuberculosis mortality continued to increase during the nineteenth century.

Countrywide, statistical data for tuberculosis mortality in the USA do not exist until after 1933, although there are reliable statistics for particular cities and states. In New York City (and in the state of Massachusetts), deaths from tuberculosis continued to increase throughout the nineteenth century and only showed a steady decline from 1882 onwards.

The reasons suggested for the decline in tuberculosis and deaths caused by it during this period in different parts of Europe and in North America have always been somewhat controversial. A widely held view is that the decline in tuberculosis mortality in those regions during the nineteenth century had little to do with medical treatment or public health measures, but was principally due to a general increase in the standard of living, including better nutrition, housing and working conditions and less crowding.

Other workers, by contrast, maintain that the association between the decline in the prevalence of tuberculosis and improving socio-economic conditions is not so straightforward. They assert that the decline in prevalence was not inevitable but resulted from the cumulative result of many public health initiatives introduced by determined and dedicated people, often in the face of considerable apathy and backsliding by politicians, the medical profession and health authorities.[9] The term 'Luddite trap' has been applied to the notion that, as poverty is the underlying cause of the spread of tuberculosis, focus on the alleviation of poverty was all that was required and specific disease control measures were unnecessary.[10] (The word Luddite is applied to nihilists who resist innovation and is derived from Lancashire textile workers, led by Ned Ludd, who opposed mechanization in the Industrial Revolution and even smashed up machines.) An important example of a specific control measure was the isolation of infectious patients in infirmaries, hospitals and sanatoria.

During the twentieth century, the decline in the number of people with tuberculosis accelerated, in both North America and Europe, this time fuelled by an understanding of its contagious nature, and from the 1950s onwards, the availability of effective antituberculosis chemotherapy and, to a lesser extent, vaccination and the eradication of bovine tuberculosis. Unfortunately, the decreasing incidence of tuberculosis in the industrially developed nations led to complacency, a sense that the disease had been 'conquered', a dismantling of the tuberculosis control services and a loss of diagnostic awareness. Indeed, the complacency set in while the prevalence, although declining, was still very high. As early as 1908, Leonard Williams bemoaned the widespread backsliding and complacency and wrote, in a paper intriguingly entitled *The worship of Moloch* and full of delightful tongue-in-cheek remarks, 'The crusade against consumption may be said to have degenerated into a pious opinion that the (tubercle) bacillus resembles the socialist in being a very wicked and obtrusive person whose existence it is well that people of refinement should forget'.[11] Williams added, 'And the pity, nay the horror of it all, is that the backsliding is most noticeable precisely where militant activity should be most conspicuous'.

Predictably, like the proverbial thief in the night, the disease returned and, following serious outbreaks, notably in New York City, the control services were hastily reassembled and the soaring incidence reversed at enormous cost. The American public health expert Lee Reichman has picturesquely termed this situation the 'U-shaped curve of concern'.[12]

TUBERCULOSIS TODAY

As indicated above, the decline in the incidence of tuberculosis that had been observed in several industrialized nations over a century or so has now reversed. (Of course, such a decline never took place, or occurred very slowly, in the developing nations, but this was generally and conveniently overlooked.) This reversal and, in particular, several widely reported cases of tuberculosis that awoke the general population and politicians to the seriousness of the risk of disease led to calls for action and, in 1993, the declaration of tuberculosis as a global emergency.

This declaration by the World Health Organization (WHO) was made immediately after a conference held in London entitled 'Tuberculosis: back to the future'.[13] This title implied that, in a sense, a historic disease was coming back, but it also implied that history was not merely repeating itself. Thus, the current pandemic of tuberculosis differs in many respects from the previous situation. For example, we now have a very powerful tool at our disposal – short-course chemotherapy – for overcoming this disease, yet because of gross misuse of this tool we are faced with the spectre of epidemics of drug-resistant tuberculosis. Additionally, we have the increasing impact of HIV infection, the most prevalent of all the factors disposing to tuberculosis. Finally, we live in a very different world politically. Until a few decades ago, tuberculosis was rife in the Western world and there was a strong incentive to develop cures for the disease, even if the cost was high. Many other countries were 'colonies' of the wealthier ones in which the remedies were developed and deployed, and were, to a very variable and generally suboptimal extent, beneficiaries of these new scientific developments. Nowadays, the world powers are not the somewhat paternalistic colonizing nations, but those who control the huge multinational companies and banks whose interest in human welfare, with a few notable and encouraging exceptions, is very far down on their agenda, except when a threat to their own health and welfare is perceived.

Pharmaceutical companies are usually unwilling to develop drugs unless there is likely to be a high financial gain. Thus, only a handful of new drugs for the treatment of widespread killers such as tuberculosis and malaria have emerged over the past decade, compared to thousands of drugs for the 'lifestyle illnesses' of those in the affluent nations. Sadly, globalization, which was meant to bring the human race together into one caring family, has had the very opposite effect, and among the first casualties was health. This situation may change for the better, however, as a result of the establishment in the year 2000 of a global alliance for tuberculosis drug development (see Chapter 13).

THE BURDEN OF TUBERCULOSIS IN THE WORLD TODAY

The number of people with active tuberculosis at a given time is just the tip of an iceberg, as many more are infected by the tubercle bacillus and are therefore at risk of developing the disease (Fig. 1.1). The WHO estimates that one-third of the world's population, around 2000 million people, are infected with *M. tuberculosis*.[14] The percentage of the population infected varies from region to region: in Europe, around 11 per cent are infected, mostly elderly people, while more than half the population may be infected in some tropical countries, a high proportion of them younger people.

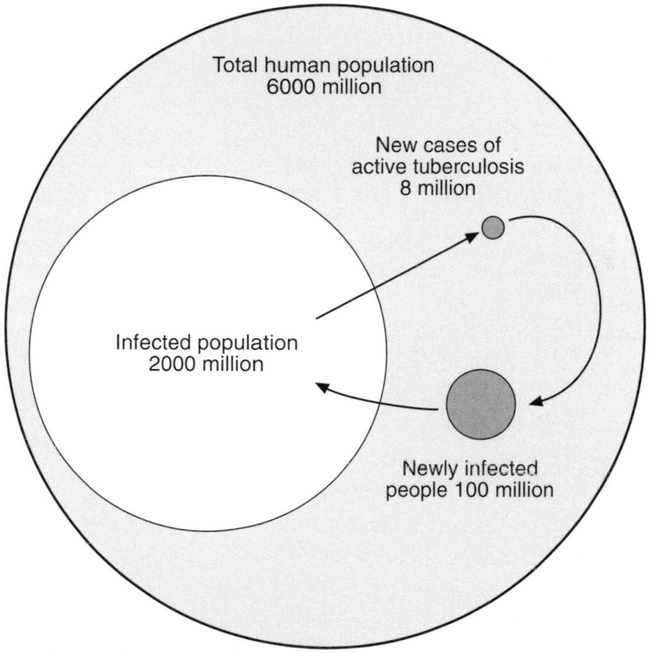

FIGURE 1.1 *The dynamics of tuberculosis in the global human population.*

A comprehensive WHO survey based on data from 1997 showed that, from this pool of infected people, 7.96 million developed active tuberculosis (range, 6.3–11.1 million) in that year.[15] Around 1.5 million cases occurred in sub-Saharan Africa, nearly 3 million in South-East Asia, and more than a quarter of a million in Eastern Europe. Although cheap and effective therapy is available, an estimated 1.87 million people (range 1.4–2.8 million) died of the disease in that year, equivalent to 23 per cent – almost a quarter – of the patients. Indeed, worldwide, tuberculosis accounts for one in seven deaths among young adults, and a quarter of all *preventable* deaths.[16]

The estimated number of new cases rose from almost 8.0 million in 1997 to 8.4 million in 1999 and 8.7 million in 2000.[17] This rise was largely due to the increase in the incidence of tuberculosis in those African countries most affected by the HIV/acquired immunodeficiency syndrome (AIDS) pandemic. The WHO expects that, if there are no changes in control efforts, there will be 10.2 million new cases in 2005, with Africa having more cases than any other WHO region. In the year 2002, 80 per cent of the world's tuberculosis patients lived in 22 countries, as shown in Table 1.1.[17] Fifty per cent of the patients lived in just five countries – India, China, Indonesia, Nigeria and Bangladesh – but this is partly explained by the huge populations of these countries.

TABLE 1.1 The estimated incidence of tuberculosis in the 22 high-burden countries, 2002

Country	Population (thousands)	Number of tuberculosis patients (thousands)	Rate per 100 000 population
India	1 008 937	1856	184
China	1 275 133	1365	107
Indonesia	212 092	595	280
Nigeria	113 862	347	305
Bangladesh	137 439	332	242
Ethiopia	62 908	249	397
Philippines	75 653	249	330
Pakistan	141 256	247	175
South Africa	43 309	228	526
Russian Federation	145 491	193	132
UR Congo	50 948	163	320
Kenya	30 669	149	484
Vietnam	78 137	148	189
Tanzania	35 119	126	359
Brazil	170 406	116	68
Thailand	62 806	88	140
Uganda	23 300	82	351
Myanmar	47 749	80	168
Mozambique	18 292	79	433
Cambodia	13 104	75	572
Zimbabwe	12 627	70	584
Afghanistan	21 765	70	321
Total	**3 781 004**	**6910**	**183**
Global total	6 053 531	8735	144

Owing to the chronic nature of the disease and the limited resources for effective diagnosis and treatment in many countries, there are at any given time approximately 20 million people with active tuberculosis. Around half of these have infectious forms of the disease and infect some 100 million people (more than 1 per cent of the world's population) annually.

Around 95 per cent of cases of tuberculosis, and 98 per cent of deaths due to it, occur among people living in the developing nations but, going hand in hand with poverty and HIV infection, this disease is (as described below) re-emerging in industrialized nations as a very ominous threat to public health. On a global scale, tuberculosis accounts for more preventable ill-health and death than any other single pathogen in existence today. Although AIDS has now replaced tuberculosis as the leading infectious cause of death, it must be borne in mind that approximately a third of AIDS-related deaths are, in fact, due to tuberculosis.[18]

The WHO estimates that, with the present level of tuberculosis control, 1 billion people will be infected between the years 2000 and 2020, 200 million will develop active tuberculosis and 35 million will die of it. Although Africa has experienced a particular increase in the incidence of tuberculosis due to the HIV pandemic, most of the cases of tuberculosis occur in the more populous Asian countries. As mentioned above, more than half the cases of tuberculosis in the world occur in just five countries – Bangladesh, China, India, Indonesia and Pakistan – and future trends will critically depend on the spread of HIV infection in those countries. The current burden of tuberculosis may be summed up as:

- at least 8 million people develop active tuberculosis every year,
- more people die from tuberculosis than from any other curable infectious disease in the world,
- every second, someone in the world is infected with the tubercle bacillus,
- someone dies of tuberculosis every 15 seconds,
- every day, 25 000 people develop active tuberculosis,
- tuberculosis costs the world an estimated US$12 billion annually,
- one person with infectious tuberculosis infects between 10 and 15 people in 1 year.

TUBERCULOSIS IN THE INDUSTRIALIZED NATIONS

After decades of decline, tuberculosis is on the increase in many parts of the industrialized world. In the USA, the incidence of tuberculosis has continued to decline over the past several decades, from more than 84 000 cases in 1953 to a nadir of approximately 22 000 cases in 1984. After that year, a resurgence occurred in the USA, especially in the age range 25–40 years, principally due to the prevalence of HIV infection in this group and homelessness.[19,20] By 1992, the numbers of reported cases had climbed to 26 673, but a massive response from the federal and state health authorities brought this down to an all-time low of 14 871 cases in 2003.[71] However, the 1.4 per cent decrease between 2002 and 2003 was the smallest since the rigorous control measures were instituted in 1992, emphasizing the important lesson that should have been learned from recent history, that sustained control efforts are essential to prevent further resurgences of the disease.[12]

In the UK, the incidence of tuberculosis declined throughout the twentieth century (except for a slight increase during the Second World War) until the late 1980s, when a slow but steady increase in the number of notified cases was observed (Figs 1.2 and 1.3). Between 1987 and 2000, the notified cases of tuberculosis rose by 21 per cent in England and Wales and by 73 per cent in London where, in the year 2000, 2938 cases (43 per cent of the total for England and Wales) occurred.[22] The distribution of cases was not uniform in London. Whereas very few cases were notified from the more affluent governmental districts (boroughs), the incidence in other boroughs approached that seen in some cities in developing nations.

Unlike the USA, there is no evidence as yet to suggest that HIV infection is responsible for the upsurge of tuberculosis in the UK. The increase in notifications of tuberculosis in Britain is mainly due to tuberculosis in people who have recently immigrated, or whose families immigrated, into the UK from the Indian subcontinent (India, Pakistan, Bangladesh), where the prevalence and incidence of tuberculosis are high. Table 1.2 shows

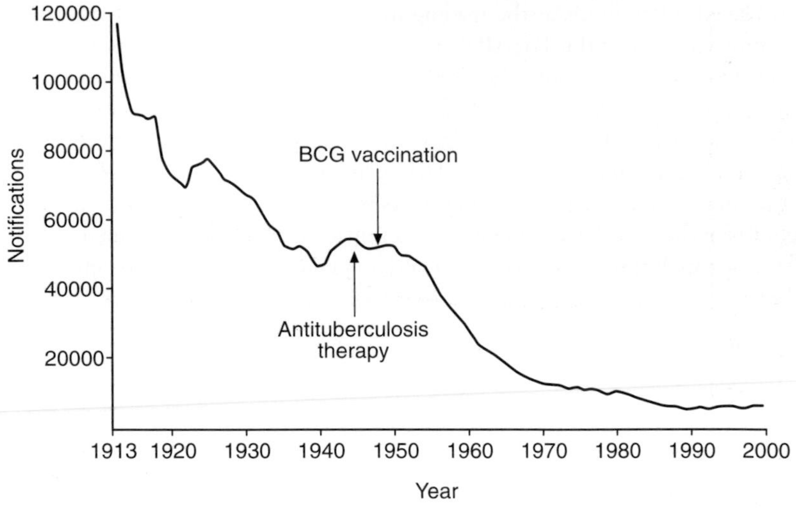

FIGURE 1.2 *Total annual number of notifications of all forms of tuberculosis, England and Wales, 1913–2000. (Data from the Public Health Laboratory Service.)*

TABLE 1.2 Number of cases of tuberculosis per 100 000 of the population in England and Wales, 1999, according to ethnic origin of the patients

Ethnic origin of patients	Number of cases per 100 000 population
Black African	226.62
Pakistani	137.17
Indian	110.56
Chinese	61.39
Bangladeshi	59.47
Black Caribbean	28.67
Black other	17.40
White	3.74
Other	43.01

the wide differences in the incidence of tuberculosis in the various ethnic groups in England and Wales.[22] Other groups in the industrially developed nations who are at an increased risk for tuberculosis include the elderly, the homeless, particularly vagrants and 'travellers', and anyone who is immunocompromised, not just those who are infected with HIV.[19]

TUBERCULOSIS AND POVERTY

The association between poverty and tuberculosis has been well recognized for centuries. Likewise, as described above, the decline in the prevalence of the disease in the industrialized nations has been linked to socio-economic development, although the precise nature of the link is open to question. There is a definite link between poverty and the prevalence of tuberculosis in the developing nations, where 95 per cent of cases of the disease and 98 per

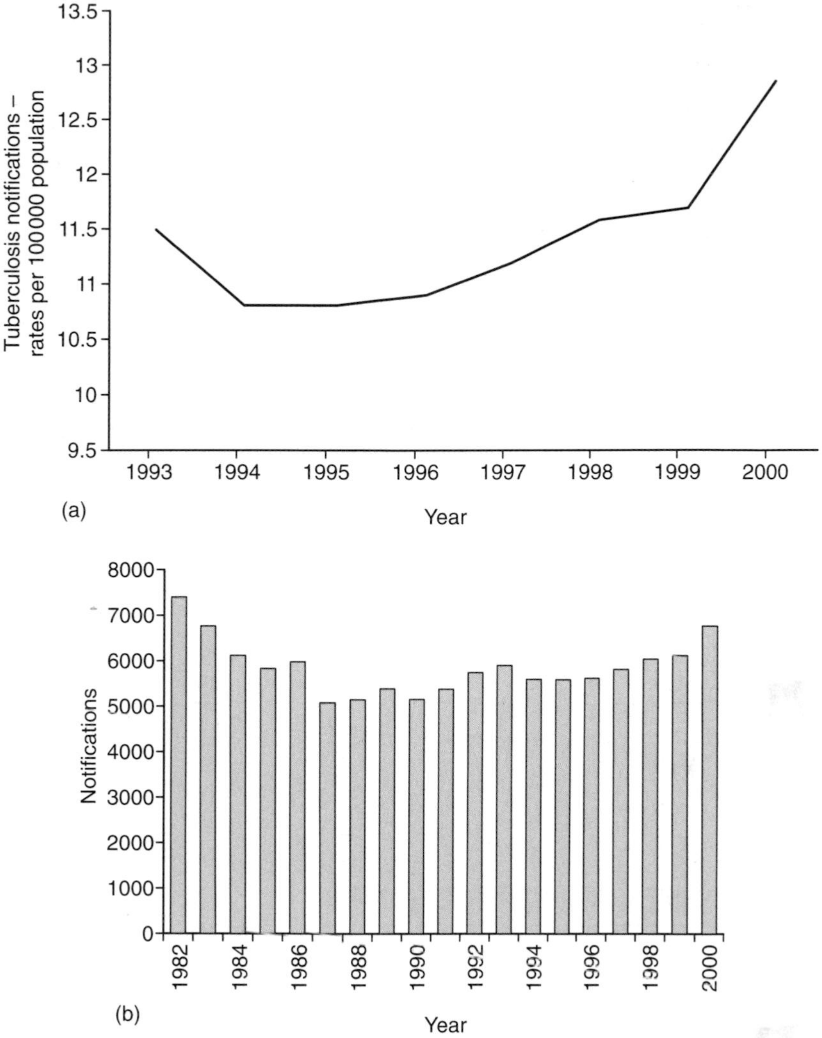

FIGURE 1.3 *Tuberculosis notification rates per 100 000 population, England and Wales, 1993–2000. (Data from the Public Health Laboratory Service Communicable Disease Surveillance Centre, based on statutory notifications.)*

cent of deaths due to it occur. Overcrowding, malnutrition and concurrent infections undoubtedly contribute to this, as does the rising incidence of HIV infection in some regions, as described below. A very important factor, however, is the poor quality of medical services resulting in a failure to detect and cure many of those with open, infectious, tuberculosis.

Not only is tuberculosis a disease affecting the poor in the developing nations, it is also a major cause of poverty. More than three-quarters of cases occur in the economically active age range of 14–54 years; on average, a case of tuberculosis in a household reduces the income by 25 per cent, and the death of an adult from this disease causes 15 years of lost income.[23]

Poverty is also rife in the so-called wealthy nations where, in fact, there is a great and growing division between those who receive an adequate and steady income and those who do not. In England and Wales, between 1980 and 1992, the incidence of tuberculosis rose by 35 per cent in the poorest 10 per cent of the population and by 13 per cent in the next poorest 20 per cent, but there was no increase in the remaining relatively better off 70 per cent.[24] In London, a clear association between risk of tuberculosis and overcrowding has been demonstrated, irrespective of the ethnic origins of the patients.

In addition to overcrowding, exposure to smoke from 'biomass' cookers, using wood or, in some regions, cow dung as fuel, is a clearly established risk factor for tuberculosis.[25] This was once a risk factor in the UK, as picturesquely described by Richard Morton in his book *Phthisiologia*, published in 1689: '... also a foggy and thick Air, and that which is filled with the Smoak of Coals, does extreamly promote a Consumption by vitiating the Animal Spirits, which are necessary to the Natural Fermentation of the Blood; and also by stuffing and weakening the Lungs that serve for Respiration, which are the Seat and Theatre of this Distemper'. Coal fires are a thing of the past in most industrialized nations but, for many, the same injurious effects are wilfully induced by the inhalation of tobacco smoke. Despite the very clear warnings issued by the WHO and various governments on the grave health hazards of smoking, many people, including young and educated people, continue to indulge in this unhealthy and antisocial habit. Several studies, notably an extensive one among Chinese public health workers, have firmly established that smoking is a major risk factor for tuberculosis, even when all confounding factors are accounted for.[26] An extensive retrospective study in India revealed that men who smoke are four to five times more likely to die of tuberculosis than non-smokers (women are largely unaffected, as, sensibly, few Indian women smoke) and that smoking leads to almost 200 000 additional tuberculosis-related deaths annually, usually of young adults.[27] Anti-smoking campaigns, stricter legislation to prevent advertising and smoking in public places and, in particular, a good example set by nurses and other tuberculosis care workers could therefore contribute substantially to a reduction of this risk.

TUBERCULOSIS AND THE HIV/AIDS PANDEMIC

In the words of the WHO, HIV infection is 'fuelling the tuberculosis epidemic' as it is now the most important predisposing factor for the development of active tuberculosis. As described above, a non-immunocompromised person who has overcome primary tuberculosis infection has about a 5 per cent chance of developing post-primary tuberculosis later in life. In a person infected with both *M. tuberculosis* and HIV, the risk of developing active tuberculosis rises to around 8 per cent *each year* – a greatly increased risk.[28] If an HIV-infected person becomes primarily infected or re-infected by the tubercle bacillus, the risk of progressing to active tuberculosis is very high, especially if he or she has had AIDS-defining conditions. Furthermore, the disease process, which usually takes years or even decades to develop, is 'telescoped' down to just a few months. Little wonder, therefore, that co-infection with *M. tuberculosis* and HIV has been termed 'the cursed duet' and that, in addition to using the term 'apocalyptic', the WHO has stated that '*HIV and TB co-infection represents an unprecedented global public health crisis*'.

At the end of the year 2003 it was estimated that there were between 34 and 46 million HIV-seropositive people worldwide.[29] The global distribution is shown in Table 1.3. Many of these people live in regions with a high incidence of tuberculosis – 28 million in sub-Saharan Africa and more than 8 million in Asian countries, notably India, China and Indonesia. As one-third of these were co-infected with tubercle bacilli and therefore had an annual 8 per

TABLE 1.3 Estimated numbers of adults and children living with HIV infection and AIDS at the end of the year 2003

Region	Number of people
Sub-Saharan Africa	25–28.2 million
South and South-East Asia	4.6–8.2 million
Latin America	1.3–1.9 million
Eastern Europe and Central Asia	1.2–1.8 million
East Asia and Pacific	700 000–1.3 million
North America	790 000–1.2 million
Western Europe	520 000–680 000
North Africa and Middle East	470 000–730 000
Caribbean	350 000–590 000
Australia and New Zealand	12 000–18 000
Total	**34–46 million**

Data from UNAIDS.

cent chance of developing overt tuberculosis, an additional million cases of this disease are estimated to have occurred in that year as a result of HIV infection. According to WHO estimates, 12 per cent of all cases of tuberculosis worldwide were HIV related in the year 2001, a massive increase from the 4 per cent in 1995.[30]

At present, the greatest impact of HIV-related tuberculosis is felt in sub-Saharan Africa, where around 70 per cent of the world's HIV-infected people live. In that region, at least 30 per cent of all cases of tuberculosis are HIV-related, with a country-to-country range of 20–70 per cent. In Zambia, for example, around two-thirds of all cases of tuberculosis are HIV related. Children are also suffering: the percentage of Zambian children with tuberculosis admitted to hospital who were found to be infected with HIV rose from 18 per cent to 67 per cent over an 8-year period up to 1995, in contrast to a constant 10 per cent in children admitted to hospital for surgical conditions.[31]

Infection with HIV is having a devastating effect on health services and societal structure in Africa. Not only is tuberculosis placing a very great burden on health services, but also many of the patients require treatment for other HIV-related infections and conditions. Healthcare workers increasingly suffer from AIDS and tuberculosis and require sick leave. The number of cases of tuberculosis among the staff of a hospital in South Africa rose from 2 in the period 1991–92 to 20 in 1993–96.[32] Twelve of 14 who were tested for HIV infection were found to be positive. Families are also affected. Among pregnant women in Zambia, a quarter of whom are infected with HIV, tuberculosis is now one of the principal causes of maternal death.[33] Table 1.4 shows that, at one major centre in Zambia, the maternal mortality ratio (defined as the number of maternal deaths for every 100 000 live births) rose from 160 in 1974–76 to 921 in 1996–97, with indirect (non-obstetric) causes of death rising from 6 per cent in the former period to 57 per cent in the latter period, thereby accounting for more deaths than obstetric causes. As shown in Tables 1.4 and 1.5, tuberculosis was second only to malaria as an indirect cause of death in 1996–97 and 70 per cent of those dying of indirect causes, and 92 per cent of those dying of tuberculosis, had HIV disease.

Unlike other AIDS-defining conditions, tuberculosis may occur fairly early in the course of HIV infection, while the immune status of the patient is still relatively good.

TABLE 1.4 Changing trends in maternal mortality, as percentage of total deaths, at the University Teaching Hospital in Lusaka, Zambia

Study period	1974–76	1982–83	1989	1996–97
Direct causes				
Abortion	8	23	24	14
Toxaemia	25	20	12	9
Haemorrhage	15	10	7	5
Puerperal sepsis	17	15	15	8
Ruptured uterus	14	7	3	2
Other	15	5	9	4
Indirect causes				
Malaria	0	5	13	17
Tuberculosis	0	0	2	14
Other	6	15	15	26
Total number of deaths	**80**	**60**	**101**	**251**
Number of maternal deaths per 100 000 live births	160	118	667	921

TABLE 1.5 Indirect (non-obstetric) causes of maternal mortality at the University Teaching Hospital in Lusaka, Zambia, 1996–1997

Cause	Total numbers (%)	Number HIV infected (%)
Malaria	43 (30)	16 (37)
Tuberculosis	36 (25)	33 (92)
Unspecified upper respiratory infection	32 (22)	31 (97)
Cryptococcal meningitis	6 (4)	6 (100)
Gastroenteritis	8 (6)	8 (100)
Kaposi's sarcoma	4 (3)	4 (100)
Other[a]	16 (11)	4 (25)
Total	**145**	**102 (70)**

[a]Bacterial meningitis, septicaemia, cardiorespiratory failure, perforated appendix, Guillain–Barré syndrome, suicide, head injury.

Unfortunately, tuberculosis also suppresses immune responses and, even if treated successfully, may lead to a significant shortening of the life spans of the patients. Several studies in Africa have shown that, despite good responses to antituberculosis therapy, patients with HIV-related tuberculosis are much more likely to die during or within a year of completing therapy than patients not infected with HIV.[34] These deaths are largely due to other opportunistic infections to which these patients are prone.

Tuberculosis is a common cause of death in those with AIDS and accounted for 30 per cent of the estimated 3 million AIDS-related deaths in 2003. Tragically, HIV infection is spreading rapidly in the Indian subcontinent and in South-East Asia, where, owing to the huge population, most of the world's cases of tuberculosis occur. Thus, unless the spread of HIV is checked by public health measures or by the advent of effective vaccination or therapeutic strategies, the problems currently facing Africa will be experienced on a much greater scale in those regions.

DRUG-RESISTANT TUBERCULOSIS

The very high hopes raised by the discovery of the first effective antituberculosis drug (streptomycin) in 1944 were soon dashed by the finding that many treated patients initially improved but then relapsed. The cause of the relapse was the development of bacterial resistance to this drug. Fortunately, other effective antituberculosis agents were soon discovered, and in a series of extensive studies in the UK led by Sir John Crofton, it was found that combination regimens not only cured the patient but prevented the emergence of drug resistance. Further extensive studies by the Medical Research Council Tuberculosis Unit in the UK and overseas played a central role in the subsequent development of the modern short-course therapeutic regimens described in Chapter 12. These regimens commence with a 2-month intensive phase with (usually) four drugs, which kills the great majority of tubercle bacilli, followed by a 4-month continuation phase with two drugs to kill the few remaining bacilli.

Two forms of drug resistance have been described: **primary** (or **initial**) **resistance** and **acquired resistance**. Primary resistance is the result of infection of a previously untreated person by a patient who has drug-resistant tuberculosis. As it is not always easy to determine with certainty that a patient who appears to have primary resistance has not in fact previously received antituberculosis medication, some prefer the term initial resistance. Acquired resistance refers to the development of drug resistance during suboptimal or poorly managed treatment. This classification of the types of drug resistance is of value in epidemiological surveys. Thus a high incidence of primary resistance indicates that the transmission of tuberculosis in the community is poorly controlled, while the continuing occurrence of acquired resistance points to inadequacies in the drug regimen or in the supervision of therapy.

Patients with resistance to a single drug usually respond to modern treatment regimens, but serious problems arise when there is resistance to two or more drugs. In particular, resistance to the two most potent drugs, rifampicin and isoniazid, makes treatment of the disease very difficult and costly. Tuberculosis caused by bacilli resistant to these two drugs, whether or not they are also resistant to other drugs, is defined by the WHO as **multidrug-resistant tuberculosis** (MDR TB).

A common cause of acquired drug resistance is the failure of the patient to take the drugs regularly and to complete the prescribed course of medication. The patient is usually blamed for this, but in the majority of cases the fault lies with the health services. The faults include prescription of inappropriate courses of therapy, provision of poor quality drugs, a failure to explain the nature of the disease and the importance of treatment, and a failure to give the patient any support and encouragement. Although the supervised administration of the drugs aids adherence and cure, and forms an important component of the WHO **DOTS** (Directly Observed Therapy, Short Course) strategy described in Chapter 13, this should constitute just part of a more comprehensive 'holistic' care of the patients, with due attention to the many problems that they and their families experience. Nurses, of course, have a prime and pivotal part to play in the provision of such comprehensive care.

In 1994, the WHO and the International Union Against Tuberculosis and Lung Disease (UNION) commenced a global survey of resistance to four commonly used antituberculosis drugs: isoniazid, rifampicin, ethambutol and streptomycin. (Pyrazinamide is also regularly used, but resistance to it is, for technical reasons, difficult to determine with accuracy.) The first survey report was published in 1997 and covered 35 settings.[35] It was clear that drug resistance was widespread, more so than previously apparent, and that there were certain 'hotspot' regions in which a very high proportion of cases were resistant. These findings were confirmed and extended to 58 settings in the second report (published in 2000),[36] and to 77 settings in the third report (published in 2004).[37] The incidence of resistance to any of the four drugs varied greatly from no reported cases in Andorra, Malta and Iceland to 57.1 per cent in Kazakhstan. The prevalence of MDR TB as defined above likewise varied enormously from setting to setting – fewer than 10 cases were reported in several Western and Central European countries but a very high incidence was found among new cases in some settings, especially the Tomsk Oblast (district) in Russia (13.7 per cent), Uzbekistan (13.2 per cent), Estonia (12.2 per cent), the Liaoning province of China (10.4 per cent) and Lithuania (9.4 per cent). Among previously treated patients, the median incidence of MDR TB was 7 per cent and some settings reported very high levels, notably Oman and Kazakhstan with 58.3 and 56.4 per cent respectively. Although many settings reported increasing numbers of cases of drug and multidrug resistance, some (Cuba, Hong Kong, South African Republic, Thailand and the USA) reported decreasing numbers.

The information on which the above surveys were based was not complete, as many countries, including half the 22 countries with the highest burden of tuberculosis, had not provided data. In the third report, it is estimated that around 300 000 new cases of tuberculosis in the world in the year 2003 were multidrug resistant.[37] Figure 1.4 shows the range of the prevalence of MDR TB in new and previously treated patients in a selection of countries (data from the second report).

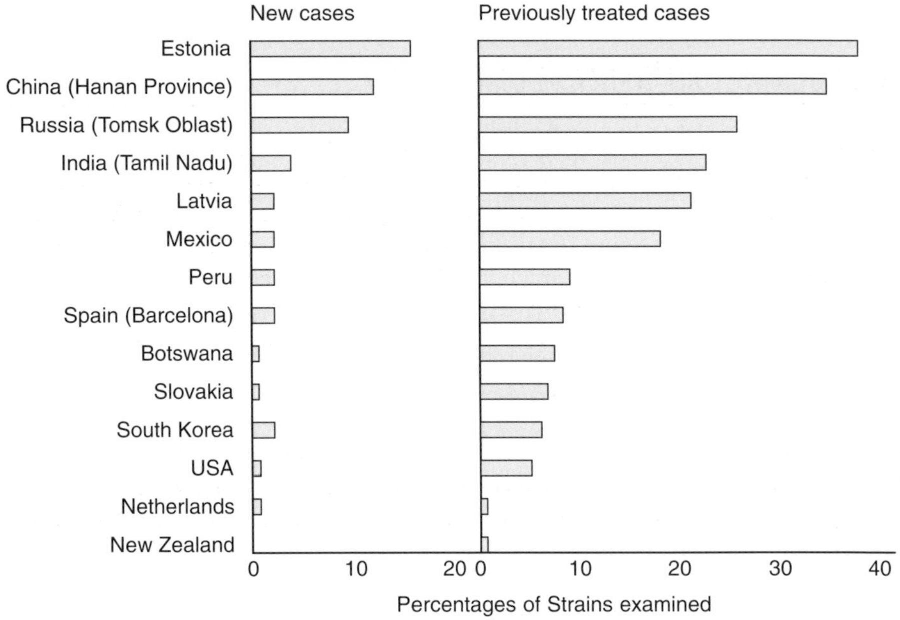

FIGURE 1.4 *The prevalence (percentage of strains examined) of multidrug resistance in new and previously treated patients in a selection of countries.*

The high incidence of MDR TB in Russia is both worrying and illustrative.[38] Under the communist regime in that country, tuberculosis had been in decline for several decades, reaching an annual incidence of 34 cases in every 100 000 of the population in 1991. Since that year, when communism collapsed, the incidence rose steadily, reaching 85 in every 100 000 of the population by 1998. This upsurge was attributed to a combination of poverty, malnutrition, poor housing, conflict and a fragmentation of health services. A particular problem of drug resistance was identified in Russian prisons, in which up to 1 million people are held and, of these, around 100 000 have active tuberculosis. Many of these prisoners have MDR TB. In one studied prison it was detected in 24.6 per cent of tuberculosis patients, and in as many as 92 per cent of those who failed to respond to therapy. Patients with active tuberculosis who are discharged from prison do not always continue to receive adequate management, and this could have serious consequences for health over a wider region. The medical aid agency Médecins Sans Frontières has remarked that: 'It is only a matter of time before multidrug-resistant tuberculosis of Russian origin becomes a daily reality world-wide. The cost of the epidemic to the world will be counted in billions of pounds and may become unmanageable'.

The presence of HIV infection does not by itself lead to an upsurge of MDR TB, and this has not occurred in most African countries that have large numbers of cases of HIV-associated tuberculosis. By contrast, several well-documented epidemics of HIV-related MDR TB have occurred in the USA, notably in New York City.[39] This is because HIV infection facilitates outbreaks of tuberculosis in hospitals, prisons and common lodging facilities where such immunocompromised individuals are crowded together. Thus, if the source case has MDR TB, a mini-epidemic of such disease will ensue. Similar outbreaks have occurred in the UK; for example, in 1995, four patients who had been exposed to the source case in April in a six-bed ward in an HIV unit in London had developed MDR TB by mid-June of that year.

TUBERCULOSIS – AN EPIDEMIC OF INJUSTICE

In J.R.R. Tolkien's fantasy epic *The lord of the rings*, Mr Bilbo Baggins disappeared in a flash of light at his 111th ('eleventy first') birthday party and was never seen in his home village again. Sadly, 111 years after Robert Koch's discovery of its cause in 1882, tuberculosis was showing no signs of disappearing. On the contrary, it was clearly on the increase, so much so that in that year (1993) the WHO declared it a global emergency. The great paradox in tuberculosis is that there is hardly a disease for which the treatment has been so perfected by a multitude of clinical trials, rendered so simple to understand by WHO guidelines, and so cheap by international co-operation – yet is so terrifyingly prevalent.

In 1907, an American public health physician, John B. Huber, wrote:[40]

> The tubercle bacillus is an index, by inversion, of the real progress of the human race. By it the claim of civilization to dominate human life may fairly be judged. Tuberculosis will decrease with the substantial advance of civilization, and the disease will as surely increase as civilization retrogrades.

It is somewhat challenging to the conscience of humankind that, in 1907, one in seven deaths among young American adults was due to tuberculosis and today, in the era of highly effective therapy which has drastically reduced its prevalence in the USA, this disease is now the cause of one in seven deaths among young adults worldwide.

A leading expert on tuberculosis at the WHO, Arata Kochi, has written:

> Tuberculosis is one of the world's most neglected health crises. In spite of its alarming danger, surprisingly little action has been taken to address the TB epidemic. Every day, I ask why this situation is allowed to continue. Is it possible that no one really cares whether 30 million people will die in the next decade from TB? How can TB be such a

> neglected priority when it is one of the most cost-effective adult diseases to treat? Can we comprehend the magnitude of this injustice? The growing TB epidemic is no longer an emergency only for those who care about health, but for those who care about justice.

In similar vein, Lee Reichman, a distinguished American public health specialist, has condemned the indolence of communities, physicians, health workers, governments, the press and international agencies, adding: '... if any of these parties did what they should do, things might be different. Especially if they were to show the wholly justified but shockingly absent outrage for which the situation cries out'.[41] The WHO has also called for religious leaders to use their stature to address inequities in health care for poor people: 'Since there is a cure for tuberculosis – a cure that is not being fully used – this disease is no longer a medical epidemic, but an epidemic of injustice'.

Medical historians may look back to the period between the discovery of the antituberculosis drugs and the advent of the HIV pandemic and the emergence of multidrug resistance as a window of opportunity in which tuberculosis could have been reduced to a shadow of its former self. In 1994, Sir John Crofton, the greatly respected pioneer of the treatment of tuberculosis, wrote:[42]

> It is a sad reflection on society's incompetence that, more than thirty years after the methods for cure and prevention were evolved and before the advent of the HIV epidemic, there were already more patients with active tuberculosis in the world than there had been in the 1950s.

The encouraging news is that, after years of advocacy by the WHO, particularly through its 'Stop TB' partnership, the international community is at last (as described in Chapter 13) showing active interest and, though perhaps with faltering steps, making material effort to right this gross injustice. This will require the efforts and dedication not only of doctors, nurses and those in the various other branches of the healthcare professions, but also of those in many other disciplines, including bioscientists, sociologists, anthropologists, health economists, politicians, educators, human rights activists, ethicists and financiers. New interdisciplinary alliances will have to be forged, with the abandonment of old axioms and dogmas. The task ahead will be highly complex and challenging but, in the words of John Porter of the London School of Hygiene and Tropical Medicine, 'Complexity should be seen as an incentive to developing novel ways of working together'.[43] Notwithstanding this extended teamwork, recent experience clearly emphasizes the very central role for the nurse in the control of tuberculosis, particularly in the fields of health education, in dispelling ignorance and stigma, and in providing the human dimension of care that is crucial to the success of case finding, case holding and the completion of treatment.

Summary

Tuberculosis is a disease of great antiquity and, in recent decades, the science of epidemiology has led to a clear understanding of its infectious nature and the way in which it is spread and maintained in a community. After decades of decline in the industrialized nations, the disease is on the increase. In the developing nations, the incidence remains high and, owing to the population explosion, there are now more cases of the disease than at any previous time in human history. Poverty and poor health services account for the high incidence in the developing nations, and neglect and loss of interest are, at least in part, responsible for the resurgence in the industrialized world. The future will not recapitulate the past. We now have the powerful tool of highly effective therapy and the WHO has set out clear principles for its use. Sadly, though, past misuse has led to the development of forms of tuberculosis that are highly resistant to the standard drug regimens. Furthermore, the HIV pandemic, by lowering resistance to the disease, poses a serious threat to the control of tuberculosis in many parts of the world. The conquest of this disease will require the participation of many workers from a wide range of disciplines, but the role of the tuberculosis nurse will be paramount.

Prologue to the next chapter

Although tuberculosis may be said to have many causes, including poverty, overcrowding, poor medical services and general inequity and injustice, the actual cause, without which there would be no disease called tuberculosis, is a bacterium. Thus, any attempt to understand this disease, its spread, diagnosis and treatment must be firmly rooted in an understanding of the nature and properties of this bacterium. This is therefore the theme of the next chapter.

REFERENCES

1. Ryan F. *Tuberculosis, the greatest story never told*. Bromsgrove, Worcestershire: Swift Publishers, 1992.
2. Waksman SA. *The conquest of tuberculosis*. London: Robert Hale Ltd/Cambridge: Cambridge University Press, 1965.
3. Dormandy T. *The white death. A history of tuberculosis*. London: Hambledon Press, 1999.
4. Dubos R, Dubos J. *The white plague: tuberculosis, man, and society*. New Brunswick, NJ: Rutgers University Press, 1952, reprinted 1992.
5. Roberts CA, Buikstra JE. The history of tuberculosis from earliest times to the development of drugs. In Davies PDO (ed.), *Clinical tuberculosis*, 3rd edn. London: Arnold, 2003, 3–20.
6. Enarson DA, Rouillon A. The epidemiological basis of tuberculosis control. In Davies PDO (ed.), *Clinical tuberculosis*, 2nd edn. London: Chapman and Hall Medical, 1998, 535–50.
7. Raviglione MC, Nunn P. Epidemiology of tuberculosis. In Zumla A, Johnson MA, Miller RF (eds), *AIDS and respiratory medicine*. London: Chapman and Hall, 1997, 117–41.
8. Rieder H. Methodological issues in the estimation of the tuberculosis problem from tuberculin surveys. *Tuber Lung Dis* 1995; **76**: 114–21.
9. Grange JM, Gandy M, Farmer P, Zumla A. Historical declines in tuberculosis – nature, nurture and the biosocial model. *Int J Tuberc Lung Dis* 2001; **3**: 208–12.
10. Farmer P, Nardell E. Nihilism and pragmatism in tuberculosis control. *Am J Public Health* 1998; **88**: 1014–15.
11. Williams L. The worship of Moloch. *Br J Tuberc* 1908; **2**: 56–62. Cited by Zumla A, Grange JM. Doing something about tuberculosis. *BMJ* 1999; **318**: 956.
12. Reichman LB. The U-shaped curve of concern. *Am Rev Respir Dis* 1991; **144**: 741–2.
13. Porter JDH, McAdam KPWJ (eds). *Tuberculosis: back to the future*. (London School of Hygiene and Tropical Medicine Third Annual Public Health Forum.) Chichester: Wiley, 1994.

14. Kochi A. The global tuberculosis situation and the new control strategy of the World Health Organization. *Tubercle* 1991; **72**: 1–6.
15. World Health Organization. *Global tuberculosis control.* WHO Report 1997. Publication WHO/TB/1997.225. Geneva: World Health Organization, 1997.
16. Murray CJ, Styblo K, Rouillon A. Tuberculosis in developing countries: burden, intervention and cost. *Bull Int Union Tuberc Lung Dis* 1990; **65**(1): 6–24.
17. World Health Organization. *Global tuberculosis control: surveillance, planning, financing.* WHO Report 2002. Publication WHO/CDS/TB/2002.295. Geneva: World Health Organization, 2002.
18. World Health Organization. *Global tuberculosis control.* Publication WHO/CDS/2001.287. Geneva: World Health Organization, 2001.
19. Grange JM, Story A, Zumla A. Tuberculosis in disadvantaged groups. *Curr Opin Pulm Med* 2001; **7**: 160–4.
20. Cantwell MF, Snider DE, Cauthen GM, Onorato IM. Epidemiology of tuberculosis in the United States, 1985 through 1992. *J Am Med Assoc* 1994; **272**: 535–9.
21. Centers for Disease Control. Trends in tuberculosis – United States, 1998–2003. *MMWR* 2004; **53**(10): 209–14.
22. Communicable Disease Surveillance Centre. *Tuberculosis update*. London: Public Health Laboratory Service, September 2001. (This and subsequent updates are available on <www.hpa.org.uk>.)
23. Needham DM, Godfrey-Faussett P. Economic barriers for tuberculosis patients in Zambia. *Lancet* 1996; **348**: 14–135.
24. Bhatti N, Law MR, Morris JK et al. Increasing incidence of tuberculosis in England and Wales: a study of the likely causes. *BMJ* 1995; **310**: 967–9.
25. Perez-Padilla R, Perez-Guzman C, Baez-Saldana R, Torres-Cruz A. Cooking with biomass stoves and tuberculosis: a case control study. *Int J Tuberc Lung Dis* 2001; **5**: 441–7.
26. Yu GP, Hsieh CC, Peng J. Risk factors associated with the prevalence of pulmonary tuberculosis among sanitary workers in Shanghai. *Tubercle* 1988; **69**: 105–22.
27. Gajalakshmi V, Peto R, Kanaka TS, Jha P. Smoking and mortality from tuberculosis and other diseases in India: retrospective study of 43,000 adult male deaths and 35,000 controls. *Lancet* 2003; **362**: 507–15.
28. Dolin PJ, Raviglione MC, Kochi A. Global tuberculosis incidence and mortality during 1990–2000. *Bull World Health Organ* 1994; **72M**: 213–20.
29. UNAIDS. *Epidemiological update, December 2003*. Geneva: World Health Organization, 2003. Also available online at <www.unaids.org/en/resources/epidemiology.asp>.
30. World Health Organization Stop TB Partnership. *The Global Plan to Stop Tuberculosis.* Geneva: World Health Organization, 2002.
31. Chintu C, Zumla A. Childhood tuberculosis and infection with the human immunodeficiency virus. *J R Coll Physicians Lond* 1995; **29**: 92–4.
32. Wilkinson G, Gilks CF. Increasing frequency of tuberculosis among staff in a South African district hospital: impact of the HIV epidemic on the supply side of health care. *Trans R Soc Trop Med Hyg* 1998; **92**: 500–2.
33. Ahmed Y, Mwaba P, Grange JM et al. A study of maternal mortality at the University Teaching Hospital. Lusaka, Zambia: the emergence of tuberculosis as a major non-obstetric cause of maternal death. *Int J Tuberc Lung Dis* 1999; **3**: 675–80.
34. Van den Broek J, Mfinanga S, Moshiro CM et al. Impact of human immunodeficiency virus on the outcome of treatment and survival of tuberculosis patients in Mwanza, Tanzania. *Int J Tuberc Lung Dis* 1998; **2**: 547–52.

35. World Health Organization/International Union Against Tuberculosis and Lung Disease. *Anti-tuberculosis drug resistance in the world*. Publication WHO/TB/97.229. Geneva: World Health Organization, 1997.
36. World Health Organization/International Union Against Tuberculosis and Lung Disease. *Anti-tuberculosis drug resistance in the world*, Report no. 2. Geneva: World Health Organization, 2000.
37. World Health Organization/International Union Against Tuberculosis and Lung Disease. *Anti-tuberculosis drug resistance in the world*. Report no. 3. Geneva: World Health Organization, 2004. Also available online at <www.who.int/gtb/publications/drugresistance/2004/drs_report_1.pdf>.
38. Perelman MI. Tuberculosis in Russia. *Int J Tuberc Lung Dis* 2000; **4**: 1097–103.
39. Simone PM, Dooley SW. Drug-resistant tuberculosis in the USA. In Davies PDO (ed.), *Clinical tuberculosis*, 2nd edn. London: Chapman and Hall Medical, 1998, 265–87.
40. Huber JB. Civilization and tuberculosis. *Br J Tuberc* 1907; **1**: 158–68. Cited in Grange JM, Zumla A. The global emergency of tuberculosis: what is the cause? *J R Soc Health* 2002; **122**: 78–81.
41. Reichman LB. Tuberculosis elimination – what's to stop us? *Int J Tuberc Lung Dis* 1997; **1**: 3–11.
42. Crofton J, Foreword. In Davies PDO (ed.), *Clinical tuberculosis*. London: Chapman and Hall Medical, 1994, xv–xvi.
43. Porter J, Grange JM. Preface. In Porter JDH, Grange JM. *Tuberculosis. An interdisciplinary perspective*. London: Imperial College Press, 1999, V–viii.

FURTHER READING

Bates B. *Bargaining for life: a social history of tuberculosis, 1876–1938*. Philadelphia: University of Pennsylvania Press, 1992.

Dubos R, Dubos J. *The white plague: tuberculosis, man, and society*. New Brunswick, NJ: Rutgers University Press, 1952, reprinted 1992.

Grange JM. The resurgence of tuberculosis. In Noah N, O'Mahony M (eds), *Communicable disease epidemiology and control*. Chichester: Wiley, 1998, 105–32.

Parsons L, Lister G (eds). *Global health: a local issue*. London: Nuffield Trust, 2000.

Porter JDH, Grange JM. *Tuberculosis. An interdisciplinary perspective*. London: Imperial College Press, 1999.

Roberts CA, Buikstra JE. The history of tuberculosis from earliest times to the development of drugs. In Davies PDO (ed.), *Clinical tuberculosis*, 3rd edn. London: Arnold, 2003, 3–20.

Ryan F. *Tuberculosis, the greatest story never told*. Bromsgrove, Worcestershire: Swift Publishers, 1992. (Published in the USA as *The forgotten plague: how the battle against tuberculosis was won and lost*. Boston: Little, Brown and Company, 1992.)

Shaw T. Tuberculosis: the history of incidence and treatment. *Nurs Times* 1995; **91**(38): 27–8.

Waksman SA. *The conquest of tuberculosis*. London: Robert Hale Ltd/Cambridge: Cambridge University Press, 1965.

Wilson LG. The historical decline of tuberculosis in Europe and America: its causes and significance. *J Hist Med* 1990; **45**: 366–96.

CHAPTER 2

The bacterial cause of tuberculosis and related diseases

Introduction

To understand, diagnose, treat and control any infectious disease, a detailed knowledge of the causative organism, whether it be a bacterium, virus, fungus, prion or parasite, is essential. This is certainly true of tuberculosis and closely related diseases. Tuberculosis is a chronic disease caused by one of the bacteria of the genus *Mycobacterium,* which have a number of very distinctive properties and characteristics. These properties contribute not only to the mode of infection, but also to the development of the disease and the serious problems encountered in its control.

Learning outcomes

After studying and reflecting on the material in this chapter, you will be able to:

- describe the distinguishing characteristics of the genus *Mycobacterium,*
- discuss the difference between an obligate mycobacterial pathogen and an environmental mycobacterium that may occasionally cause disease,
- outline the basic principles and methods by which mycobacterial species were and are identified,
- identify the mycobacteria causing tuberculosis and leprosy and the more frequently encountered environmental mycobacteria that cause human disease,
- outline the characteristic 'acid-fast' staining property that enables mycobacteria to be detected microscopically in clinical specimens.

BACKGROUND

Until the late nineteenth century, the cause of tuberculosis was unknown. Although many theories of causation existed, including the concepts that it was a hereditary disease or due to nutritional factors, its contagious nature was suspected as long ago as the time of the ancient Greek philosophers and physicians, more than 300 years before Christ.[1]

In the middle of the nineteenth century, the French chemist Louis Pasteur firmly established that 'germs' were the cause of many diseases of humans and animals. In 1868, following Pasteur's pioneering work, Jean-Antoine Villemin, a French Army surgeon, published his extensive studies conclusively demonstrating that tuberculosis was caused by an unknown but infectious agent which could be transmitted by the inoculation of tuberculous material from human tissue to animals and, subsequently, from animal to animal.[2]

Less than 20 years later in Berlin, on 24th March 1882, Robert Koch stunned the scientific world when he described for the first time the microorganism that caused tuberculosis.[3] Using a special technique for staining infectious material on slides, Koch was able to demonstrate this microorganism in lesions and, equally important, in the sputum of people with active tuberculosis. Shortly afterwards, another famous German bacteriologist, Paul Ehrlich, discovered the so-called acid-fast property of the tubercle bacillus; namely, the ability of the bacillus to retain certain dyes after treatment with dilute mineral acids. For this reason, the microorganisms causing tuberculosis and its related species discussed below are often termed **acid-fast bacilli** (AFB). Ehrlich discovered AFB in his own sputum but fortunately recovered from tuberculosis, a recovery he attributed to a course of Koch's tuberculin therapy and a year's holiday. Modifications of Ehrlich's technique, notably by Ziehl and Neelsen, whose names the staining procedure now bears, are routinely used for detecting these microorganisms in sputum and tissues today and are among the most important diagnostic tests used in identifying people with active tuberculosis.

MYCOBACTERIA

The microorganism that Robert Koch so brilliantly discovered and conclusively associated with the aetiology of tuberculosis more than 100 years ago is a bacterium that belongs to the genus *Mycobacterium*. (This is the only genus in the family *Mycobacteriaceae*, which itself is within the broad and rather loosely defined order *Actinomycetales*.) *Mycobacterium* is the 'official' name, but members of this genus are often termed mycobacteria. (Note that, by convention, the official name starts with a capital M and is in italics.) The name *Mycobacterium* is derived from the Greek words *mukês*, meaning fungus, and *baktêrion*, meaning 'little rod', and is in reference to the characteristic mould-like growth of members of this genus on the surface of liquid culture media. This in turn is due to the fact that mycobacteria have very complex and thick cell walls composed largely of fatty acids that render the cells water repellent, or hydrophobic.

The genus *Mycobacterium* contains the causative agents of tuberculosis – a group of very closely related bacteria collectively termed the *Mycobacterium tuberculosis* complex. Members of this complex are often called tubercle bacilli. (In this context, it should be noted that the term bacillus, meaning a rod, refers to any rod-shaped bacterium, such as the anthrax bacillus and the tetanus bacillus, which are not related to the tubercle bacilli.) The genus also contains the leprosy bacillus, *M. leprae*, and many other species of mycobacteria that normally live freely in the environment. The latter, of which there are currently more than 100 named species and undoubtedly many more to be named in the future, normally live in watery environments such as marshes, wet soil, streams and lakes. Many species colonize pipes supplying water to homes and public facilities such as hospitals – sometimes at a high density. Contact with these mycobacteria by drinking water, washing or inhaling aerosols while showering is thus an everyday occurrence. In the great majority of cases, this contact is harmless although, as described in Chapter 5, they may have effects on immune responses to tuberculosis and leprosy that are not always beneficial.

The mycobacteria living in the environment are, not surprisingly, called **environmental mycobacteria** (EM) and, in some publications, particularly in the USA, **non-tuberculous mycobacteria** (NTM). Older terms include 'atypical' and MOTT (mycobacteria other than typical tubercle) bacilli. As described in Chapter 11, some species of EM may, under some circumstances, cause disease in humans and animals.

Characteristics of mycobacteria

Mycobacteria have several important features (Box 2.1), including the following.

BOX 2.1 Characteristics of mycobacteria

- Thick, tough, complex, lipid-rich and waxy cell wall
- Hydrophobic
- Gram positive, although weakly stained by this method
- Acid-fast or acid–alcohol-fast
- Slow growing: even so-called rapid growers grow slowly relative to many other bacteria encountered in clinical practice
- Environmentally hardy, but they do not form spores
- Non-motile, short to moderately long, straight or slightly curved non-capsulate, sometimes beaded rods measuring 0.2–1.0 μm in diameter and 1.0–10 μm in length; filamantous and occasionally branching forms may be seen in clinical material
- Aerophilic (obligate aerobes or microaerophiles)
- Mostly mesophilic; prefer moderate temperatures (25 °C to 41 °C) for growth; a few species are thermophilic, surviving at high temperatures

Size

Like all bacteria, the mycobacteria are very small, being 0.2–1.0 micrometres (μm) in diameter and 1.0–10 μm in length.

Shape

Mycobacteria do not have an external capsule, i.e. they are non-capsulate. Most are either straight or slightly curved and slender rods, although some species are almost circular and others are long and filamentous, and cultural conditions make great differences to the shape of the bacterial cells. They usually stain evenly, although *M. tuberculosis* in sputum from patients given various antibiotics, and some of the environmental mycobacteria, may have a beaded appearance. Mycobacteria do not have flagellae and are therefore non-motile; nor do they possess heat-resistant spores and are thus killed by temperatures below boiling, as in the heat treatment or pasteurization of milk.

Cell structure

The genetic material of a mycobacterium, termed the **genome**, is contained within a single, tightly wrapped, circular chromosome that forms the so-called nuclear body. This, in common with all bacteria but unlike mammalian or plant cells, is not separated from the cytoplasm by a nuclear membrane. Additionally, some mycobacteria, e.g. members of the *M. avium* complex described below, contain additional small, circular chromosome-like units of deoxyribonucleic acid (DNA) called **plasmids**. The chromosome, or genome, lies within the cytoplasm, which is surrounded by a cell membrane, which, in turn, is surrounded by a tough cell wall.

Cell membrane

This is similar to that found in all living cells and consists of a double layer of phosphate-containing lipid molecules. The cell membrane is closely associated with various enzymes involved in energy processes in the cell and it contains the pigments responsible for the orange and yellow colour of some species of mycobacteria, as described below.

Cell wall

The mycobacterial cell wall is the most complex one known in all of nature. It is particularly rich in high-molecular-weight fats and waxes, which are responsible for many of the distinguishing properties of this genus. The cell wall of a mycobacterium principally consists of an inner layer of peptidoglycan (murein), which is a high-molecular-weight polymer composed of interlacing chains of polysaccharides and peptides. This tough and rigid structure is found in all bacteria, except for a small minority of species that lack cell walls. Outside the murein layer is another interlaced layer, a polysaccharide composed of the carbohydrates arabinose and galactose and therefore called arabinogalactan. Exterior to this is a thick layer composed of long-chain fatty acids (mycolic acids) with long and short arms containing, respectively, around 60 and 30 carbon atoms. The outer cell wall layer is composed of mycosides – complex molecules containing sugars, amino acids and lipids, which vary from species to species and in some cases show considerable variation within species. This variation allows some species to be divided according to their reaction with specific antibodies, although nucleic acid-based typing methods are more generally used today. The tough, thick, fatty and waxy cell wall renders mycobacteria water repellent (hydrophobic) and resistant to drying and to the bactericidal action of antibodies, complement and many chemical disinfectants (including acids and alkalis) and detergents. The structure of the mycobacterial cell wall is shown diagrammatically in Fig. 2.1.

Temperature requirements

Mycobacteria grow best within a limited temperature range between 25 °C and 41 °C. Tubercle bacilli have an even more limited temperature range of growth and fail to grow at either 25 °C or 41 °C. Bacteria which have a fondness for moderate temperatures, such as tubercle bacilli, are known as **mesophiles**. A few mycobacterial species, including *M. xenopi*, are called **thermophiles** as they prefer a higher temperature. One species, *M. ulcerans*, which causes a disease known as Buruli ulcer (see Chapter 11), has a very restricted temperature range of growth – just a degree or two either side of 32 °C. Temperature ranges of growth are a useful aid to the identification of mycobacterial species.

Growth characteristics

The time required for a bacterial cell to divide and its population to double is called the **generation time**. In common with other bacteria, mycobacteria replicate by binary fission, i.e. they split into two daughter cells. While some bacteria, such as *Staphylococcus aureus*, have a generation time of around 20 minutes, mycobacteria replicate much more slowly, some with a generation time of 20 hours or longer. Various culture media are used to grow tubercle bacilli

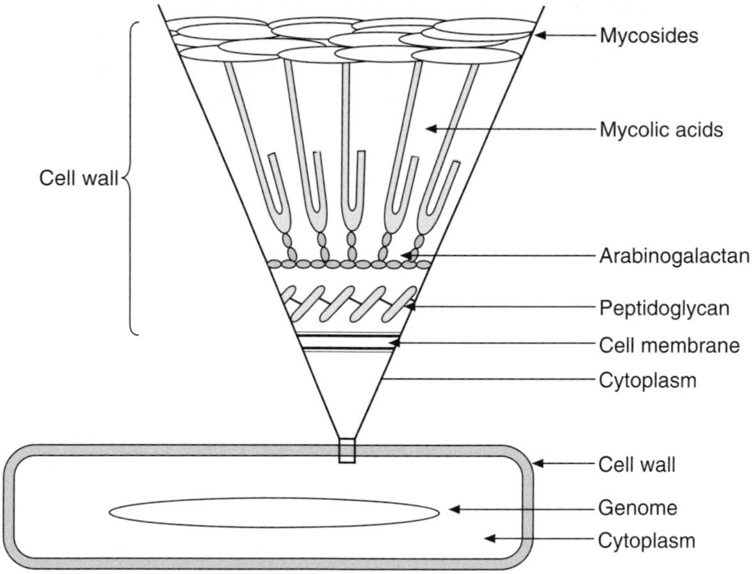

FIGURE 2.1 *Diagrammatic structure of the mycobacterial cell wall.*

and the most widely used, such as Löwenstein–Jensen (LJ) medium, are essentially heat-coagulated egg preparations containing glycerol and various mineral salts. They also contain a dye, malachite green, which, by mild disinfectant activity, helps protect against contamination and also provides a green background against which the mycobacterial colonies are more readily seen. Growth of tubercle bacilli and many of the environmental mycobacteria is first visually apparent on LJ medium after 2–8 weeks at 37 °C. Some mycobacteria are termed rapid growers, although they still grow slowly compared to many bacteria, and, on subculture, their growth is visible on egg-based medium within a week of inoculation. Colonies of tubercle bacilli on egg-based medium are of an off-white or cream-like colour and are usually rough and dry, resembling small cauliflowers or breadcrumbs. Some of the environmental mycobacteria have a similar appearance, but others produce smooth colonies and some have a bright orange or yellow pigment. In some cases, this pigment develops in the dark (**scotochromogens**), whereas in others, pigment only develops during or after exposure to light (**photochromogens**). Mycobacteria also grow in various liquid media and, on microscopy, *M. tuberculosis* may form twisted, rope-like micro-colonies termed 'serpentine cords'.

Differential staining characteristics

A variety of staining techniques are used to visualize bacteria in clinical material. One of the most widely used is the **Gram stain**, developed by the Danish bacteriologist Hans Christian Gram in 1884. This allows bacteria to be divided into two major groups: Gram positive and Gram negative. Mycobacteria are Gram positive, although they are not easily stainable by this method. Accordingly, they are detectable on the basis of their acid-fastness.

Acid-fast staining

In this procedure, the red dye carbol fuchsin (one of the arylmethane dyes) is poured over a heat-fixed film of the specimen, usually sputum, and the slide is then heated until steam rises, but not until boiling occurs (boiling detaches the material from the slide). After the slide has cooled, it is washed with water and is then decolourized with a weak mineral acid such as 3 per cent hydrochloric acid in water or alcohol. (Some texts state that the use of alcohol rather than water differentiates tubercle bacilli from EM. This is not the case: all mycobacteria are acid–alcohol-fast and the use of alcohol merely gives a cleaner picture and avoids staining artefacts.) After rinsing, a counterstain (usually malachite green or methylene blue) is then applied to the smear. Some bacteria will not retain the red stain when decolourized by acid and will then take up the green or blue colour of the counterstain; these are referred to as **non-acid-fast** bacteria. As discussed previously, mycobacteria are acid-fast bacilli as they retain the red stain after acid treatment. This property is almost unique to the mycobacteria, although members of closely related genera such as *Nocardia* and bacterial spores as are found in, for example, *Clostridium tetani* (the cause of tetanus) are weakly acid-fast.

Oxygen requirements

Most bacteria grow best in the presence or oxygen and are termed **aerobes**, with those having an absolute requirement for oxygen being called **obligate aerobes**. Some, termed **facultative anaerobes**, also grow in the absence of oxygen. Others will not grow in, and are often harmed by, the presence of oxygen and are known as **obligate anaerobes**. All mycobacteria, including tubercle bacilli, are obligate aerobes and therefore require oxygen for growth. Two members of the *M. tuberculosis* complex, *M. bovis* and *M. africanum* (described below), prefer lower oxygen tensions and are termed **microaerophiles**.

Pathogenicity and virulence

The term **pathogenicity** refers to the ability of an organism to cause disease. Bacteria were once divided into pathogens and non-pathogens, but this distinction is blurred, especially in patients with immunosuppression. Some bacteria, e.g. the *M. tuberculosis* complex and *M. leprae*, can only cause infection and disease and are termed obligate pathogens; whereas others, termed opportunist pathogens, normally live harmlessly as environmental saprophytes or as commensals in, for example, the human gastrointestinal and upper respiratory tracts but can cause disease under some circumstances. **Virulence** is a more specific measurement of the 'power' of a microorganism to cause disease. Thus members of the *M. tuberculosis* complex are all pathogens but vary in their virulence. In practice, determination of the virulence of tubercle bacilli is very difficult, but there is some evidence for the existence of 'wimpy' and 'burly' variants.[4]

More detailed descriptions of the properties of the mycobacteria are given in standard textbooks.[5–7]

The genome of the mycobacterium

As mentioned above, the genetic element (or **genome**) of a mycobacterium is, in common with that of all bacteria, a single circular chromosome composed of a 'double helix' of DNA. Some mycobacteria have small additional closed rings of DNA called **plasmids** or episomes. In some bacterial genera, plasmids carrying important genes determining, for example, resistance to antibiotics have been identified. In the case of the mycobacteria, however, no important genetic function has convincingly been ascribed to them.

Each mycobacterial genome contains many genes that are found in all mycobacteria and, indeed, in all bacteria. Some of the genes are in fact structurally closely related to some found in higher animals, including human beings. (In this context, there is much more genetic similarity between species than might at first be apparent. Human beings, for example, share about 98 per cent of their genes with the gorilla and some, perhaps, give the impression of sharing even more![8]) Other genes are more specific to groups within the genus *Mycobacterium*. Thus, the slowly growing and rapidly growing mycobacteria have genetic differences that are reflected in differences in proteins in their cytoplasm. Finally, some genes are unique to each mycobacterial species and to variants within those species.

Accordingly, identification of these various pieces of DNA in the genome makes it possible to prepare **DNA probes** that may be used to identify cultivated mycobacteria at the generic, specific or subspecific level. Furthermore, as described in Chapter 7, very small numbers of mycobacterial genomes in clinical specimens may be rapidly amplified by a technique called the **polymerase chain reaction** (PCR) into millions of copies so that they may be readily detected.[9] As in the case of DNA probes, the PCR may be used to detect mycobacteria at the generic, specific or subspecific level. The same technique may be used to detect mutations in the genes responsible for resistance to antituberculosis drugs, and kits are commercially available for the rapid detection of strains resistant to rifampicin, the most important of the drugs used in modern treatment regimens.[10]

A characteristic of all genomes is the presence of so-called **insertion sequences** (IS) or 'jumping genes'. These sequences, which are usually but not invariably unique to each species, have the strange property of replicating and inserting themselves in various parts of the genome. Bacilli within the *M. tuberculosis* complex as defined below usually contain between one and more than 20 copies of an insertion sequence, IS6110, although a very few strains do not contain any. Furthermore, even if two epidemiologically unrelated strains have the same number of insertion sequences, their position in the genome differs considerably. Thus, if genomes of tubercle bacilli are extracted, digested into fragments with enzymes termed endonucleases, the fragments separated according to size on a gel by means of an electric current (electrophoresis) and 'probed' with DNA of the IS6110, bands varying in number and position are observed. Despite the fact that insertion sequences jump around the genome, their position is constant enough to allow strains to be compared for epidemiological purposes.[11] This technique, known as **restriction fragment length polymorphism** (RFLP) typing, is the basis of DNA fingerprinting and is shown diagrammatically in Fig. 2.2. Alternative methods that can be used after PCR amplification of DNA in clinical specimens, thus avoiding the need for isolation of the bacilli by culture, are now available.

In addition to the genome composed of DNA, bacteria also have small cytoplasmic bodies called **ribosomes**, which are responsible for the synthesis of proteins. These contain units of ribonucleic acid (RNA) with nucleic acid sequences that differ from one species to another. Typing of mycobacteria according to differences in these sequences, or in the DNA coding for them – a process termed **ribotyping** – is making an important contribution to the classification or taxonomy of the mycobacteria, and in recent years several new species have been identified in this manner.[12]

The entire genome of *M. tuberculosis* has been mapped and this is already leading to fascinating and important advances in the understanding of this organism and its interaction with its human host.[13]

The species of mycobacteria

Since Robert Koch's isolation of the tubercle bacillus in 1882, numerous mycobacteria have been isolated from clinical specimens and the environment and have been given a variety of

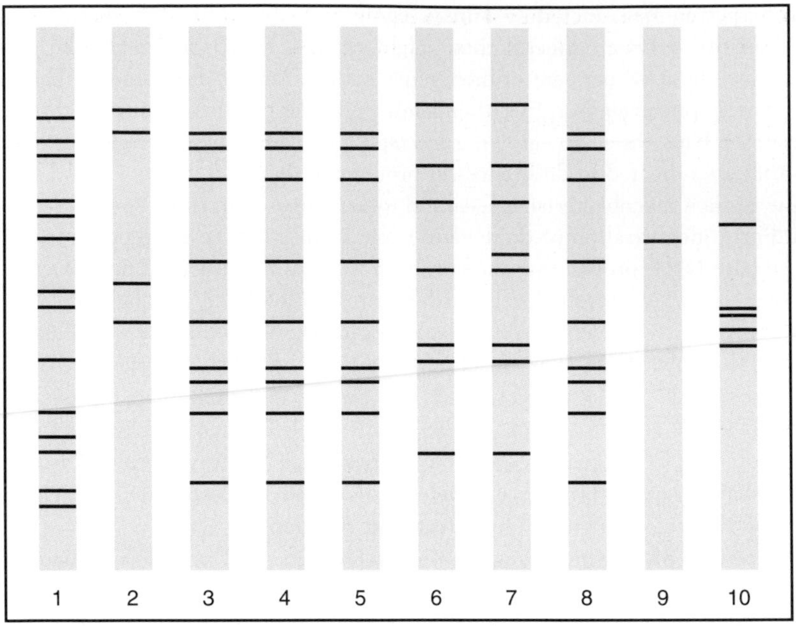

FIGURE 2.2 *DNA fingerprinting (RFLP). A diagrammatic representation of electrophoretic gels showing variation between strains of* Mycobacterium tuberculosis. *Strains in lanes 3, 4 and 5 are identical. Strains in lanes 6 and 7 differ in the presence of one additional band in lane 7, indicative of a recent 'jump' of an insertion sequence.*

names. In the 1950s, despite the fact there were a huge number of published names, the classification was so confusing that it was almost impossible to allocate many isolates other than classical tubercle bacilli to described species and accordingly they were sometimes termed 'anonymous mycobacteria'. Before 1980, the earliest published name was, by international agreement, the valid one, and confusion often occurred when an earlier name for a well-known species was unearthed in an old and obscure journal. In 1980, in an attempt to bring order into chaos, lists of approved bacterial names were drawn up by working groups and were intended to serve as the reference for all subsequent classification and nomenclature. In the case of the mycobacteria, 41 species were listed,[14] but many new species have been described subsequently and the number currently exceeds 100. (A regularly updated list of valid bacterial species is available on the Society for Systematic and Veterinary Bacteriology websites – <www.bacterio.cict.fr> and <www.bacterio.net>) Many of these species are, however, rare and obscure and in this chapter only the well-documented species are described. Until recently, mycobacteria were allocated to species by doing large numbers of tests, such as growth at various temperatures, pigment production, growth on various media and enzymic activity, calculating the degree of similarity between isolates and determining 'cut-off' levels of similarity to distinguish genera, species and variants within species. Today, as mentioned above, classification is based more on homology of the DNA and RNA, but some of the older tests are widely used for identification purposes in clinical laboratories.

The *Mycobacterium tuberculosis* complex

The species that cause tuberculosis in mammals, *M. tuberculosis*, *M. bovis*, *M. africanum* and *M. microti*, are members of the *M. tuberculosis* complex. Strictly speaking, these are members of a single species, as demonstrated by analysis of their DNA and ribosomal RNA, as described above, but the traditional nomenclature is universally used (Table 2.1).

TABLE 2.1 Members of the *M. tuberculosis* complex

Variant or 'species'	Oxygen preference	Susceptibility to pyrazinamide	Susceptibility to TCH[a]	Nitratase activity[b]
M. tuberculosis				
Classical	Aerobic	Susceptible	Resistant	Positive
Asian	Aerobic	Susceptible	Susceptible	Positive
M. africanum				
Type I	Microaerophilic	Susceptible	Susceptible	Negative
Type II	Microaerophilic	Susceptible	Susceptible	Positive
M. bovis	Microaerophilic	Resistant	Susceptible	Negative
BCG vaccine	Aerobic	Resistant	Susceptible	Negative

[a]Thiophen-2-carboxylic acid hydrazide, an analogue of isoniazid.
[b]Reduction of nitrate to nitrite ions.
BCG, Bacille Calmette–Guérin.

Human tuberculosis is caused by three members of the complex: *M. tuberculosis*, *M. bovis* and *M. africanum*.[15]

M. tuberculosis

M. tuberculosis is the principal cause of tuberculosis in humans, and infectious individuals can transmit this infection to other people and, more rarely, to a variety of animals which they are in close contact with, for example cattle, captive primates, dogs and cats. Although cattle can be infected with human tubercle bacilli, they very rarely develop disease as a result of this infection and they do not transmit bacilli to other cattle or back to human beings.

Some geographical variations in the characteristics of *M. tuberculosis* have been described. Thus, for example, there are minor differences between strains isolated in Europe and south India, but all isolates are virulent in human beings.[16] A very rare variant, *M. canetti*, forms smooth colonies on egg-based medium.[17] Molecular analysis has confirmed that *M. tuberculosis* shows genetic variation and four major genotypes have been described and appear to differ in their virulence in mice.[18] The most virulent is the Beijing genotype, prevalent in Asia and the former USSR, but further studies are required to relate the relative virulence of these genotypes in a mouse model to that in human beings.

M. bovis

M. bovis is also referred to as the 'bovine tubercle bacillus' and infects, and causes tuberculosis in, cattle and in a wide variety of other domestic and wild animals, including sheep, pigs, non-human primates, dogs and cats.[19] It also causes tuberculosis in humans. A variety of wild animals are natural reservoirs of *M. bovis*, including the badger (UK and Ireland), opossum (New Zealand), marsh antelope (Zambia) and bison (Canada). Strains of *M. bovis* are divisible by DNA analysis into the classical bovine type, *M. bovis* subspecies *bovis*, and a variant, termed *M. bovis* subspecies *caprae*, originally isolated from goats and a cause of disease in some veterinary surgeons. This variant may be commoner than previously realized, as a third of strains of *M. bovis* isolated from cases of human tuberculosis in Germany between 1999 and 2001 were of the *caprae* subspecies.[20]

It is difficult for many laboratories to differentiate bovine from human tubercle bacilli in culture, although this can be done in most large reference laboratories.[15] An important difference with relevance to therapy between *M. bovis* and *M. tuberculosis* is that the former is naturally resistant to pyrazinamide, one of the first-line antituberculosis drugs.

M. africanum

M. africanum was first isolated from humans in equatorial Africa. It consists of a group of strains with variable properties and, genetically, it bridges the gap between the human and bovine tubercle bacilli. On the basis of biochemical differences, two subtypes, I and II, have been described,[15] and these have subsequently been shown to differ at the genomic level. *M. africanum* is a cause of human tuberculosis throughout equatorial Africa, where, in Kampala, Uganda, subtype II is the commonest causative organism, having been found in one study to be responsible for 157 of 234 cases.[21]

M. africanum causes tuberculosis in humans and in goats, but apparently not in cattle.[19] Strains are isolated in other parts of the world, including the UK, principally in immigrants from Africa.[22] Although having many features in common with *M. bovis*, strains of *M. africanum* resemble *M. tuberculosis* in being susceptible to the antituberculosis drug pyrazinamide.

M. microti

M. microti was first identified in field voles in 1937 and causes tuberculosis in voles, wood mice, shrews and other small mammals.[19,23] It is generally regarded not to be a cause of disease in humans, although a few cases of tuberculosis due to an organism closely resembling, if not identical to, *M. microti* have been described in recent years.

Bacille Calmette–Guérin (BCG) vaccine was originally derived from a tubercle bacillus isolated from a cow with mastitis and therefore assumed to be *M. bovis*. It was weakened (attenuated) by serial cultures over many years by the French scientists Albert Calmette and Camille Guérin. By 1921, this strain had lost its ability to cause tuberculosis in experimental animals and to this day is the vaccine used to protect against tuberculosis. As shown in Table 2.1, it differs in certain respects from *M. bovis*. For further details, see Chapter 6.

Other mycobacteria

M. leprae

After tuberculosis, leprosy (also known as Hansen's disease) is the most prevalent mycobacterial disease and is caused by *M. leprae*.[24] Leprosy is a chronic infectious disease which mainly affects the skin, peripheral nerves, mucosa of the upper respiratory tract and the eyes, and may therefore lead to disfigurement and blindness. For this reason, a particular stigma has become associated with the disease, and those suffering from it have often had to endure the additional burdens of ostracism and isolation.[24] Leprosy dates back in history to between 600 and 400 BC. Biblical leprosy was not leprosy as now defined but was probably a fungal disease or, possibly, chronic skin tuberculosis. When the leprosy bacillus was discovered by the Norwegian physician Gerhard Henrik Armauer Hansen in 1873, it was the first bacterium to be definitely identified as the cause of a human disease. It is impossible to calculate how many human beings have been affected by leprosy throughout the course of human history, but the number must run into hundreds of millions. With the introduction of dapsone in the 1940s, effective treatment for leprosy became available and at the present time multidrug therapy, usually based on dapsone, rifampicin and clofazimine, is used with great success. Despite effective therapy, leprosy is still an important cause of human morbidity and mortality throughout the world today, especially in India, Indonesia, Myanmar, Africa and Brazil.

The exact prevalence of leprosy is unknown, but in recent years approximately 600 000 new patients each year have been registered and treated.[25] Unlike other mycobacteria, *M. leprae* cannot be grown on culture media in the laboratory, although it grows in immunodeficient mice and in the armadillo. This failure to grow on culture media has been attributed to the loss of many of its functional genes except, unfortunately, those that permit it to continue as a human pathogen.[24]

Environmental mycobacteria

As mentioned above, more than 100 species of EM have now been identified and new species are continuously being described. Some species have often been identified as the cause of disease of humans or animals but most are rarely or never the cause. There is, however, no clear distinction between those that cause disease and those that do not and it is possible that any species could cause disease given the opportunity, such as in a patient with severe immunosuppression. Diseases caused by these mycobacteria are often termed opportunistic mycobacterial diseases or **mycobacterioses**.

The most common EM causing human disease are described below and summarized in Table 2.2. More details on these and the less frequently encountered species are given in standard textbooks,[5–7] and the diseases they cause are reviewed in Chapter 11.

TABLE 2.2 Principal environmental mycobacteria of clinical interest

Mycobacterium	Notes
M. abscessus	A rapid grower, previously classified as a subspecies of *M. chelonae*, causing post-injection and other superficial infections, and pulmonary and disseminated disease
M. avium	Included with *M. intracellulare* in the MAC; a common cause of disseminated AIDS-related disease
M. celatum	Principally a pulmonary pathogen; a closely related species is *M. branderi*
M. chelonae	A rapid grower, causing lesions similar to those of *M. abscessus*
M. fortuitum	A rapid grower, causing lesions similar to those of *M. abscessus* and *M. chelonae* (some strains are now placed in the separate species *M. peregrinum*)
M. genevense	A cause of disseminated disease in AIDS patients
M. gordonae	Previously termed *M. aquae*, it is a common isolate from water and a contaminant of specimens and a very rare pulmonary pathogen
M. haemophilum	A cause of skin lesions in renal transplant patients and lymphadenitis
M. intracellulare	Usually included with *M. avium* in the MAC
M. kansasii	Principally a pulmonary pathogen
M. malmoense	A species isolated with increasing frequency in Europe; principally a pulmonary pathogen
M. marinum	The cause of swimming pool granuloma or fish tank granuloma
M. scrofulaceum	A cause of cervical lymphadenopathy (scrofula) and also, occasionally, pulmonary disease; less common now than in the past
M. simiae	Principally a pulmonary pathogen
M. terrae complex	This complex contains three species: *M. terrae*, *M. triviale* and *M. nonchromogenicum*; *M. terrae* has caused a few infections in agricultural workers with injuries contaminated by soil
M. szulgai	Principally a pulmonary pathogen
M. ulcerans	The cause of Buruli ulcer
M. xenopi	A species of limited geographical distribution, but common in southern England

MAC, *M. avium* complex; AIDS, acquired immunodeficiency syndrome.

M. avium complex

***M. avium* complex** (MAC) contains the species formerly termed *M. avium*, *M. intracellulare*, *M. lepraemurium* and *M. paratuberculosis*. As in the case of the *M. tuberculosis* complex, these are really variants of a single species and are thus now generally referred to as variants of *M. avium*, for example *M. avium* var. *paratuberculosis*. The avian tubercle bacillus *M. avium* var. *avium* causes tuberculosis in birds, lymphadenitis in pigs and various manifestations of disease in a variety of other wild and domestic animals. *M. avium* var. *intracellulare* is very similar in many respects to *M. avium* var. *avium*, and the two are not readily separated except by an analysis of their nucleic acids. Accordingly, they are usually grouped together as *M. avium–intracellulare* (MAI). In human medicine, the term *M. avium* complex (MAC) is usually used synonymously with MAI. This complex is the most common cause of non-tuberculous human opportunistic mycobacterial disease throughout the world, causing lymph node infection of children and pulmonary disease of adults. It is by far the most common cause of localized and disseminated mycobacterial disease in those infected with the human immunodeficiency virus (HIV). Indeed, for unknown reasons, HIV-infected people are particularly prone to disease caused by *M. avium* var. *avium* rather than other environmental mycobacteria.

The other members of the complex, *M. avium* var. *lepraemurium* and *M. avium* var. *paratuberculosis*, are principally of veterinary interest. The former, which causes a leprosy-like condition in rats and, occasionally, cats, is quite different from *M. leprae*, the human leprosy bacillus, and does not cause human disease. The latter causes hypertrophic enteritis or Johne's disease, an intestinal disease of cattle and other ruminants. Some workers have claimed that it causes Crohn's disease, a chronic intestinal disease of humans, but the evidence is circumstantial and further studies are required.

M. kansasii

M. kansasii is, after the MAC, the commonest cause of pulmonary infection due to EM. It is one of the photochromogenic species, forming pigment only on exposure to light. Non-pigmented variants are occasionally encountered. On microscopy, cells are often elongated and show a distinct beaded or banded appearance, which is due to lipid storage granules in their cytoplasm.

M. marinum

M. marinum is another photochromogen and is the cause of superficial skin lesions resembling chronic skin tuberculosis following grazes or other minor injuries usually acquired in swimming pools or while handling aquaria. The disease is therefore called swimming pool granuloma or fish tank granuloma (or, occasionally, fish fancier's finger). Microscopically, it resembles *M. kansasii*.

M. xenopi

M. xenopi was originally isolated from a tumour-like lesion on a *Xenopus* toad in the days when that animal was used for pregnancy testing. Unlike MAC, it is only seen in certain geographical regions. It is particularly common in southern England – along the Thames estuary and the south coast. It is a so-called thermophile and survives in hot water. It has been isolated from the hot-water systems of hospitals and has, on more than one occasion, contaminated specimen containers and endoscopes that were washed but not sterilized, thereby leading to false diagnosis of disease. Most cases of human disease due to this species involve the lung.

M. malmoense

M. malmoense is another species with a limited geographical distribution and, in contrast to *M. xenopi*, is most often seen in the north of England and other parts of northern Europe. It was first described in 1977 and since then has, for unknown reasons, increased in prevalence as a cause of human disease in areas where it is encountered.

M. scrofulaceum

M. scrofulaceum is, in contrast to *M. malmoense*, less often seen nowadays than in the past. As the name suggests, it has been isolated from cases of scrofula and it is also an occasional pulmonary pathogen. Formerly it was grouped with MAC in the *M. avium–intracellulare–scrofulaceum* (MAIS) complex but is now recognized as being a distinct species.

M. gordonae

M. gordonae is a rare cause of pulmonary and other human disease but is commonly found in water and thus frequently contaminates clinical specimens. It was previously known as *M. aquae* or the 'tap water scotochromogen'.

M. haemophilum

M. haemophilium derives its name (meaning 'blood-loving') from its unusual property, for a mycobacterium, of requiring medium enriched with blood or other sources of iron for its cultivation in the laboratory. It is a cause of skin lesions in patients with immunosuppression due to renal dialysis and transplantation, but has also been isolated from cases of cervical lymphadenitis in otherwise healthy children.

M. ulcerans

M. ulcerans is the cause of Buruli ulcer, a serious and crippling skin disease seen in certain tropical and sub-tropical countries. It grows very slowly on conventional media, with colonies taking 10–12 weeks to appear. It also has a narrow temperature range of growth in culture – just a degree or two either side of 32 °C. The species *M. shinshuense*, a very rare cause of skin ulcers in China and Japan, is a variant of *M. ulcerans*.

Other slowly growing environmental mycobacteria

Other slowly growing EM have been isolated from cases of human disease, notably pulmonary disease. These include *M. celatum*, *M. branderi*, *M. simiae* and *M. szulgae*. The species *M. genevense* has been isolated from acquired immunodeficiency syndrome (AIDS) patients with disseminated mycobacterial disease resembling that due to MAC. It is not easily cultivated and has also been isolated from pet and zoo birds, which could therefore be sources of infection.

Rapidly growing environmental mycobacteria

Many EM are rapidly growing, but only a minority are of clinical importance. The species *M. abscessus*, *M. chelonae*, *M. fortuitum* and (uncommonly) *M. peregrinum* cause a range of infections, including post-injection abscesses, accidental and surgical wound infections, pulmonary and disseminated disease. The nomenclature is rather confusing. Originally, *M. abscessus* and *M. chelonae* were separate species; they were then combined under the single name *M. chelonae*, but are now separate again. Likewise, *M. fortuitum* and *M. peregrinum* were separated until they were united as *M. fortuitum*, but they are also now separate again. Post-injection abscesses and wound infections have, very rarely, been caused by other species, including *M. terrae* which, as the name suggests, is found in soil and has been isolated from lesions following gardening injuries.

Summary

The genus *Mycobacterium* contains more than 100 known species, and probably many more as yet undescribed ones. A few of these, the members of the *M. tuberculosis* complex and *M. leprae*, are obligate pathogens but the many others live freely in the environment and some may cause human disease under certain circumstances. The mycobacteria have several distinguishing characteristics, notably their thick, complex cell walls that impart the diagnostically useful property of acid-fastness. Mycobacteria are divided into slow growers and rapid growers, though the latter still grow slowly relative to many other bacteria encountered in clinical practice. The various mycobacterial species have traditionally been defined and identified by a range of simple tests, but methods showing differences in their DNA and RNA are increasingly being used.

Prologue to the next chapter

Before they can cause disease, the mycobacteria must enter the human body and, in the case of tuberculosis, the great majority of the infecting bacilli enter the lung. Thus an understanding of the anatomy of the lung and related structures in the thorax leads to an appreciation of the nature of the commonest form of tuberculosis. This is the theme of the next chapter.

REFERENCES

1. Meachen A. *A short history of tuberculosis*. New York: AMS, 1978.
2. Villemin JA. *Études sur la tuberculose*. Paris: Baillière, 1868. Relevant sections translated in Major RH. *Classic descriptions of disease*, 3rd edn. Springfield, IL: Charles C Thomas, 1959, 66–8.
3. Koch R. Die Aetiologie der Tuberculose. *Berliner Klinische Wochenschrift* 1882; **19**: 221–38. Translated by Pinner B, Pinner M. *Am Rev Tuberc* 1932; **25**: 285–323.
4. Small PM. Tuberculosis in the 21st century: DOTS and SPOTS. *Int J Tuberc Lung Dis* 1999; **3**: 949–55.
5. Collins CH, Grange JM, Yates MD. *Tuberculosis bacteriology. Organization and practice*, 2nd edn. Oxford: Butterworth Heinemann, 1997.
6. Jenkins PA. The microbiology of tuberculosis. In. Davies PDO (ed.), *Clinical tuberculosis*, 2nd edn. London, Chapman and Hall Medical, 1998, 69–79.
7. Grange JM. *Mycobacteria and human disease*, 2nd edn. London: Arnold, 1996.
8. Barrett DS. Are orthopaedic surgeons gorillas? *BMJ* 1988; **297**: 1638–9.
9. Foulds J, O'Brien R. New tools for the diagnosis of tuberculosis: the perspective of developing countries. *Int J Tuberc Lung Dis* 1999; **2**: 778–83.

10. De Beenhouwer H, Lhiang Z, Jannes G et al. Rapid detection of rifampicin resistance in sputum and biopsy specimens from tuberculosis patients by PCR and line probe assay. *Tuber Lung Dis* 1995; **76**: 425–30.
11. Van Soolingen D. Molecular epidemiology of tuberculosis and other mycobacterial infections: main methodologies and achievements. *J Intern Med* 2001; **249**: 1–26.
12. Rogall T, Flohr T, Böttger EC. Differentiation of mycobacterial species by direct sequencing of amplified DNA. *J Gen Microbiol* 1990; **136**: 1915–20.
13. Young DB. Blueprint of the white plague. *Nature* 1998; **393**: 537–44.
14. Skerman VDB, McGowan V, Sneath PHA. Approved lists of bacterial names. *Int J Syst Bacteriol* 1980; **30**: 225–420.
15. Grange JM, Yates MD, de Kantor IN. *Guidelines for speciation within the Mycobacterium tuberculosis complex*, 2nd edn. WHO/EMC/ZOO/96.4. Geneva: World Health Organization, 1996.
16. Yates MD, Collins CH, Grange JM. 'Classical' and 'Asian' variants of *Mycobacterium tuberculosis* isolated in South-East England, 1977–1980. *Tubercle* 1982; **63**: 55–61.
17. Pfyffer GE, Auchenthaler R, van Embden JD, van Soolingen D. *Mycobacterium canetti*, the smooth variant of *M. tuberculosis* isolated from a Swiss patient exposed in Africa. *Emerg Infect Dis* 1998; **4**: 631–4.
18. Lopez B, Aguilar D, Orozco H et al. A marked difference in pathogenesis and immune response induced by different *Mycobacterium tuberculosis* genotypes. *Clin Exp Immunol* 2003; **133**: 30–7.
19. Reilly LM, Daborn CJ. The epidemiology of *Mycobacterium bovis* infections in animal and man: a review. *Tuber Lung Dis* 1995; **76**(Suppl.): 1–46.
20. Kubica T, Rusch-Gerdes S, Niemann S. *Mycobacterium bovis* subsp. *caprae* caused one-third of human *M. bovis*-associated tuberculosis cases reported in Germany between 1999 and 2001. *J Clin Microbiol* 2003; **41**: 3070–7.
21. Niemann S, Rusch-Gerdes S, Joloba ML et al. *Mycobacterium africanum* subtype II is associated with two distinct genotypes and is a major cause of human tuberculosis in Kampala, Uganda. *J Clin Microbiol* 2002; **40**: 3398–405.
22. Grange JM, Yates MD. Incidence and nature of human tuberculosis due to *Mycobacterium africanum* in South East England: 1977–1987. *Epidemiol Infect* 1989; **103**: 127–32.
23. Wells AQ. Tuberculosis in wild voles. *Lancet* 1937; **232**: 1121.
24. Grange JM, Lethaby JI. Leprosy of the past and today. *Semin Respir Crit Care Med* (Tuberculosis and Other Mycobacterial Infections, Guest Editor L Heifets) 2004; **25**: 271–81.
25. World Health Organization Leprosy Group. Leprosy. In Cook GC, Zumla A (eds), *Manson's tropical diseases*, 21st edn. Edinburgh: Saunders (Elsevier), 2003, 1065–84.

FURTHER READING

Grange JM. *Mycobacteria and human disease*, 2nd edn. London; Arnold, 1996.

Jenkins PA. The microbiology of tuberculosis. In Davies PDO (ed.), *Clinical tuberculosis*, 2nd edn. London: Chapman and Hall Medical, 1998, 69–79.

Levi MH. The microbiology of tuberculosis. In Lutwick LI (ed.), *Tuberculosis: a clinical handbook*. London: Chapman and Hall Medical, 1995, 153.

CHAPTER 3

The respiratory system

Introduction

Most people are infected with *Mycobacterium tuberculosis* as a result of airborne exposure and it may be useful at this point briefly to review the structure and function of the respiratory tract and relate it to the clinical consequences of infection. In most cases, infection with *M. tuberculosis* occurs by inhalation of droplet nuclei containing tubercle bacilli. These travel through the upper and then the lower respiratory tracts and eventually reach the alveoli of the lungs, where infection may be established and, in some susceptible individuals, overt disease will ensue.

Learning outcomes

After studying and reflecting on the material in this chapter, you will be able to:

- discuss the essential function of the respiratory system,
- describe the basic anatomy of the upper and lower respiratory tracts, the lung and the mediastinum,
- outline the route by which tubercle bacilli reach the terminal bronchioles and alveolae of the lung,
- discuss the organs and structures principally involved in pulmonary tuberculosis – the lung, hilar lymph nodes and the pleurae.

BACKGROUND

Respiration facilitates the exchange of oxygen (O_2) and carbon dioxide (CO_2) between the atmosphere and the cells of the body. The processes of respiration include pulmonary ventilation, transport of respiratory gases in the blood, external respiration and internal respiration. These processes are controlled by collections of specialized cells in the brain known as respiratory centres.

Pulmonary ventilation is the movement of air in and out of the lungs, a continuous process of respiratory inspiration and expiration – namely, breathing. During inspiration, we breathe in (inhale) air because it contains O_2, which all cells in the body constantly require for their cellular metabolism and energy production. During expiration, we breathe out (exhale) as a means of eliminating CO_2, a waste product of cellular metabolism. The amount of air moved in and out of the lungs each minute is known as the minute ventilation (V_E) and this varies according to how much work is being performed. As the workload increases, more energy is needed, increasing the demand for O_2, which increases the rate of pulmonary ventilation. At rest, the average rate of breathing (respiratory rate) is 12–15 breaths (or respirations) per minute. The average amount of air breathed during each respiration (the tidal volume) is 0.5 litres (L), giving a minute ventilation of 6–7.5 L. During heavy work or strenuous exercise, however, the volume of air breathed is greatly increased and can be as much as 180 L/min.

External respiration is the exchange of gases (O_2 and CO_2) between the alveoli and the capillary network that closely surrounds them. **Internal respiration** is the exchange of gases between the capillaries and the tissue cells in every part of the body. The **transport of respiratory gases** takes place in the blood. The atmospheric air we inhale contains approximately 20 per cent O_2 and 80 per cent nitrogen (N_2) plus water vapour (H_2O), small amounts of CO_2 and traces of some other gases. We exhale a gas mixture that is much the same as that we inhaled, except it contains less O_2 (16 per cent) and slightly more CO_2 and water vapour. Most of the O_2 (97 per cent) we absorb is transported in the blood combined with haemoglobin (forming oxyhaemoglobin); the remaining 3 per cent of O_2 is transported dissolved in plasma. Although some CO_2 (7 per cent) is also transported in the blood dissolved in plasma and a further 23 per cent is transported combined with haemoglobin, most (70 per cent) is transported as carbonic acid (H_2CO_3). In the plasma H_2CO_3 dissociates (separates) to hydrogen ions (H^+) and bicarbonate ions (HCO_3^-). Hydrogen ions create a more acidic environment and the body needs to regulate the acid–base balance by neutralizing or buffering this effect of hydrogen ions. This is achieved by combining the hydrogen ions with haemoglobin, which acts as a major buffer within the blood. The buffering of CO_2 in the blood and its elimination from the body by the respiratory and renal systems are the principal means by which the pH of the blood is regulated and kept within the narrow limits of 7.35 to 7.45. This is an essential physiological function of these two systems, which ensures that an internal equilibrium (homeostasis) conducive to life is maintained.

The respiratory system needs to harmonize with the actions of the cardiovascular system to ensure efficient delivery of O_2 to the cells and the removal of CO_2 from them. Respiration must also react to the changing metabolic requirements of the body. Breathing is under the control of the **respiratory centres** in the brainstem (pons and medulla), which are composed of different types of specialized sensor neurones. These monitor the pH of the extracellular fluid within the brain, the partial pressures of O_2 and CO_2 (pO_2 and pCO_2) in the blood, and mechanical changes in the chest wall. In response to this information, the respiratory centres modify ventilation to ensure that both the amount of O_2 delivered to the tissues and the amount of CO_2 removed from them matches their metabolic requirements.[1]

The airway that is involved in breathing is known as the respiratory system and is made up of an upper respiratory tract, which consists of a variety of air passages, the lower respiratory tract, consisting of the lower part of the trachea and bronchi, and the lungs (Fig. 3.1). In this chapter, we focus on those structures involved in pulmonary ventilation and external respiration and follow the anatomic pathway of tubercle bacilli from exposure to pulmonary infection.

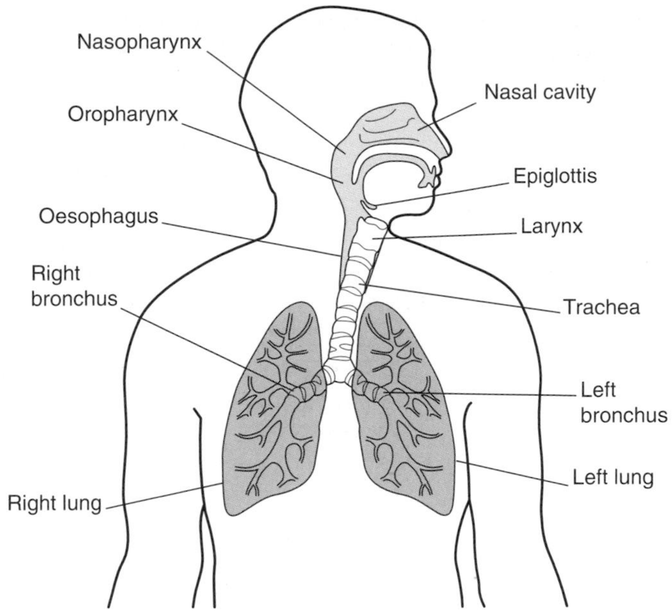

FIGURE 3.1 *The respiratory system.*

THE UPPER RESPIRATORY TRACT

The upper respiratory tract includes the nose and the mouth, through which air is both inhaled and exhaled, and the pharynx and larynx and the upper part of the trachea (Fig. 3.2) Following exposure, tubercle bacilli in the form of aerosolized respiratory droplets of different sizes are first inhaled into the upper respiratory system.

Nose

Air enters the body through the nose or mouth. The nose consists of the outwardly visible external nose and an internal part known as the nasal cavity. The nose is used for breathing and for smelling. It has a good blood and nerve supply, and nasal lymphatic vessels drain into the submandibular lymph nodes and then into the cervical lymph nodes. Because of its rich blood supply, air is warmed as it passes through the nose. The openings of the nose (the anterior nares or 'nostrils') lead into the nasal cavity, which is divided by a vertical separation known as the nasal septum. This cavity is formed by several bones: the nasal bone forms the roof, and the sides of the cavity are formed by the ethmoid and maxillary bones. These bones contain cavities (sinuses) that communicate with the nasal cavity.

The nasal cavity is lined with ciliated mucous membranes which filter out inhaled particles, such as dust and aerosolized respiratory droplets larger then 5 micrometres (μm) in diameter. (Formerly called a micron, a micrometre is one-millionth (10^{-6}) of a metre.) To increase the surface area within the nasal cavity, thereby maximizing its filtering capacity, each side of the nasal cavity contains three curved bony projections, called turbinates or conchae, covered with ciliated mucous membranes.

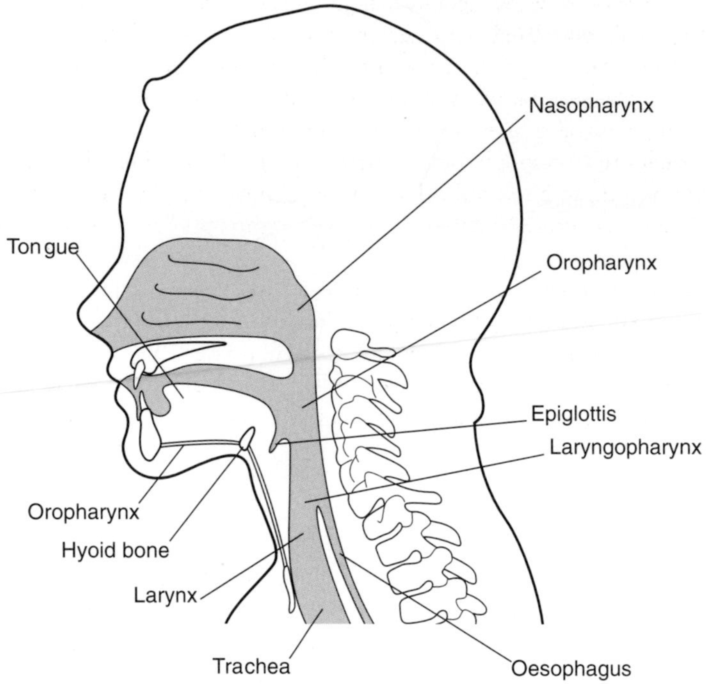

FIGURE 3.2 *The upper respiratory system.*

Two important structures lie within the nasopharynx: the adenoids, which are collections of lymphatic tissue beneath the epithelium of the roof and posterior wall of the nasopharynx, and the openings into the Eustachian canal, which lie on the side walls of the nasopharynx, level with the floor of the nose. The posterior nares terminate the nasal cavity as it continues as the nasopharynx.

Pharynx

Air passes from the nose and flows into the pharynx (throat), the upper portion of both the respiratory and digestive tracts. The pharynx is a musculo-membranous passage that extends from the base of the skull until it divides into the oesophagus (a long flexible tube which carries food into the stomach) and the larynx. There are two parts of the pharynx. The upper portion consists of the nasopharynx, a continuation of the nasal cavity from the posterior nares and lying above the soft palate of the mouth, which separates it from the rest of the pharynx when food or liquids are being swallowed. The lower portion of the pharynx consists of two sections: the oropharynx, which lies behind the mouth and tongue, between the soft palate and the upper edge of the epiglottis, and the laryngopharynx (or hypopharynx), which lies behind the larynx, below the upper edge of the epiglottis and opening into the larynx and oesophagus. The tonsils, important collections of lymphatic tissue, are found within the oropharynx. At the bottom of the pharynx, air is conducted through the larynx and food is directed down the oesophagus.

Although the nasal mucosa is inherently highly resistant to the tubercle bacillus, trauma and atrophic changes associated with ageing increase the risk of the bacilli successfully lodging within the nasal lining.[2,3] In most cases, the bacilli originate from foci of tuberculosis elsewhere in the respiratory system. Notwithstanding, tuberculosis of the nose, nasopharynx and paranasal sinuses is rare, even in populations in which there is a high incidence of pulmonary tuberculosis.[2,4] Miliary tuberculosis (discussed in Chapter 9), now seen mainly in immunocompromised individuals such as those with human immunodeficiency virus (HIV) disease, may produce lesions in any part of the upper respiratory tract, especially in the nasopharynx.[2]

Tuberculosis of the peripheral lymph nodes, especially the cervical lymph nodes, is a common form of extrapulmonary tuberculosis. Cervical lymphadenitis, also known as scrofula (discussed in Chapters 2 and 9), may be the result of primary tuberculosis of the pharynx or tonsils acquired by drinking unpasteurized milk contaminated with *Mycobacterium bovis* or it may be part of the lymphatic component of primary pulmonary tuberculosis (as described in Chapter 8).

Larynx

The larynx is a valve which has three functions. When this valve is open, it provides an entry for air to be inhaled into the lower respiratory tract. When partially closed, it provides an orifice that can be modulated in phonation (speaking or singing), and when closed, it protects the lower respiratory tract during swallowing.

The larynx ('voice box') contains the elastic vocal cords which allow speech and other sounds to be made when air is passed over them, causing them to vibrate. The space between the vocal cords through which air flows into the lower respiratory tract is known as the glottis. Several cartilaginous structures make up the larynx, including the cricoid cartilage and the epiglottis. The firm, signet-ring-shaped cricoid cartilage helps to keep the trachea open, while the flap-like epiglottis closes the larynx when food or fluids are being swallowed.

In the days before antituberculosis chemotherapy, tuberculosis of the larynx was a distressing and not uncommon consequence of active pulmonary tuberculosis (usually in those with extensive cavitary lesions). Infection spread to the larynx via sputum loaded with tubercle bacilli that directly invaded the laryngeal mucosa. Patients experienced pain on swallowing and speaking, ear pain (mediated by the superior laryngeal nerve), persistent hoarseness leading to aphonia (loss of voice) and, often, upper airway obstruction due to prolific tuberculous granuloma formation. Most patients with this condition died of it.[2] Laryngeal tuberculosis almost disappeared in Europe and the USA after the 1950s, although, concomitant with the increase in pulmonary tuberculosis, this condition may still be encountered, especially in HIV-infected individuals and in the developing nations, and it is often misdiagnosed.[5,6] Laryngeal tuberculosis responds well to antituberculosis drugs.

As mentioned above, any large inhaled respiratory droplets are filtered out in the nose or entrapped by the sticky mucous membranes of the pharynx or larynx. As discussed in the next chapter, smaller aerosolized respiratory droplets evaporate quickly and the dried residua, the 'droplet nuclei,' measuring only 1–5 µm in diameter, may escape entrapment in the upper respiratory tract and be inhaled deep into the alveoli.

THE LOWER RESPIRATORY TRACT

Trachea

The trachea (or 'windpipe') is a tube through which air is inhaled into the lungs. It is approximately 11 cm (4.5 inches) in length and almost 2.5 cm (1 inch) in diameter. It commences at the lower end of the cricoid cartilage at around the level of the sixth cervical vertebra (C6). It is separated from the pharynx by the larynx and terminates between the fourth and sixth thoracic vertebrae (T4–T6) by dividing (bifurcating) into two main (primary) bronchi – the right and left bronchi (see Fig. 3.5). It is composed of a series of 15–20 U-shaped cartilages resting flat against the oesophagus, the patency of the trachea being completed by smooth muscle and fibrous tissue. It is lined with cilated mucous cells that help to filter out dust and other contaminants from the inspired air. The continuous action of this 'mucociliary escalator' carries mucus, together with debris including many microorganisms, upward into the pharynx, from where it is swallowed or expectorated.

Bronchi

Before entering the lungs, the trachea bifurcates (divides) into the left and right main bronchi. Each enters its respective lung at the hilum (see below), where it divides into smaller bronchi which serve the major lobes and then again to serve the segments of the lungs. The bronchi continue to divide and subdivide into smaller and smaller branches, called bronchioles, forming a tree-like structure (the 'bronchial tree') that extends throughout the spongy tissues of the lungs. The bronchioles eventually divide to form the terminal (respiratory) bronchioles, which lead into small clusters of spaces termed atria, which open into several sac-like dilatations known as the alveoli, where gases, mainly O_2 and CO_2, diffuse across the thin respiratory epithelium (Fig. 3.3).

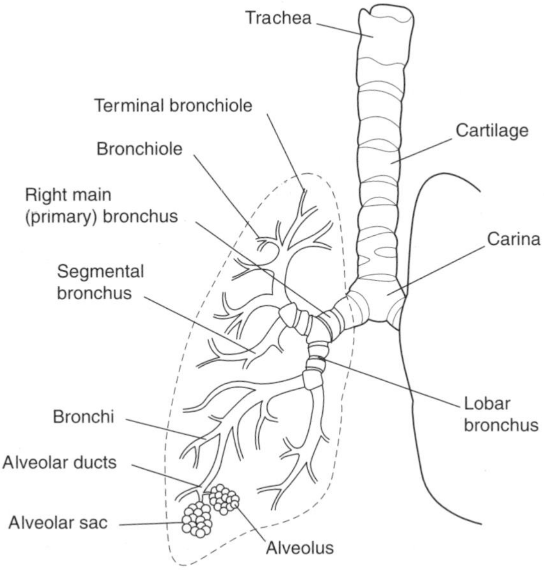

FIGURE 3.3 *The tracheobronchial tree.*

The lungs

The two lungs are spongy, sac-like structures composed of the continuously branching bronchial tree, the alveoli and an extensive blood and nerve supply. Each lung is somewhat cone shaped, with the top (or apex) extending above the sternal end of the first rib and a concave base lying over the diaphragm. The surfaces of the lungs are exactly moulded to the form of the inner aspects of the chest wall and the surfaces of the central mediastinum (described below). The lungs are divided into lobes by grooves or clefts known as fissures (Fig. 3.4).

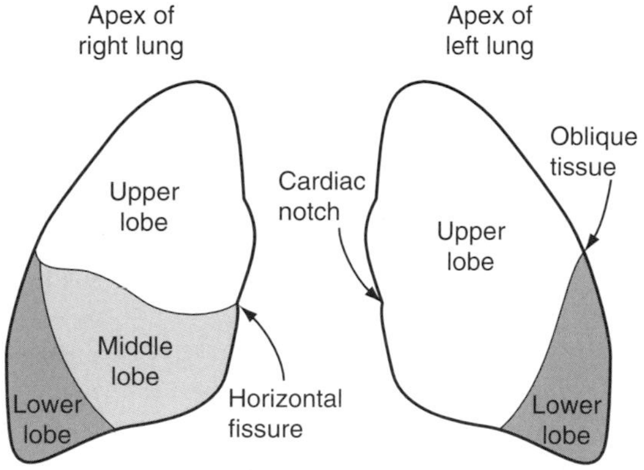

FIGURE 3.4 *The lungs (lateral aspects): outer surfaces show impression of the ribs: (A) right lung, (B) left lung.*

The right lung is slightly larger than the left and is divided by two fissures (horizontal and oblique) into three lobes: the upper, middle and lower lobes. The left lung is divided by an oblique fissure into just two lobes.

The lobes of the lungs are further subdivided into several wedge-shaped bronchopulmonary segments, each of which has its own blood, bronchial, nerve and lymphatic supplies. Each lung usually contains ten bronchopulmonary segments. Because each is anatomically and functionally distinct, a segment can be surgically removed, and this is sometimes done in the treatment of tuberculosis.[7]

Each lung is surrounded by a serous membrane called the pleural membrane that lines the pleural cavity, as discussed below.

The mediastium

The mediastium refers to the potential space that is situated in the midline of the thorax (chest), between the two lungs and between the sternum in front and the vertebral column behind (Fig. 3.5). The mediastium is only a 'potential' space in that it is completely full of vital organs and structures, including the heart contained in the pericardium, the great blood vessels, loose aerolar tissue, lymphatic vessels, the bifurcation of the trachea into the two main bronchi, the oesophagus and important nerves, including portions of the vagus, splanchnic and phrenic nerves.

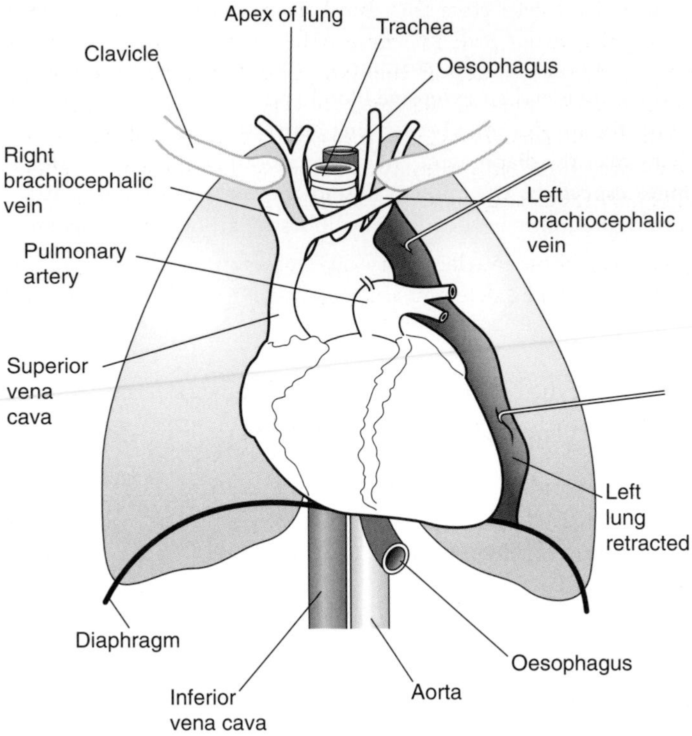

FIGURE 3.5 *Mediastinum: organs associated with the lungs.*

The mediastium is divided into a superior (top) and inferior (bottom) region and the inferior region is further divided into the anterior mediastium (the area in front of the pericardium), the middle mediastium (the area which contains the pericardium and great vessels) and the posterior mediastium (the area between the pericardium and the lower eight thoracic vertebrae).

Importantly, each lung is attached and anchored to the mediastium and rests upon the diaphragm below. In the mediastium, the medial (middle) surface of each lung has an opening (or aperture), which is known as the hilum (pleural: hila), through which the bronchi, nerves and blood and lymphatic vessels pass. The mediastinum contains several lymph nodes; those situated at the hilum of each lung are particularly involved in the disease process in primary pulmonary tuberculosis (see Chapter 5) and, especially in children, may become greatly enlarged.

Alveoli

Each large alveolar sac is like a cluster of grapes and contains several small alveoli, each with thin, distensible cell walls (see Fig. 3.3). Each alveolus is surrounded by an extensive network of capillaries, and gases (O_2 and CO_2) are exchanged through the thin, semi-permeable cell walls separating the alveolus from these capillaries. If the alveoli become inflamed as a result of infection, white blood cells cross this thin barrier and participate in essential defence mechanisms. The price to be paid for these defence mechanisms is that cells and fluid exuding from the capillaries fill the alveoli and prevent air from entering them. If inflammation is extensive, large areas of the lung become consolidated, leading to diminished oxygenation of the blood. Alveolar cells secrete a detergent-like substance, known as surfactant, which lines the alveoli and respiratory air passages and which reduces the surface tension of pulmonary fluids and, consequently, contributes to the elastic properties of pulmonary tissue.

As discussed above, droplet nuclei consisting of tubercle bacilli are small enough to reach the alveoli, where they will be detected and engulfed by alveolar macrophages.

Alveolar macrophages

Macrophages are phagocytic cells derived from blood monocytes and are found throughout the body. They differ in their properties according to the tissue or organ in which they settle; those in the lung are termed alveolar macrophages and are well adapted to the high O_2 levels in the airways. In a sense, they are 'outside' the body, as they reside in the alveoli and terminal bronchioles, exposed to the inhaled atmosphere, and ingest inhaled particulate matter, including microorganisms. Macrophages may be able to destroy engulfed tubercle bacilli but when, as is often the case, they fail so to do, the bacilli multiply, leading to the formation of the primary pulmonary complex of tuberculosis (as discussed in Chapter 5).

Diaphragm

The diaphragm is a sheet of muscle with a central fibrous portion that separates the thoracic and abdominal cavities. It resembles a dome extending upwards into the chest. It is a major muscle of respiration and moves up and down, rather like a piston, with respiration. It is principally supplied by the phrenic nerve, which arises from nerves in the neck and passes down to the diaphragm through the mediastinum. The peripheral parts of the diaphragm are also supplied by the nerves supplying the muscles between the six or seven lower ribs.

Pleura

The lung and the cavity occupied by the lung (formed by the inner surface of the thoracic wall and the upper surface of the diaphragm) are lined by a thin serous membrane termed the pleura (plural: pleurae). The portions of the pleura lining the lung and the thoracic cavity are, respectively, termed the pulmonary (or visceral) and the parietal pleurae. In health, the pulmonary and parietal pleurae are in close contact, with only a thin film of serous fluid between them. This pleural fluid holds the two membranes together and acts as a lubricant, reducing friction. If the chest wall is punctured, air may enter and fill the pleural cavity, causing the lung to collapse. This condition is termed **pneumothorax**. In the time before the antituberculosis drugs were introduced, attempts were made to rest the affected lung by artificially inducing a pneumothorax (as described in Chapter 12). Alternatively, a pneumothorax may develop if a tuberculous cavity open to a bronchus erodes into the pleural cavity to form a **bronchopleural fistula**. Inflammation of the pleura (pleurisy) causes an excessive secretion of serous fluid, which compresses the lung. If the normally clear serous exudate becomes infected, it may become purulent – this is termed **empyema**.

Summary

The principal function of breathing is to facilitate the exchange of O_2 and CO_2 between the atmosphere and the cells of the body. The respiratory system, which makes breathing possible, consists of the upper and lower respiratory tracts and the lungs. The repeatedly dividing air passages (the bronchi and bronchioles) terminate in the alveoli, where gaseous exchange occurs. The lungs are bounded by the chest wall and, on the lower aspect, by the diaphragm and are separated from these structures by the pleurae. In health, the pleural membranes on the lungs, chest wall and diaphragm are close together, but in abnormal states they may become filled with air or fluid, causing the lung to collapse. The mediastinum is the central structure between the lungs and contains the heart and other vital structures as well as lymph nodes that are often involved in the pathological process of pulmonary tuberculosis.

Prologue to the next chapter

An understanding of the anatomy of the lung enables us to understand how inhaled tubercle bacilli are able to reach the terminal bronchioles and alveoli of the lung. There is, however, much more to the process of transmission of disease, without which there would be no such thing as tuberculosis. In the next chapter we look at the mechanisms of transmission in more detail, both through inhalation and by other modes of infection.

REFERENCES

1. Jefferies A, Turley A, Horton-Szar D. *Respiratory system*. London: Mosby, 1999, 5–88.
2. Mignogna FV, Garay KF, Spiegel R. Tuberculosis of the head and neck and oral cavity. In Rom WN, Stuart G (eds), *Tuberculosis*. Boston: Little, Brown & Co., 1996, 567–75.
3. Hyams VJ. Pathology of the nose and paranasal sinuses. In English GM (ed.), *Otolaryngology*. Philadelphia: Lippincott, 1991, 24–5.
4. Lau SK, Kwan S, Lee J, Wei WI. Source of tubercle bacilli in cervical lymph nodes: a prospective study. *J Laryngol Otol* 1991; **105**: 558–61.
5. Singh B, Balwally AN, Nash M et al. Laryngeal tuberculosis in HIV-infected patients: a difficult diagnosis. *Laryngoscope* 1996; **106**: 1238–40.
6. Rizzo PB, Da Mosto MC, Clari M et al. Laryngeal tuberculosis: an often forgotten diagnosis. *Int J Infect Dis* 2003; **7**: 129–31.
7. Goldstraw P. The surgery of tuberculosis. In Davies PDO (ed.), *Clinical tuberculosis*, 3rd edn. London: Arnold, 2003, 224–41.

FURTHER READING

Jefferies A, Turley A, Horton-Szar D. *Respiratory system*. London: Mosby, 1999.

CHAPTER 4

The transmission of mycobacteria

Introduction

Human tuberculosis is an infectious disease with the causative organism being transmitted from person to person, or occasionally from animal to human beings. This seems so obvious today but, like many of the obvious scientific facts that we now take for granted, it was arrived at via a slow and tortuous pathway. Even today, the exact mode of transmission is not always clear in all cases. Although mostly acquired by inhalation of cough spray containing tubercle bacilli, other modes of transmission occur, such as drinking milk containing *Mycobacterium bovis* or accidentally injuring the skin with instruments contaminated with tubercle bacilli. Some very rare modes of transmission have been described and some of these are very bizarre and, if human suffering was not caused, would be comical.

Learning outcomes

After studying and reflecting on the material in this chapter, you will be able to:

- give a brief historical account of the events and discoveries that led to the scientific acceptance that tuberculosis is an infectious disease,
- discuss the difference between infection and disease,
- describe the principal modes by which tubercle bacilli are spread in the community and how people become infected,
- identify the potential for nosocomial transmission of tuberculosis in healthcare settings.

During the midst of the great European and American tuberculosis pandemics at the beginning of the nineteenth century, no one knew with any real degree of certainty exactly how (or even if) tuberculous was transmitted from person to person. At that time, two major European theories of causation had evolved. One theory was that tuberculosis was a hereditary disease, and the other was that it was an infectious disease, transmitted from one person with the disease to others.

The words *infection* and *infected* are often used loosely. Thus a person may be said to be infected, but so may inanimate objects, such as surgical instruments or clinical laboratory waste. Also, there is a distinct difference between infection and disease, yet active tuberculosis is sometimes but wrongly termed tuberculous infection. Infectious diseases are sometimes termed contagious diseases, although, strictly speaking, this means transmission by touch, from the Latin *tangere* – to touch.

The concept that tuberculosis was a hereditary disease was principally attributed to physicians in northern Europe who, observing that tuberculosis frequently occurred in families, believed that many individuals were born with an inherited constitutional defect (a weakness or 'diathesis') which predisposed them to develop the disease. By contrast, physicians in southern Europe, especially in Italy and Spain, believed quite the opposite. They were convinced that tuberculosis was an infectious condition, being spread from person to person.

TUBERCULOSIS AS AN INFECTIOUS DISEASE

Aristotle (384–322 BC), the Greek philosopher and scientist, postulated an infectious basis of phthisis (tuberculosis), as did Galen in Rome (AD 129–c.199), the most outstanding physician of antiquity after Hippocrates. The concept of infection was elaborated in sixteenth-century Italy by the Florentine physician, philosopher and poet Hieronymus Fracastorius (AD 1483–1553). At that time, certain epidemic diseases, such as smallpox, typhus and syphilis, were thought by many to be communicable to other people. In his book *De Contagione* (1546), Fracastorius described three different ways in which people could become infected by tiny **germs** (invisible infectious particles) from an infectious person: namely, by direct contact (touching the person with the disease), by contact with inanimate objects or substances (**fomites**) which had been contaminated by the sick person, such as clothing and eating utensils, and by breathing in air which had been contaminated by the person with the disease. Fracastorius laid the foundations for the 'germ theory', i.e. a doctrine holding that certain diseases are caused by the activity of microorganisms and these can be transmitted from one person to another.[1]

The germ theory had a profound effect on southern European physicians and was further elaborated in late seventeenth and early eighteenth-century Britain. In his book *Phthisiologia*, or *A treatise of consumption*, published in 1689, Richard Morton (1637–1698), physician to the King, wrote: 'This Disease (consumption of the lungs) is also propagated by infection. For this Distemper (as I have observed by frequent Experience) like a Contagious Fever does infect those that lye with the Sick Person with a certain taint'. Soon after, in 1722, another English physician, Benjamin Marten (c. 1690–c. 1752), proposed that 'animalcules' (microorganisms) were the cause of tuberculosis. Notwithstanding, the idea that tuberculosis was a contagious disease met with considerable resistance.

A variety of microbiological discoveries from the seventeenth century onwards would need to take place before the true infectious nature of tuberculosis was recognized and accepted. Foremost among these were the invention of the compound microscope and discovery of plant cells by Robert Hooke (1635–1703) in 1665 and further improvements in microscopy by Anton van Leeuwenhoek (1632–1723) in 1673, which enabled living microorganisms, including bacteria, to be seen. Gradually, the theory that a variety of 'germs', today referred to as pathogenic microorganisms or **pathogens**, could cause different diseases became accepted. In the middle of the nineteenth century, the 'Golden Age of Microbiology' was ushered in by the brilliant discoveries of the French chemist Louis Pasteur

(1822–1895), who conclusively demonstrated that fermentation, putrefaction and, subsequently, infectious diseases of humans and animals were caused by microorganisms. Armed with Pasteur's new techniques, a number of distinguished physicians and scientists, including Paul Ehrlich, Robert Koch, Joseph Lister and Ignaz Semmelweis, laid the foundations of modern microbiology. Indeed, it has been said of Robert Koch that if he returned to life today and entered a modern microbiology laboratory, he would simply roll his sleeves up and get on with his work!

The first conclusive proof that tuberculosis was indeed infectious was provided by a French military surgeon, Jean-Antoine Villemin (1827–1892), who, in 1865, demonstrated that healthy rabbits developed tuberculosis after receiving an injection of diseased tissue from the lungs of a man who had died of tuberculosis.[2] Villemin also demonstrated that the sputum of people with tuberculosis contained the infectious agent of tuberculosis, whatever it was. (He also showed that rabbits developed identical lesions when inoculated with diseased tissue from cattle with a tuberculosis-like condition, thereby adding to the growing evidence that tuberculosis in cattle and humans was very closely related, if not identical.) Here, then, was the ultimate proof that germs, not hereditary factors, caused tuberculosis. It was only left for Robert Koch (1843–1910), in a series of brilliant observations published in 1882, to identify the microorganism that was the cause of the oldest and, arguably, one of the most devastating diseases in human history.[3]

During his previous work on anthrax, and strongly influenced by his teacher Jacob Henlé (1809–1885), Koch realized the importance of proving that an organism isolated from a patient with a disease really was causing the disease and was not just a contaminant or secondary invader of diseased tissues. He therefore developed a series of principles for confirming the microbial causation of an infectious disease:

1. detection of the microorganism in all cases of the disease according to the distribution of the lesions;
2. isolation of the microorganism in pure culture and its passage through several subcultures;
3. reproduction of the disease in experimental animals by inoculation of the isolated microorganism and its re-isolation from the lesions of such animals.

These criteria became known as **Koch's postulates** (or Koch–Henlé postulates) and their importance is still recognized today. The detailed and painstaking work of Koch, including the careful application of his postulates, proved that tuberculosis was indeed infectious, firmly established the cause, and quickly overcame the few residual doubters.

INFECTION AND DISEASE

It is very important to distinguish between infection and actual disease. As described in detail in Chapter 1, only a minority of those infected by a tubercle bacillus actually develop the disease known as tuberculosis.

Infection takes place in a series of steps. First, the bacilli enter the body, which, in the case of tuberculosis, is usually by inhalation. Second, the bacilli must establish themselves in the tissues of the body and commence replication. If this is successful, there will be sufficient bacilli for their presence to be recognized by the immune system, with a corresponding detectable response. This has been termed 'immunologically effective contact' and, in the case of tuberculosis, reveals itself by the development of a positive tuberculin test, as described in the next chapter. Finally, the replication of the bacilli must be sufficient to establish clinically evident disease.

In practice, it is not easy to identify or determine these events. It would, for example, be very difficult to determine how many people inhale tubercle bacilli but destroy them before they can replicate sufficiently to cause tuberculin conversion. Thus, for practical purposes, infection by tubercle bacilli is defined as an event leading to tuberculin conversion. As described in Chapter 1, the ratio of those infected (thus defined as those who react positively on tuberculin testing) to those who develop the disease is termed the **disease ratio** and is influenced by many factors, especially immunosuppression.

THE TRANSMISSION OF MYCOBACTERIA

There are three possible ways in which tubercle bacilli and other mycobacteria can infect people: **inhalation** (by far the most common route of infection), **ingestion** and **inoculation** (Table 4.1).

TABLE 4.1 Methods of transmission of tuberculosis

Vector	Transmission	Frequency
Cough spray	Human to humans	Common
Cough spray	Cattle to cattle or humans	Sporadic, where cattle tuberculosis persists
Aerosols	Specimens and cultures in laboratories, cadavers in autopsy rooms; carcases in abattoirs to humans	Rare
Milk	Cattle to humans	Sporadic, where cattle tuberculosis persists
Contaminated sharp instruments	Skin injuries in humans	Rare
Urine	Human to cattle, by the former urinating in cowsheds	Very rare

Inhalation

Tuberculosis is transmitted from person to persons (and animal to animals) almost exclusively by airborne transmission. This requires a mechanism by which tubercle bacilli enter the sputum and are coughed out. Not all cases of pulmonary tuberculosis are infectious, as, for infectiousness to occur, the disease process and therefore the bacilli must be in direct contact with the air passages. This usually occurs when, as a result of the dysregulated immune responses described in the next chapter, there is gross tissue necrosis in the lung and the formation of cavities communicating with the bronchi. As described in Chapter 8, children with pulmonary tuberculosis are rarely infectious because such gross tissue necrosis and cavity formation are uncommon early in life. Patients with tuberculous laryngitis also cough out large numbers of tubercle bacilli.

Patients with tubercle bacilli in their sputum, and who are therefore potentially infectious, are said to have **open tuberculosis**. Detection of acid-fast bacilli in the sputum by microscopy is an important way of detecting potentially infectious patients, who are termed 'sputum smear positive'. A negative smear does not, however, mean that the patient is not infectious; however, the risk of infection from them is considerably lower. Accordingly, in control programmes, priority is given to finding the smear-positive patients by microscopy and starting them on treatment, which rapidly renders them non-infectious.

When people with 'open', infectious, pulmonary or laryngeal tuberculosis cough (or talk, sneeze, shout or sing), they produce airborne particles of different sizes, known as **respiratory droplets**, which contain the much smaller tubercle bacilli. Many respiratory droplets are quite large, whereas others are very small.

Large respiratory droplets do not disperse widely, but remain within the immediate vicinity of their source and quickly settle onto surfaces where they aggregate with dust. Even if briefly re-suspended by air currents produced by normal room activity, they remain too large to be able to carry tubercle bacilli into the alveolus of the lung on inhalation. As discussed in the next chapter, the alveolus is the principal target for tubercle bacilli. There is no real evidence that *M. tuberculosis* can be transmitted by dust particles or by fomites. When (and if) large respiratory droplets containing tubercle bacilli are inhaled, they will almost certainly become entrapped by the sticky mucous membranes of the upper respiratory tract, where local non-specific defence mechanisms usually prevent them from establishing infection. Consequently, these large droplets are not involved in the respiratory transmission of tubercle bacilli. Large respiratory droplets are, however, involved in the transmission of other pathogenic microorganisms (e.g. staphylococci, streptococci), spreading infection as an extension of direct person-to-person contact.

Smaller respiratory droplets evaporate almost instantly once they have been expelled from the mouth and nose. The dried residua which remain after the evaporation of these small aerosolized respiratory droplets are known as **droplet nuclei**. These are very buoyant and settle slowly. Normal air currents can keep droplet nuclei airborne for long periods of time and can spread them throughout a room or building. Droplet nuclei containing a few tubercle bacilli are the infectious units of tuberculosis and are approximately 1–5 micrometres (μm) in diameter.

A susceptible person becomes infected, and may develop disease, as a result of inhaling these small infectious droplet nuclei deep into the alveoli. The risk of inhalation depends on the environment in which expectoration of bacilli occurs. Traditionally, tuberculosis is associated with overcrowding, poor ventilation and limited sunlight, as the bacilli are killed by ultraviolet radiation. The risk of infection is enhanced in environments in which unfiltered air is re-circulated. In passenger aeroplanes, atmospheric air (which is extremely cold at high altitudes) is heated in radiators surrounding the jet engines before entering the cabins, but, to save fuel, cabin air is often partly re-circulated, and infection by tubercle bacilli, including multidrug-resistant strains, has occurred on airplane flights.[4] Guidelines for the prevention and control of the spread of tuberculosis during air travel have been published by the World Health Organization (WHO).[5]

Other sources of infection are aerosols generated while handling clinical specimens or cultures, performing autopsies or working with diseased animal carcases in abattoirs. The bovine tubercle bacillus is also usually transmitted from cattle to cattle by the aerosol route.[6] Human beings working directly with cattle can also be infected in this manner.

Ingestion

Before the widespread heat treatment (**pasteurization**) of milk, and the eradication of bovine tuberculosis, many people, but especially children, became infected by the ingestion of contaminated milk from tuberculous cows. In fact, only a small minority of tuberculous cows (around 1 per cent) develop tuberculosis of the udder, but it was (and still is) common practice to put the milk from an entire herd, or even several herds, into large tankers for transport to dairies for bottling and distribution. Thus a large quantity of milk could be contaminated by the milk from just a few diseased animals.

Infection of humans from contaminated milk causes lesions in the tonsils and associated lymph nodes and the gastrointestinal tract, with spread to other extrapulmonary sites such as bones and joints. As bovine tuberculosis has been brought under control in most parts of the developed world, it is currently no longer a significant cause of human mycobacterial disease in these regions. In the USA, only 0.1 per cent of human tuberculosis is currently caused by *M. bovis*, a rate similar to that in other countries where bovine tuberculosis has been brought under control. In those areas near the Mexican border where bovine tuberculosis remains widespread, however, the prevalence of tuberculosis caused by *M. bovis* rises to 3 per cent.[7]

A very low and diminishing incidence of tuberculosis due to *M. bovis* is likewise seen in other industrially developed regions, including Europe, but a survey of isolation techniques used in regional laboratories in the UK suggests that the disease may be under-diagnosed.[8]

In most parts of the developing world, information concerning the incidence and prevalence of tuberculosis caused by *M. bovis* is limited because of the difficulty of differentiating *M. bovis* from *M. tuberculosis* in the laboratory. The limited data reveal, however, that bovine tuberculosis is widespread in developing countries, even though the exact impact on human health and the economic burden remain uncertain.[9]

In addition to transmission of *M. bovis* from infected animals to humans, the reverse may occur, and several herds have been infected by attendants.[10] In some cases, cattle have been infected by attendants with renal tuberculosis due to *M. bovis* urinating on the hay in cowsheds. This is said to be a common practice based on the folklore belief that it adds salt to the animals' diet.

Human-to-human spread of tuberculosis due to *M. bovis* is extremely uncommon, although transmission of this form of tuberculosis leading to small outbreaks among people infected with human immunodeficiency virus (HIV) has been reported, including multidrug-resistant pulmonary tuberculosis.[11] In some parts of the developing world, such as sub-Saharan Africa and Asia, where both infections are common, *M. bovis* could therefore re-emerge as an important cause of tuberculosis in people co-infected with HIV.

Inoculation

Accidental inoculation of tubercle bacilli into the skin is an uncommon but long-recognized occupational hazard of pathologists, anatomists and butchers. In the past, tuberculous skin lesions were known as Prosectors' or Butchers' warts. The French physician René Laënnec (1781–1826), the inventor of the stethoscope, developed a tuberculous lesion of his left forefinger following an injury sustained while sawing through the vertebrae of a patient who had died of spinal tuberculosis. Accidental inoculation by sharp needles and other instruments is an occupational hazard among medical laboratory workers, and self-inoculation with suicidal intent has been reported.[12]

Some very rare and bizarre cases of inoculation tuberculosis have been described, including cases involving the penis following ritual circumcision by a Rabbi with pulmonary tuberculosis who spat on the knife before honing it to the required sharpness. Other cases have been associated with ear piercing and tattooing and in one outbreak associated with the latter, the tattooist's brother, who had open pulmonary tuberculosis, used his saliva to make up the pigments.

Brawl chancre is the name given to traumatic inoculation tuberculosis of the knuckle acquired by punching a person with open tuberculosis in the teeth. This is, fortunately, an extremely rare condition!

Other mycobacteria

M. leprae

The portal of entry of *M. leprae* into the human body is unknown. Although it has long been assumed that the leprosy bacillus is principally spread by direct skin-to-skin contact with a person who has the disease, it is more likely that most susceptible individuals become infected with *M. leprae* by inhaling infectious droplets, shed from the nose of a person with multibacillary leprosy, into their upper respiratory tract. Inoculation, including insect and animal bites and tattooing, may also be rarely implicated.[13,14]

Environmental mycobacteria

As discussed in Chapter 11, a variety of environmental mycobacteria can cause disease in susceptible individuals, especially those who are immunocompromised. These mycobacteria are ubiquitous in the environment, being present in dust, soil and water, as well as in wild and domestic animals and birds.[15] Pipes for supplying water to homes and institutions, including hospitals, are frequently and persistently colonized by environmental mycobacteria. Exposure to these organisms by drinking and bathing and through inhalation of aerosols while showering therefore regularly occurs. Thus the ratio of infection to disease – the disease ratio – is extremely low. Some disease due to environmental mycobacteria results from inoculation into the skin by injection of contaminated material or abrasions caused by contaminated objects.

Nosocomial transmission of tuberculosis

Potential nosocomial transmission of tuberculosis is a recognized risk in healthcare settings – from patient to patient, from patient to healthcare personnel and, more rarely, from healthcare personnel to patient. Residents of nursing homes for the elderly are at increased risk relative to similarly aged people living at home, and employees in such homes are also at increased risk compared to individuals in other employment matched for age, race and sex.[16] Special vigilance is also required in preventing nosocomial transmission in those healthcare settings which care for immunocompromised patients.

In recent years, the emergence of multidrug-resistant tuberculosis has added a new and worrying dimension to the subject of transmission of the disease in hospitals and other institutions. Understandably, those in the healthcare profession are concerned for their safety and rightly demand the best available protection. On the other hand, extreme forms of barrier nursing, with staff wearing fully protective clothing and respirators and avoiding all but essential contact with patients, are very dehumanizing and demoralizing for the patients and raise serious ethical issues in the management of patients with HIV disease who may be terminally ill. Infection prevention and control measures to minimize the risk of transmitting *M. tuberculosis* complex in healthcare settings are discussed in Chapters 19 and 20.

Summary

After centuries of conflicting views, the transmissible nature of tuberculosis was firmly established in the late nineteenth century by the detailed and pioneering work of Villemin and Koch. Overt disease requires entry of the causative organism into the human body, its establishment and replication in the tissues and production of clinically evident lesions. The ratio of infection (for practical purposes detected by conversion to tuberculin reactivity) to overt disease is termed the disease ratio. Infection is usually by the respiratory route, but some cases follow ingestion of bacilli (particularly *M. bovis* in milk) or accidental inoculation into the skin. Infection by environmental mycobacteria also occurs by these routes.

Prologue to the next chapter

Once the tubercle bacillus enters the tissues of the host, by whatever route, it meets the formidable defences of the immune system. Not only do the induced immune responses determine whether or not the disease becomes established, sometimes progressing to death, they also play a very crucial role in the generation of the lesions characteristic of the disease. They thereby determine the clinical and radiological features of the disease and the environment in which the antituberculosis drugs act. The processes that facilitate the transmission of tubercle bacilli from person to person are brought about by particular immune responses. Furthermore, an appreciation of the immune responses in tuberculosis is essential for an understanding of the problems surrounding vaccination against this disease and the use of the tuberculin test for its diagnosis. Before considering the clinical features of tuberculosis, its immunological characteristics is the theme of the next chapter.

REFERENCES

1. Dormandy T. *The white death. A history of tuberculosis*. London: Hambledon Press, 1999.
2. Villemin JA. *Études sur la tuberculose*. Paris: Baillière, 1868. Relevant sections translated in Major RH. *Classic descriptions of disease*, 3rd edn. Springfield, IL: Charles C Thomas, 1959, 66–8.
3. Grange JM, Bishop PJ. 'Über tuberculose'. A tribute to Robert Koch's discovery of the tubercle bacillus, 1882. *Tubercle* 1982; **63**: 3–17. Also published, in part, in *Bull Int Union Tuberc* 1982; **57**: 116–21.
4. Kenyon TA, Valway SE, Ihle WW et al. Transmission of multidrug-resistant *Mycobacterium tuberculosis* during a long airplane flight. *N Engl J Med* 1996; **334**: 933–8.
5. World Health Organization. *Tuberculosis and air travel: guidelines for prevention and control*. Publication WHO/TB/98.256. Geneva: World Health Organization, 1998.
6. Fanning EA. *Mycobacterium bovis* infection in animals and humans. In Davies PDO (ed.), *Clinical tuberculosis*. London: Chapman and Hall Medical, 1994, 351–64.
7. Dankner WM, Waecker NJ, Essey MA et al. *Mycobacterium bovis* infections in San Diego: a clinicoepidemiologic study of 73 patients and a historical review of a forgotten pathogen. *Medicine* 1993; **72**: 11–37.
8. Drobniewski F, Strutt M, Smith G et al. Audit of scope and culture techniques applied to samples for the diagnosis of *Mycobacterium bovis* by hospital laboratories in England and Wales. *Epidemiol Infect* 2003; **130**: 235–7.

9. Cosivi O, Grange JM, Daborn CJ et al. Zoonotic tuberculosis due to *Mycobacterium bovis* in developing countries. *Emerg Infect Dis* 1998; **4**: 59–70.
10. Grange JM. *Mycobacterium bovis* infection in human beings. *Tuberculosis (Edinburgh)* 2001; **81**: 71–7.
11. Bouvet E, Casalino E, Mendoza-Sassi G et al. A nosocomial outbreak of multidrug-resistant *Mycobacterium bovis* among HIV-infected patients. *AIDS* 1993; **7**: 1453–60.
12. Grange JM, Noble WC, Yates MD, Collins CH. Inoculation mycobacterioses. *Clin Exp Dermatol* 1988; **13**: 211–20.
13. World Health Organization Leprosy Group. Leprosy. In Cook GC, Zumla A (eds), *Manson's tropical diseases*, 21st edn. Edinburgh: Saunders (Elsevier), 2003, 1065–84.
14. Grange JM, Lethaby JI. Leprosy of the past and today. *Semin Respir Crit Care Med* (Tuberculosis and Other Mycobacterial Infections, Guest Editor L Heifets) 2004; **25**: 271–81.
15. Falkinham JO. Nontuberculous mycobacteria in the environment. *Clin Chest Med* 2002; **23**: 529–51.
16. Stead WW. Tuberculosis among elderly persons, as observed among nursing home residents. *Int J Tuberc Lung Dis* 1998; **2**(Suppl. 1): S64–70.

CHAPTER 5

Immunity and immunopathology in tuberculosis

Introduction

The symptoms, clinical signs and course of tuberculosis, and, indeed, whether an infected person develops active disease, are critically dependent on the nature of the immune responses of the infected person. Although the term 'immunity' is usually associated with protection, the immune system can do more harm than good under certain circumstances. In fact, the tissue damage seen in tuberculosis, leading, for example, to cavity formation in the lung, is due more to inappropriate or poorly regulated immune responses than to any property of the causative organism. Thus, in tuberculosis, as in many other infectious diseases, a distinction must be made between protective immune responses and those responses that damage the host and assist the disease to progress – a phenomenon termed **immunopathology**.

Learning outcomes

After studying and reflecting on the material in this chapter, you will be able to:

- understand the basic structure and function of the human immune system,
- understand the difference between non-specific and specific immune responses,
- describe how immune responses generate the granuloma, the characteristic lesion of tuberculosis,
- describe the immunological basis of the difference between primary and post-primary tuberculosis,
- describe how inappropriate immune responses contribute to the infectiousness of tuberculosis,
- describe the origin of the tuberculin skin test and the nature and significance of a positive test,
- describe the effect of immunosuppression on the nature and course of tuberculosis,
- describe the genetic factors that affect susceptibility to tuberculosis.

As described in Chapter 1, only a minority of people infected by the tubercle bacillus develop active tuberculosis. Indeed, unless the infected person's immune responses are severely suppressed, as in, for example, human immunodeficiency virus (HIV) infection, the risk of developing active tuberculosis after infection is quite small – around 10 per cent. This implies that the other 90 per cent of infected people have lifelong effective protective immunity. The nature of this protective immunity, the way in which it differs from the immune phenomena responsible for immunopathology in those who develop active tuberculosis, the best way of inducing protective immunity by vaccination, and the ways in which responses causing immunopathology can be switched off therapeutically have all been major challenges to researchers for more than a century. The fact that tuberculosis remains a major public health problem clearly shows that the answers to these questions still remain elusive.

NON-SPECIFIC AND SPECIFIC IMMUNE RESPONSES

Millions of years of evolution have provided human beings with many ways of protecting themselves from potentially serious and lethal infections. These consist of non-specific protective mechanisms such as an intact skin, enzymes and other proteins in tears, other secretions and tissue fluids that destroy bacterial cell walls, gastric acidity, cilia lining the upper respiratory tract, and alveolar macrophages that patrol and sweep the respiratory tract like vacuum cleaners. These mechanisms deal with the numerous minor invasions by microorganisms that occur every day, but if the invader establishes itself in the tissues and commences replication, the much more powerful specific immune defences need to be activated.

The way in which the body is able to switch on specific immune responses to the many thousands of different microorganisms – bacteria, viruses, fungi and protozoa – baffled the early immunologists. Clearly, a mechanism for recognizing the vast array of different chemical structures found on the multitude of potentially invading microorganisms is required. Chemical structures (principally proteins and polysaccharides) that are recognized by the immune system are termed **antigens**. Furthermore, several different parts of a large antigenic molecule such as a protein may be recognized – each 'recognition site' is termed an **antigenic determinant**. These determinants are quite small, a sequence of five or six amino acids (the basic 'building blocks' of proteins), or simple sugar molecules.

Certain cells of the immune system bear receptors that recognize just one antigenic determinant, so there must be numerous, many thousands, of different antigen-recognizing cells. Some early immunologists thought that there must be genes for every antigen-specific cell, but this would require a huge number of genes, far more than are found in the entire set of human chromosomes. Other immunologists therefore suggested that a vast array of different antigen-recognizing cells would arise by random mutation during fetal development so that there would be a cell able to respond to every conceivable 'foreign' microorganism, even one arriving from the depths of outer space on a meteorite! The serious problem with this hypothesis is that random mutation would also result in cells recognizing antigens within the body as well as in the outside world. Such 'self-antigens' would be expected to direct the immune responses against the person's own tissues and organs – an occurrence that early immunologists realized would be incompatible with health or even life. The famous German pathologist Paul Ehrlich, a colleague of Robert Koch, termed this possibility *horror autotoxicus*.

It is now realized that self-recognizing cells are indeed generated, but are kept in check by regulatory systems. When the normal regulation of self-recognizing cells is disturbed, these cells mediate tissue damage and thereby cause the so-called autoimmune diseases such as rheumatoid arthritis, psoriasis and systemic lupus erythematosus. Despite Ehrlich's *horror autotoxicus*, it is now evident that regulated self-recognition plays an important role in facilitating certain immune responses. Thus, although numerous different antigen-recognizing cells arise during fetal development, there is a selective mechanism for 'weak self-recognizing' cells so that each person has a 'repertoire' of such cells reflecting their unique genetically determined antigenic make-up. Such 'weak self-recognizing' cells are also able to recognize certain structurally related antigens on invading microorganisms. Just as the human brain has an internal image of the body termed the homunculus – the 'little man' – so, through such 'weak self-recognition', the immune system has an internal image of the body, giving it a surveillance mechanism for internal problems such as malignant transformation of cells as well as for external invaders.[1] Thus various forms of immunosuppression, such as that seen in HIV infection, render people more susceptible not only to a range of opportunistic infections but also to certain cancers.

As we all differ genetically in our tissue antigens – a fact well known to transplant surgeons – we all have different repertoires of antigen-recognizing cells and therefore differ in the ways in which we respond to a given microorganism. In recent years there has been great interest in the way that the genes responsible for our unique tissue types determine our susceptibility and resistance to a disease such as tuberculosis, as described below.

With so many thousands of different populations of antigen-recognizing cells, there will only be a few cells able to recognize each antigen. Thus, during the early stages of a response to an antigen, a few cells recognizing it replicate to form an expanded population of identical cells – a process termed **clonal expansion** – giving a sufficient number of cells to mediate an effective immune response. As this requires several cycles of cell division, there will always be a delay between the initial infecting event and the onset of effective immune responses, a delay that may allow the infection to progress and even prove fatal. After the infection has resolved, some of the cells in the expanded clone persist as **memory cells**, so that any future, or secondary, response to the same antigenic challenge will require fewer cycles of cell division and will therefore be more rapid and effective. The purpose of vaccination is to generate such memory cells without actually causing the disease, so that the subsequent encounter with the virulent microorganism will elicit a rapid and effective secondary response.

THE STRUCTURE AND CELLS OF THE IMMUNE SYSTEM

As the immune system must be able to protect the whole body, the cells that mediate the various immune reactions are scattered throughout the various organs and tissues and many are found in the bloodstream and in the lymphatic vessels. Nevertheless, there are small organs called **lymph nodes** in which these cells are particularly concentrated and which are usually strategically placed to intercept infection spreading from the organs and limbs. They are found, for example, in the axilla, the groin, the root or hilum of the lung, the mesenteric root of the intestine and in proximity to the tonsils and pharynx. Thus, in tuberculosis that principally affects the lung, the hilar lymph nodes are often involved in the disease process and their enlargement may be evident on chest X-ray. The spleen is another large reservoir of cells of the immune system, particularly those involved in antibody formation.

The cells of the immune system are formed in the bone marrow from stem cells that, under suitable influences, develop into any of the several cell types forming this system (Fig. 5.1). The resulting cells are divisible into two major classes: the **lymphocytes**, which are involved in the generation and regulation of immune response; and cells of the **monocyte** and **granulocyte** class, which engulf (phagocytose) and kill microorganisms. Cells of the immune system are often termed leucocytes, as, when seen in blood films, they are colourless, unlike the red erythrocytes.

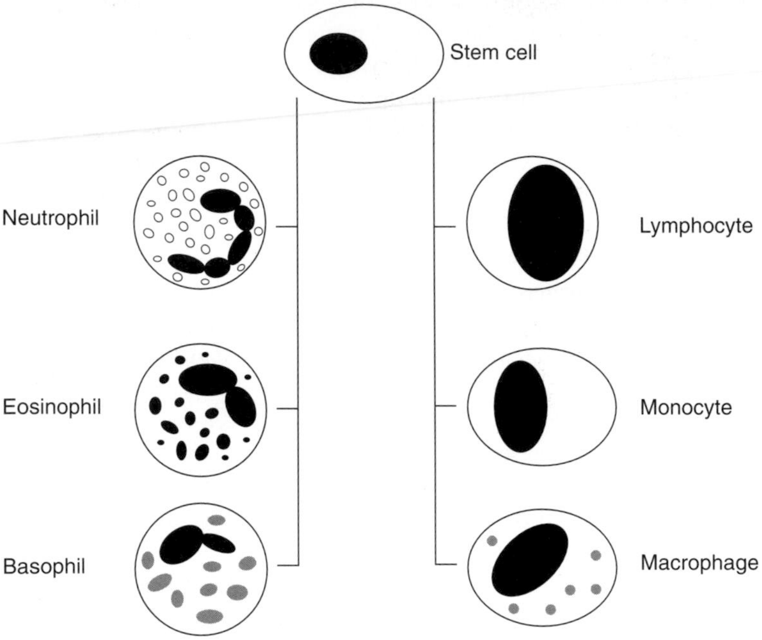

FIGURE 5.1 *The principal sets of white blood cells.*

The T and B lymphocytes

The lymphocytes are further divisible into two classes, the T and B lymphocytes, usually termed T and B cells (Fig. 5.2). The T cells are thus called because the thymus gland is involved in the maturation of undifferentiated lymphocytes into these cells. The T cells are responsible for the initial recognition of antigen, for controlling the various immune responses of the so-called 'cell-mediated' type and initiating the production of antibody by the B cells. The B cells are so named because, in birds, they mature in a structure (part of the intestinal tract) called the bursa of Fabricius. This bursa is not found in mammals – instead, B cells mature in various sites, including the bone marrow. When activated by antigen challenge and signals from T cells that also recognize the antigen, B cells mature into plasma cells, which produce and secrete antibody.

The phagocytic cells

The other major class of cells of the immune system, the phagocytic cells, is divided into two types: the granulocytes and the monocytes. Granulocytes derive their name from their very

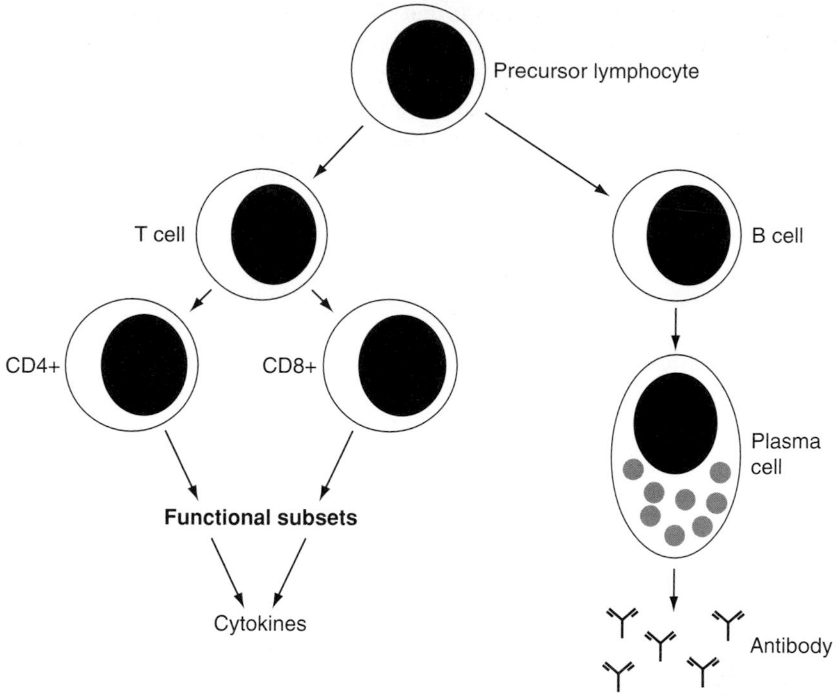

FIGURE 5.2 *The sets and subsets of the lymphocytes.*

granular cytoplasm and are further divided into three forms according to the colour of these granules after being stained with the mixture of haematoxylin and eosin that is routinely used to examine blood films. The commonest granulocyte in the bloodstream is the **neutrophil**, which has very faintly stained granules. The nucleus of this cell is quite unusual, consisting of several connected lobes, sometimes up to five. These cells are thus also known as **polymorphonuclear leucocytes**, often shortened to 'polymorphs' or 'polys'. The other granulocytes are the **basophils**, with dark blue granules, and the **eosinophils**, with red granules. These also have lobular nuclei, though the lobulation is not as marked as in the neutrophils.

The neutrophils are released from the bone marrow in large numbers in an active form in response to acute febrile infections, and thus examination of a blood film of such patients reveals a neutrophilia – a greatly elevated number in circulation. They ingest (or phagocytose) microorganisms and kill them by means of various toxic substances within their cytoplasmic granules. Neutrophils are, however, short lived, dying within around 48 hours of their release form the bone marrow. The basophils and eosinophils are involved in immunity to worm infestations, still a major health problem in many countries, and also in allergic reactions such as asthma, hay fever and urticaria.

The other main group of phagocytes is the cells of the **monocyte–macrophage** series. The name monocyte implies that they have a spherical or oval nucleus, distinctly different from that of the polymorphonuclear cells described above, while the term macrophage implies that they are bigger than granulocytes. (Some workers differentiate between monocytes and macrophages, but any difference is rather academic.) Although phagocytic, a key difference between these cells and the granulocytes is that they are long-lived and, in the absence of an immunological challenge, they are metabolically relatively inactive. They are found in many parts of the body, where they become modified according to local conditions. The alveolar macrophages are well adapted to the high oxygen tension of the lung and crawl around the alveoli and bronchioles scavenging microorganisms and dust particles. They are almost certainly the first cells to encounter inhaled tubercle bacilli. Before functioning effectively in an immune reaction, macrophages must be *activated* by specific T cell-mediated responses. As described below, specific macrophage activation is the key component of protective immunity in tuberculosis.

Phagocytosis was first observed by the Russian biologist Ilya Ilich Mechnikov (1845–1916) in the same year (1882) that Koch discovered the tubercle bacillus. When Mechnikov showed Koch his stained preparations of phagocytosis, he initially met with a very cold response: 'I do not care where the microbes are, whether they are inside or outside the cells'. Subsequently, though, Koch realized the importance of the discovery and he and Mechnikov became good friends and both received Nobel prizes.

ANTIBODY-MEDIATED IMMUNE REACTIONS

The immunity mediated by antibody is termed **humoral immunity** (a rather quaint term derived from the ancient concept of bodily humours), as distinct from **cell-mediated immunity** (described later). Antibody is involved in defence against infection in several ways. It destroys certain membrane-coated viruses and bacteria with thin cell walls by attaching to surface antigens on the pathogen and thereby facilitating the binding and activation of a cascade of serum and tissue proteins termed **complement**. Activated components of complement are then able to punch holes in the cell membrane or wall, thereby killing the pathogen. Antibody alone, or with complement components bound to it, on the surfaces of bacteria makes it much easier for phagocytic cells to engulf the bacteria so that they may be destroyed within these cells. This process is termed **opsonization**, derived from an ancient Greek word meaning to prepare a meal. In the case of tuberculosis, however, neither of these two immune defence mechanisms is effective, as the mycobacterial cell wall is too thick and complex to be lysed by complement and, in contrast to most bacteria, tubercle bacilli are at an advantage when within phagocytic cells, particularly macrophages. Tuberculosis, therefore, is an example of 'intracellular parasitism'. In fact, binding of complement to the tubercle bacillus is beneficial to this organism as it aids its entrance into the phagocytic cell.

A third role of antibody is to neutralize bacterial toxins that cause tissue damage. The classical examples are diphtheria and tetanus. Although some components of the tubercle bacillus have toxic properties, these seem to be of little importance in the development of tuberculosis. For these various reasons, antibody plays at most a minor role in protection against tuberculosis.

The various types of T cells and their functions

The T cells may be considered the 'middle management' of the immune system and, like bureaucrats, they are given fancy titles that supposedly reflect their functions. In practice, also like bureaucrats, their titles do not always accurately reflect what they actually do or are capable of doing in a given circumstance, and what they do may in fact be counterproductive and damaging rather than beneficial and helpful.

In the 1980s, techniques for the production of highly specific antibodies from single clones of B cells, and thus termed **monoclonal antibodies**, were developed and these enabled the detection of antigenic surface markers on cells of the immune system. Numbers 4 and 8 in a set of monoclonal antibodies were found to divide T cells into two main subsets, initially termed T4 and T8, but subsequently referred to as CD (cluster differentiation) 4 and 8. Although the distinction is not as clear cut as once thought, CD4 cells are principally involved in the initiation and induction of immune reactions. These are called helper/inducer T cells. The CD8 cluster contains cells that are involved in suppression of responses and are also one of the types of cells involved in the destruction of cells that are 'flagged up' by certain unusual antigens on their surfaces. These 'sick' cells include those containing viruses and certain bacteria, such as the tubercle bacillus. Such CD8 cells also detect and, in many cases, destroy cells altered by malignant change and they thwart the efforts of transplant surgeons by attacking cells in grafted organs unless they are very closely matched to the tissues of the recipient. For these reasons, CD8 cells are termed suppressor/cytotoxic cells. In health, there is a balance between the CD4 and CD8 cells, which may be thought of as the accelerators and brakes of immune responses. A major problem in the HIV-infected patient is the progressive loss of the helper/inducer CD4 cells but not of the suppressor/cytotoxic CD8 cells, until late in the course of HIV disease, leading to a severe immune imbalance as well as an immune deficiency.

Th1 and Th2 T cells

In the mid-1970s, it became clear that protective immunity and immunopathology in tuberculosis were quite distinct and antagonistic phenomena, yet both were mediated by lymphocytes. While some workers claimed that they were the result of essentially the same mechanism but differing in degree or intensity, others postulated that they were caused by different lymphocyte populations or lymphocytes at different stages of maturation.

The answer to the question of how apparently identical lymphocyte populations mediate quite different immune responses under different circumstances was provided in the early 1990s by a further important discovery. It was found that T helper (Th) cells could mature along at least two different pathways, resulting in functionally different populations termed Th1 and Th2 (Fig. 5.3).[2] The difference in function of these cell subpopulations is the result of the different types of chemical messengers, or **cytokines** (the word means 'cell energizers'), that they directly or indirectly produce. The different sets of cytokines from the Th1 and Th2 cells are said to mediate, respectively, Type 1 and Type 2 immune reactions. As will become apparent, the pattern of such immune reactivity is of key importance in the outcome of infection by a tubercle bacillus.

With an understanding of the cells involved in the immune responses, it is now possible to consider how tuberculosis develops, why primary infections resolve in many cases, why some patients develop forms of the disease with massive lung destruction, how immune reactions generate the conditions for the transmission of bacilli to others, and why the presentation of the disease is different in those immunosuppressed by HIV infection and other disorders than those with intact immune responses.

Primary tuberculosis

The outcome of infection by the tubercle bacillus and the various stages of human tuberculosis are summarized in Figure 5.4. Owing to technical problems and ethical issues, little is known of the early events following the inhalation of tubercle bacilli by humans. We can

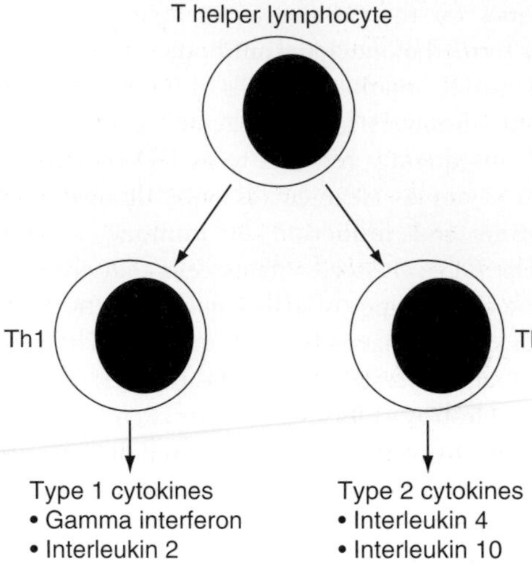

FIGURE 5.3 *The Th1 and Th2 T helper cells.*

only extrapolate from extensive experimental studies in the rabbit. The infective particle in pulmonary tuberculosis is the minute cough spray droplet (see Chapter 4) containing one or a few tubercle bacilli. These reach a terminal bronchiole or alveolus where the bacilli are engulfed by an alveolar macrophage, which may be able to prevent their growth and remove them from the lung on the ciliary escalator.

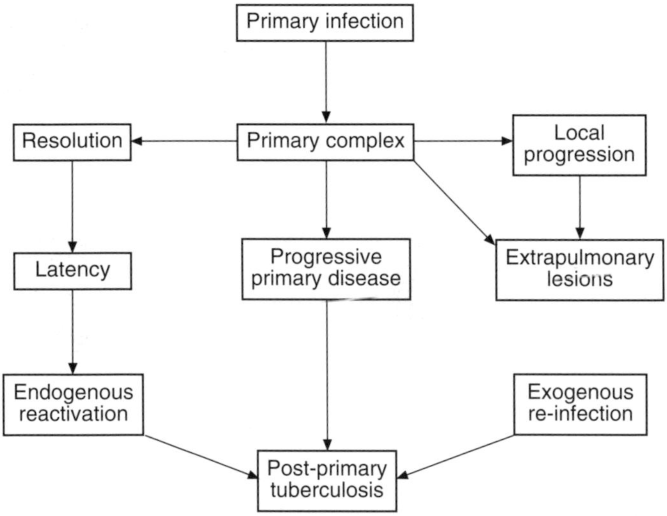

FIGURE 5.4 *The stages and evolution of human tuberculosis.*

If, however, the bacilli replicate and kill the alveolar macrophage, they are taken up by other such cells, but they also initiate local inflammation, which renders the thin alveolar and adjacent capillary walls more permeable. Phagocytic cells in the blood, both neutrophils and macrophages, pass through this permeable barrier and participate in the local struggle.

As a result, a cluster of tissue-derived and blood-derived leucocytes is formed, similar to that seen around a thorn in the finger. The resulting early lesion of tuberculosis is termed a **foreign body granuloma** and, at this stage, does not involve any specific immune responses.

Some tubercle bacilli are transported, probably within phagocytic cells, to the lymph nodes at the root or hilum of the lung, where secondary foci of disease develop. The initial focus of disease in the lung together with the secondary focus in the lymph nodes at the hilum of the lung is termed the **primary complex**. Within the lymph nodes, tubercle bacilli are engulfed by specialized cells called **antigen-presenting cells** (APCs), which partly digest the bacilli and present some of their antigens on the cell surface in such a manner that they are recognized by T cells with corresponding antigen receptors. Interactions and signalling between the APC and the T cell cause the latter to undergo proliferation, yielding clones of T cells of the various types mentioned above responding to various antigens of the tubercle bacillus.

The important T cells for protective immunity in tuberculosis are Th1 helper/inducer T cells, which surround the granulomas of the primary complex and secrete cytokines, notably gamma interferon (IFNγ), which attracts macrophages to the granuloma and activates them so that they are more able to engulf and destroy tubercle bacilli (Fig. 5.5).[3] The process of activation of the macrophages also requires vitamin D, which explains why people with low levels of this vitamin are particularly susceptible to tuberculosis, and why a combination of cod liver oil and ultraviolet light appeared to be of benefit to some patients in the days before effective drug therapy was available.[4]

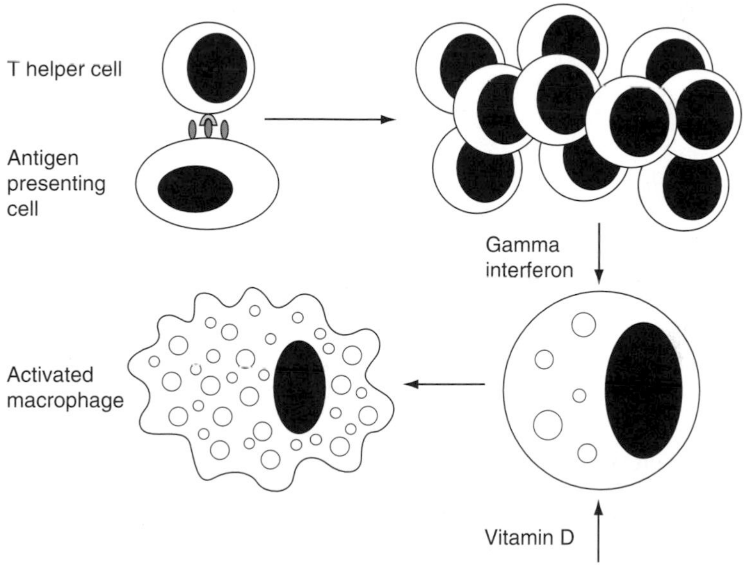

FIGURE 5.5 *The principal components of cell-mediated immunity: antigen presentation, clonal expansion of antigen-specific T cells and macrophage activation.*

Activated macrophages have very motile cell membranes (seen microscopically as 'membrane ruffling' in fixed preparations), many more intracellular vacuoles containing substances toxic to microorganisms, and a high metabolic rate and oxygen consumption. The granuloma changes from the 'foreign body granuloma' to a much more dynamic structure, the 'high turnover granuloma of immunogenic origin'.

Microscopically, the mature and activated macrophages in the granuloma superficially resemble the epithelial cells of the skin and are thus termed 'epithelioid cells'. These form a zone, many cells deep, around the infective core of the lesion.

Being metabolically highly active, the macrophages in the granuloma avidly consume oxygen diffusing into the lesion so that the centre, containing the bacilli, becomes anoxic and necrotic. As the material in the centre of the granuloma resembles cottage cheese, this necrotic process is termed **caseation** and, although seen in some other granulomatous disorders, it is particularly evident in tuberculosis. Some of the activated macrophages fuse to form Langhans' giant cells with as many as 20 nuclei in a characteristic horse-shoe arrangement. These giant cells are very characteristic of, though not completely specific to, tuberculosis. The presence of granulomas showing central caseous necrosis and Langhans' giant cells in biopsies from patients with compatible histories, signs and symptoms strongly supports a diagnosis of tuberculosis. However, confirmation requires detection of the causative organism by microscopy, culture or amplification of specific DNA. The cellular structure of the granuloma is shown diagrammatically in Figure 5.6.

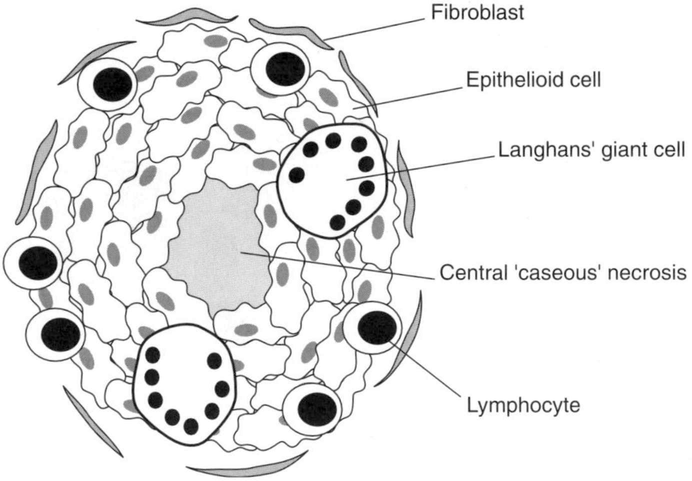

FIGURE 5.6 *Diagrammatic representation of the structure of the tuberculous granuloma, or tubercle.*

The anoxic, acidic and necrotic centre of the granuloma provides a very hostile environment for the tubercle bacilli and many die. Others are killed within macrophages by various active oxygen and nitrogen metabolites and digestive enzymes. As a result, the active disease process resolves in the great majority of cases. The quiescent lesion is then encased by fibrous scar tissue and may later show cartilaginous change and calcification.

Latent tuberculosis

Unfortunately, this is not the end of the story, as not all the tubercle bacilli are eradicated by this healing process. A few remain in the tissues in a poorly understood **persister** state for months, years and even decades and are the cause of reactivation tuberculosis.[5] In the industrially developed nations, small numbers of elderly patients with tuberculosis due to

Mycobacterium bovis, which they probably acquired before the cattle tuberculosis control schemes were completed, are notified each year. In the UK, bovine tuberculosis was virtually eradicated by 1960, so these cases indicate that infection may remain dormant for over 40 years. Until recently, it was thought that these persisting bacilli are really dormant and are trapped in the densely scarred and calcified primary lesions. It is now known that DNA specific for the tubercle bacillus is widely distributed in apparently normal lung tissue of infected people,[6] and there are strong theoretical reasons for thinking that persisting bacilli are not truly dormant but are in a cycle of replication and destruction.[7] Thus, isoniazid only kills replicating tubercle bacilli, and yet preventive therapy with this agent alone (see Chapter 12) significantly reduces the risk of reactivation tuberculosis in those shown to be infected by means of the tuberculin test. In view of this property of isoniazid, no protection would be expected if the bacilli were truly dormant. In addition, latently infected people remain tuberculin positive for long periods, suggesting the continued generation of antigen by replicating bacilli.

Post-primary tuberculosis

If the immune response of a person with latent infection is weakened by, for example, HIV infection, other intercurrent infections such as measles, renal failure, cancer, old age, corticosteroid or post-transplant immunosuppressive therapy, reactivation of disease leading to so-called **post-primary tuberculosis** occurs. In many cases, however, there is no obvious cause for reactivation. In some cases, especially when the primary infection occurs in adolescents or adults rather than in children, the primary lesion progresses and eventually takes on the characteristics of post-primary lesions without an intervening period of latency – this is termed **progressive primary tuberculosis**.

For many decades it was widely held that post-primary tuberculosis was always the result of endogenous reactivation of latent disease. Recent studies, however, particularly those based on DNA 'fingerprinting', have revealed that some cases are caused by exogenous re-infection.[8] In regions where tuberculosis was common but is now uncommon, new cases are likely to be due to endogenous reactivation, but where the prevalence of the disease, and thus the risk of infection, is high, proportionally more cases are due to exogenous re-infection. Even in countries with a low prevalence of tuberculosis, exogenous re-infection is not uncommon. In a recent study in Holland, roughly one in six new disease episodes among patients with a history of tuberculosis or evidence of past infection were attributed to recent re-infection.[9] Also, the latter is particularly common in populations in which the immunity of many is compromised by HIV infection.

In the absence of immunosuppressive conditions such as HIV infection, the risk of people who have successfully overcome their primary infection – and that is most infected people – subsequently developing post-primary tuberculosis is small, around 5 per cent. The clinical presentation and course of post-primary tuberculosis are (as described in Chapter 8) quite different from those of primary disease. Wherever the site of the primary lesion, most post-primary lesions develop in the upper zones of the lung.[10] A number of rather unconvincing explanations for the preference for this site have been given.

The lesions of post-primary tuberculosis differ in several important ways from the primary lesions. Although granuloma formation and central caseous necrosis occur, the necrotic element is much more evident than in primary disease. The lesions may reach enormous size, even filling the entire upper zone of a lung, and because of their tumour-like appearance are called **tuberculomas**. Protein-digesting enzymes secreted by activated macrophages in the wall of the granuloma soften and liquefy the necrotic material in the centres of the lesions. Thus when, as often happens, the lesions eventually erode into the air passages (the bronchi), the liquefied necrotic material enters the bronchial tree and is either coughed up or percolates to other parts of the lung. The result of this process is the formation of a **pulmonary cavity**.

Cavity formation and its effect on bacillary growth are shown in Figure 5.7. Before the cavity is formed, the centre of the tuberculoma is anoxic, acidic and full of free fatty acids, high levels of which are toxic to tubercle bacilli. Accordingly, few viable bacilli are present in the hostile environment of the interior of the lesion. Once the cavity is formed, the fatty acids are largely voided and the walls are exposed to the atmosphere of the lung – air enriched with carbon dioxide – the ideal gaseous environment for growth of tubercle bacilli. There is accordingly a prolific growth of bacilli on the cavity walls, and the bacilli readily enter the sputum and are expectorated. The patient now has open or infectious tuberculosis, and bacilli are usually seen in the sputum on microscopical examination of acid-fast stained smears.

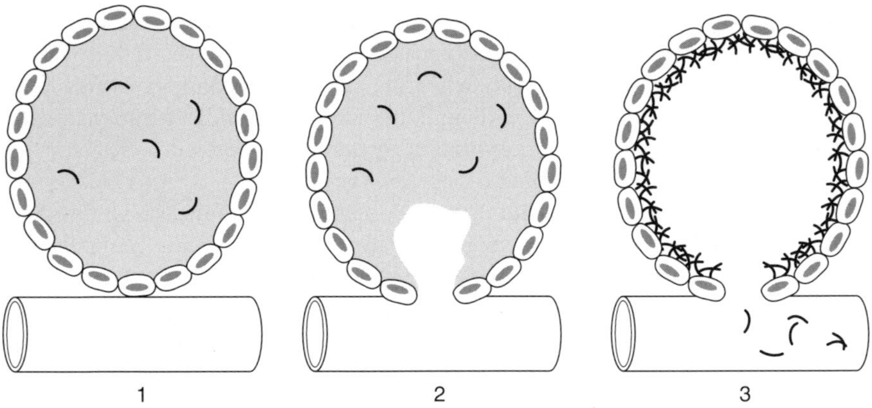

FIGURE 5.7 *The development of the pulmonary cavity and its effect on bacillary growth.*

The tubercle bacilli in post-primary pulmonary tuberculosis may be regarded as being in three physiological 'compartments' (Fig. 5.8):[11] first, actively replicating bacilli in the slightly alkaline, well-oxygenated cavity wall; second, slowly replicating bacilli in acidic, anoxic closed caseating lesions; and, third, those within macrophages. This functional division is of great relevance to therapy, as described in Chapter 12.

In contrast to primary lesions, there is little spread of bacilli by the lymphatics or blood vessels from the lesions of post-primary tuberculosis, probably because the necrotic process and the accompanying dense scarring destroy the vessels in the region of the lesions. Instead, bacilli spread within the lumen of the bronchi throughout the affected and the opposite lung; they may lodge in the larynx causing tuberculous laryngitis (a very painful and distressing complication in the pre-chemotherapy era) or may be swallowed and cause indurating ulcers in the gastrointestinal tract.

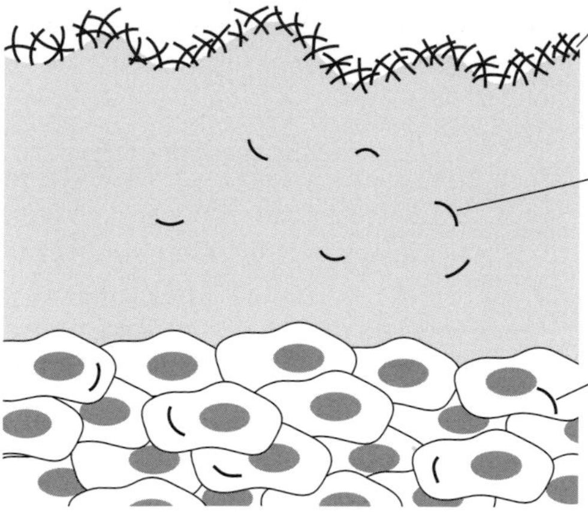

FIGURE 5.8 *The three 'compartments' of tubercle bacilli in post-primary human tuberculosis.*

The immunological basis of the difference between primary and post-primary tuberculosis

The difference between primary and post-primary tuberculosis has an immunological basis. In resolving primary lesions, Th1 T cells facilitate protective responses as described above, but in post-primary lesions Th2 T cells are responsible for the extensive necrosis. This appears to be due to the faulty regulation of the activity of a cytokine called **tumour necrosis factor-alpha** (TNFα).[12,13] In the presence of Th1 (Type 1) cytokines, TNFα plays a key role in the formation and function of the granuloma, but Th2 (Type 2) cytokines, directly or indirectly, render tissues exquisitely susceptible to killing by TNFα (Fig. 5.9). Thus, whenever a protective granuloma develops, it is destroyed by this adverse immunological response and the process continues to spread through the lung tissue until the huge post-primary lesions have developed, with eventual cavity formation and the onset of infectiousness.

A characteristic of advanced and untreated post-primary tuberculosis is extreme wasting (**cachexia**) of the patient, as well described and portrayed by Victorian novelists, poets and artists. This phenomenon is due to excessive release of TNFα (termed cachectin in earlier literature) from the tuberculous lesions.

It is important to realize that the characteristics of post-primary pulmonary tuberculosis, notably cavity formation and infectiousness, are the direct consequence of the activity of the immune system. As described below and in Chapter 10, severely immunosuppressed patients, such as those with HIV infection and a low CD4 T cell count, show little or no cavity formation and are, as a rule, less infectious. Unfortunately, their granuloma-forming protective immune responses are also suppressed, so that the bacilli spread unrestricted through the lungs and the disease often becomes disseminated throughout the body.

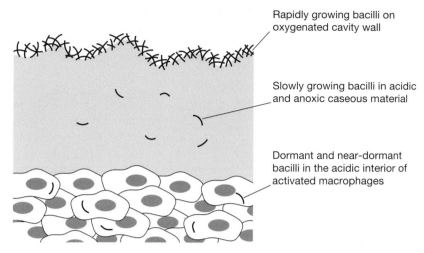

The reason for the adverse forms of immune regulation resulting in inappropriate Th2 T cell-mediated activity in those who develop post-primary tuberculosis is unclear. It was originally thought that Th1 and Th2 T cells were mutually antagonistic so that a person was either in a Th1 or Th2 mode, like being up or down on a see-saw. Others likened the two modes to the opposite *Ying* and *Yang* energies in Chinese philosophy. While such mutual

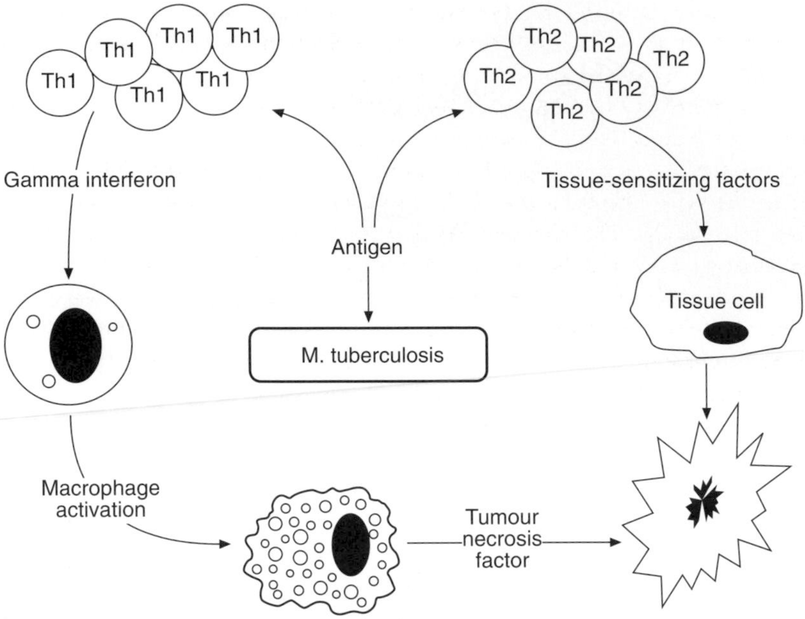

FIGURE 5.9 *The contrasting effects of Th1-mediated and Th2-mediated immune responses in tuberculosis leading, respectively, to macrophage activation and tissue necrosis.*

antagonism does occur to some extent, both activities may be present simultaneously in a lesion. It appears that the proportion of the Th1 and Th2 cells and their activity are controlled by a complex and poorly understood system or network of regulatory T cells. Some conditions, such as old age and cancer, both of which predispose to activation of latent tuberculosis, cause a 'Th2 drift'. Endocrine activity also affects T cell maturation. Thus the adrenal hormones dehydro-epiandrosterone (DHEA) and corticosteroids favour, respectively, Th1 and Th2 activity.[14] Conditions of stress cause excess release of corticosteroids from the adrenal glands and this supports the claims from the pre-chemotherapy days that stress was a causative factor in the activation of latent tuberculosis and the progress of the disease.

The description of the immune reactions and their inappropriate regulation responsible for the manifestation of post-primary tuberculosis has led to research efforts to develop therapies that will switch off unwanted Th2 responses, boost useful Th1 responses or correct underlying regulatory pathways. Preliminary studies with bacterial components, termed adjuvants, that have 'switch-like' activities in these respects, have led to guarded confidence that new therapies will be developed.[15]

THE TUBERCULIN TEST

Few topics in the field of tuberculosis have caused more misunderstanding and confusion than the nature of the tuberculin test and the interpretation of positive skin test reactions. Even the history, dating back to Robert Koch, is bizarre. Koch was attempting to find a cure for tuberculosis and, during his many investigations, observed that viable tubercle bacilli injected into the skin of a guinea-pig with previously induced active tuberculosis caused a necrotic dermal reaction at the injection site with destruction of the injected bacilli. He then found that an injection of a bacteria-free filtrate of the broth in which the bacilli had been grown, after concentration by evaporation, elicited an identical necrotic dermal reaction. He named his preparation Tuberculinum, or Tuberculin, later changed to Old Tuberculin to distinguish it from New Tuberculin, which he prepared by grinding bacilli to release their cytoplasmic antigens. Koch concluded that as the reaction appeared to kill tubercle bacilli injected into the skin, tuberculin would likewise kill bacilli in the deep lesions of tuberculosis if given systemically. This therapy was first tested for safety on a human volunteer – Hedwig Freiberg, a 17-year-old art student and model who Koch married after divorcing his first wife – a cause of a great scandal at that time. In her diary she recorded that Koch had told her that the tuberculin injection '... might make you feel quite ill, but it probably won't kill you!' She survived, but unfortunately Koch's attempts to treat pulmonary tuberculosis by systemic injection of Old Tuberculin gave very variable and unpredictable results and a few patients died of 'tuberculin shock'.[16]

That would have been the end of the tuberculin story had it not been for the work of the Austrian physician Clemens von Pirquet (1874–1929) – a man of extraordinary intellect and industry – who pioneered the subject of **allergy** and its detection by skin-prick testing. Indeed, von Pirquet introduced the word allergy (from the Greek *allos ergos* – altered energy) to refer to altered immune reactivity on second or subsequent exposure to an antigen. The word therefore had a broader import than it now has. He also introduced the word **anergy** (Greek *an ergos* – a lack of energy). On hearing of Koch's work, von Pirquet used Old Tuberculin as skin-prick test reagent in an extensive series of studies that established that a positive reaction indicated past infection by the tubercle bacillus.[17] Von Pirquet made one (forgivable) error: he found that measles (a disease predisposing to active tuberculosis in children) suppressed tuberculin reactivity and also that the test was weak or negative in those with very advanced and progressive tuberculosis. He therefore concluded, mistakenly, that tuberculin reactivity was an indicator of protective immunity.

Tuberculin reactivity usually develops 3–7 weeks after initial infection. It is said to be the classical example of cell-mediated **delayed-type hypersensitivity** reactivity. Delayed-type hypersensitivity is a rather vague expression, merely distinguishing it from a number of antibody-mediated hypersensitivity reactions that develop much more rapidly. To this day, the relation between tuberculin reactivity and immunity remains unclear. All that can be said is that the induration seen in a positive tuberculin test is the result of a number of differing immune reactions and that it merely indicates what von Pirquet would have termed 'bacterial allergy'. Thus a positive tuberculin reaction may indicate active tuberculosis, past infection by the tubercle bacillus, past vaccination with Bacille Calmette–Guérin (BCG) or, in some circumstances, sensitization by exposure to environmental mycobacteria. Although there is some evidence suggesting that small and non-indurated reactions indicate protective immunity while large and indurated ones correlate more with immunopathology,[18] tuberculin testing cannot be used reliably to assess the immune status of an individual person. Details on techniques for performing the tuberculin test and its interpretation are given in Chapter 7.

GENETICS OF RESISTANCE TO TUBERCULOSIS

Certain human populations appear more susceptible to tuberculosis than others, but it is very difficult to separate genetic from environmental and socio-economic factors.

Tuberculosis was once rife in the industrialized nations such as the UK and the USA, and there has been considerable debate as to whether the steep decline in incidence, evident long before the introduction of effective therapy, is the result of natural selection leading to 'herd immunity' or to improving socio-economic conditions.

Early extensive studies on identical and non-identical twins clearly point to the contribution of genetic factors to resistance to tuberculosis. Subsequently, a number of specific genetic factors affecting resistance to tuberculosis, including tissue types and genes regulating vitamin D metabolism and macrophage activation, have been identified.[19] On the other hand, resistance to this disease appears to be determined by many factors and it appears unlikely that genetic factors are as important as socio-economic and environmental factors in determining the risk and prevalence of tuberculosis in a community. The principal genetically determined factors that appear to affect susceptibility to tuberculosis are listed in Table 5.1.

TABLE 5.1 Some genetically determined factors that appear to affect host susceptibility to tuberculosis

Factor	Mode of action
Tissue typing (HLA) determinants	Antigen presentation
Vitamin D receptor	Macrophage activation
Natural resistance-associated macrophage protein (NRAMP1)	Regulation of bactericidal molecules in phagocytic cells
Loci on chromosome 15 and the X chromosome	Unknown
Immunoglobulin allotypes	Unknown; they may possibly affect the extent of autoimmune tissue damage
Genes regulating cytokine production and function	Affect patterns of immune responsiveness

Adapted from Davies and Grange.[19]
Human leucocyte antigens (HLA) – also called major histocompatibility complex (MHC) molecules – are a group of molecules on the surface of all cells (except erythrocytes) that are unique to specific individuals and allow the body to distinguish between 'self' and 'non-self'.

As the tissue-typing determinants – the human leucocyte antigen (HLA) types – are involved in antigen presentation and therefore determine the antigens of the tubercle bacillus to which T cells respond, much interest has been shown in a possible link between them and susceptibility or resistance to tuberculosis. Although some links have been demonstrated, non-HLA determinants appear equally, or more, important. Some genetically regulated determinants of susceptibility or resistance are only expressed under certain restrictive circumstances. Thus, while genes regulating vitamin D activity have been implicated in resistance to tuberculosis, the expression of this effect is only significant when dietary and environmental factors lead to low serum levels of this vitamin. This effect is seen, for example, in certain ethnic minority groups in the UK who are strict vegetarians and who are deprived of sunlight by the gloomy English weather.[20]

TUBERCULOSIS AND IMMUNOSUPPRESSION

As discussed in Chapters 1 and 10, immunosuppression greatly increases the chance of those people infected by the tubercle bacillus developing active tuberculosis. In the past two decades, HIV disease has emerged as the greatest threat to the global control of tuberculosis and a leading factor in the resurgence of this disease in many countries. Of all the forms of immunosuppression seen in patients with tuberculosis, that caused by HIV infection has been the most thoroughly studied and gives a clear insight into the role of the immune system in generating both protective immunity and immunopathology.

The clinical and radiological features of tuberculosis in HIV-infected patients with a relatively high CD4 count and low viral load resemble the classical features seen in those not infected by HIV. As the CD4 count drops, usually to levels below $50/mm^3$, and the viral load rises, unusual presentations are increasingly common.[21] In particular, cavities are smaller or absent and clear-cut radiological lesions are replaced by diffuse, spreading opacities of non-specific appearance. The reduction or absence of cavity formation in the more profoundly immunosuppressed patients is a clear indication that this phenomenon, though destroying lung tissue and facilitating infectivity, is mediated by immune responses. Indeed, as a result of the reduced formation of cavities, a less than expected number of patients with HIV-related tuberculosis are sputum smear positive.

Intrathoracic lymphadenopathy, uncommon in post-primary tuberculosis, is often seen in HIV-infected patients and there may be widespread asymmetrical lymph node enlargement due to dissemination of the disease. In other cases, numerous minute lesions teeming with tubercle bacilli are found in many organs. Owing to the lack of immune reactivity and granuloma formation, these lesions lack the characteristic millet seed appearance of miliary tuberculosis (defined in Chapter 9) and, in contrast, are very difficult to see on radiology or ophthalmoscopy. This condition, which is also seen in elderly patients and in those with immunosuppression due to other causes such as renal failure, is termed **cryptogenic disseminated tuberculosis**.[22]

While HIV infection clearly has an adverse effect on the course of tuberculosis, the latter likewise has an adverse effect on the course of HIV infection, as it leads to HIV replication and dissemination throughout the body.[23] As a result, tuberculosis in HIV-positive patients, even if successfully treated, is accompanied by a high mortality in the ensuing months, usually due to other opportunistic infections.[24] Interestingly, those with smear-negative pulmonary tuberculosis have a worse prognosis than smear-positive patients, probably as a result of diagnostic delays and more severe immunosuppression.

A possible reason for this adverse effect of tuberculosis on the course of HIV disease is that the former, as well as the latter, induces a degree of immunosuppression and a drop in the CD4 T cell count, although this recovers on effective antituberculosis therapy.[25] Another likely cause is the release from the tuberculous lesions of excess TNFα, which activates the transcription of the DNA provirus of the HIV and leads to viral replication. Whatever the cause, tuberculosis, whether pulmonary on extrapulmonary, is accordingly now classified as an acquired immunodeficiency syndrome (AIDS)-defining condition.

Summary

Cell-mediated immune responses in tuberculosis are a ‘two-edged sword’, as they afford protection but are also the cause of clinical features and progression of the disease. Unravelling the various immune responses in this disease has, since the pioneering work by Koch, Mechnikov and others in the late nineteenth century, been a huge challenge to researchers, but the discovery of the major maturation pathways of T cells has added greatly to this understanding. In particular, the considerable clinical differences between primary and post-primary tuberculosis can now be largely explained. The HIV pandemic has stressed how crucial immune responses are in preventing those infected by the tubercle bacillus from developing active tuberculosis and also in determining the clinical and radiological features of the disease and the development of infectivity in an individual patient.

Despite great strides forward in our understanding of the complex interactions between the tubercle bacillus and its human host, there are still large gaps in our knowledge. Nevertheless, there are grounds for optimism that further and greater strides forward will soon be taken as the genomes of both the human being and the tubercle bacillus have been successfully mapped, and it is to be hoped that this will have an enormous and beneficial impact on research.

Prologue to the next chapter

Despite our advancing understanding of the immunology of tuberculosis, there have been relatively few practical outcomes. The skin test reagent used for tuberculin testing, though with minor modifications, dates back to the late nineteenth century and the only available vaccine, BCG, was introduced more than 80 years ago. Indeed, few vaccines are less well understood and beset with so many practical questions than BCG, which therefore is worthy of a whole chapter on its own, and it is to this intriguing topic we turn in the next chapter.

REFERENCES

1. Cohen IR, Young DB. Autoimmunity, microbial immunity and the immunological homunculus. *Immunol Today* 1991; **12**: 105–10.
2. Dong C, Flavell RA. Th1 and Th2 cells. *Curr Opin Hematol* 2001; **8**: 47–51.
3. Flynn JL, Chan J, Triebold KJ. An essential role for interferon gamma in resistance to *Mycobacterium tuberculosis* infection. *J Exp Med* 1993; **178**: 2249–54.
4. Davies PDO. Vitamin D and tuberculosis. *Am Rev Respir Dis* 1989; **139**: 1571.
5. Orme IM. The latent tubercle bacillus (I'll let you know if I ever meet one). *Int J Tuberc Lung Dis* 2001; **5**: 589–93.
6. Hernandez-Pando R, Jeyanathan M, Mengistu G et al. Persistence of DNA from *Mycobacterium tuberculosis* in superficially normal lung tissue during latent infection. *Lancet* 2000; **356**: 2133–8.
7. Grange JM. Would you know one if you met one? *Int J Tuberc Lung Dis* 2001; **5**: 1162–3.
8. Lambert ML, Hasker E, Van Deun A et al. Recurrence in tuberculosis: relapse or reinfection? *Lancet Infect Dis* 2003; **3**: 282–7.
9. de Boer AS, Borgdorff MW, Vynnycky E et al. Exogenous re-infection as a cause of recurrent tuberculosis in a low-incidence area. *Int J Tuberc Lung Dis* 2003; **7**: 145–52.
10. Balasubramanian V, Wiegeshaus EH, Taylor BT, Smith DW. Pathogenesis of tuberculosis: pathway to apical localisation. *Tuber Lung Dis* 1994; **75**: 168–78.
11. Mitchison DA. The role of individual drugs in the chemotherapy of tuberculosis. *Int J Tuberc Lung Dis* 2000; **4**: 796–806.
12. Rook GAW, Zumla A. Advances in the immunopathogenesis of pulmonary tuberculosis. *Curr Opin Pulm Med* 2001; **7**: 116–23.
13. Hernandez-Pando R, Rook GAW. The role of TNFα in T cell-mediated inflammation depends on the Thl /Th2 cytokine balance. *Immunology* 1994; **82**: 591–5.

14. Baker RW, Walker BR, Shaw RJ et al. Increased cortisol:cortisone ratio in acute pulmonary tuberculosis. *Am J Respir Crit Care Med* 2000; **162**: 1641–7.
15. Johnson JL, Kamya RM, Okwera A et al. Randomised controlled trial of *Mycobacterium vaccae* immunotherapy in non-human immunodeficiency virus-infected Ugandan adults with newly diagnosed pulmonary tuberculosis. *J Infect Dis* 2000; **181**: 1304–12.
16. Dormandy T. Tuberculin. In *The white death. A history of tuberculosis*. London: Hambledon Press, 1999, 139–46.
17. Bothamley GH, Grange JM. The Koch phenomenon and delayed hypersensitivity 1891–1991. *Tubercle* 1991; **72**: 7–12.
18. Shastri AR, Serane VT, Mahadevan S, Nalini P. Qualitative tuberculin response in the diagnosis of tuberculosis in apparently healthy schoolchildren. *Int J Tuberc Lung Dis* 2003; **7**: 1092–6.
19. Davies PDO, Grange JM. The genetics of resistance and susceptibility to tuberculosis. *Ann N Y Acad Sci* 2001; **953**: 151–6.
20. Wilkinson RJ, Llewelyn M, Toossi Z et al. Influence of vitamin D deficiency and vitamin D receptor polymorphism on tuberculosis among Gujarati Asians in west London: a case-control study. *Lancet* 2000; **355**: 618–21.
21. Ustianovsky A, Mwaba P, Zumla A. Tuberculosis and HIV – perspectives from sub-Saharan Africa. In Porter JDH, Grange JM (eds), *Tuberculosis. An interdisciplinary perspective*. London: Imperial College Press, 1999, 283–311.
22. Proudfoot AT. Cryptic disseminated tuberculosis. *Br J Hosp Med* 1971; **5**: 773–80.
23. Whalen C, Horsburgh CR, Hom D et al. Accelerated course of human immunodeficiency virus infection after tuberculosis. *Am J Respir Crit Care Med* 1995; **151**: 129–34.
24. Toossi Z. Virological and immunological impact of tuberculosis on human immunodeficiency virus type 1 disease. *J Infect Dis* 2003; **188**: 1146–55.
25. Pilheu JA, De Salvo MC, Gonzalez J. CD4+ T-lymphocytopenia in severe pulmonary tuberculosis without evidence of human immunodeficiency virus infection. *Int J Tuberc Lung Dis* 1997; **1**: 422–6.

FURTHER READING

Grange JM. Immunophysiology and immunopathology of tuberculosis. In Davies PDO (ed.), *Clinical tuberculosis*, 3rd edn. London: Arnold, 2003, 88–104.

Lucas S. Histopathology. In Davies PDO (ed.), *Clinical tuberculosis*, 3rd edn. London: Arnold, 2003, 74–87.

Rook GAW, Zumla A. Advances in the immunopathogenesis of pulmonary tuberculosis. *Curr Opin Pulm Med* 2001; **7**: 116–23.

Schluger NW. Recent advances in our understanding of human host responses in tuberculosis. *Respir Dis* 2001; **2**: 157–63.

CHAPTER 6

Vaccination against tuberculosis

Introduction

If there was a totally effective vaccine against tuberculosis, the disease could be eradicated. The fact that we have more cases of this disease today than at any previous time in human history is clear evidence that vaccine strategies are not contributing to disease control. The tuberculosis vaccine – **Bacille Calmette–Guérin** (BCG) – has been in widespread use for more than 80 years and given to billions of people, yet it is the least well understood of all vaccines and has a history that is, to say the least, bizarre and confusing. Of all the aspects of tuberculosis management and control, few generate more questions, yet receive fewer clear-cut and unambiguous answers, than vaccination. Many questions surround the mode of action of BCG, its protective efficacy in various geographical regions, populations and age groups, and its optimal use. All that can be said for certain is that while it contributes little to the overall control of tuberculosis, it prevents some of the most terrible manifestations of the disease in children and this alone fully justifies its continued widespread use.

Learning outcomes

After studying and reflecting on the material in this chapter, you will be able to:

- give a brief account of the bizarre history of BCG vaccination,
- describe how BCG resembles and differs from other vaccines,
- discuss why BCG contributes little to the overall control of tuberculosis,
- outline the use of, and contraindications to the use of, BCG vaccine,
- describe the complications of BCG and their management.

It was long realized that people recovering from certain acute infectious diseases such as diphtheria and smallpox had lasting, often lifelong, protection against a second bout of the disease. These protected people were said to be immune (from the Latin *immunis* – exemption from a public service). The first attempt to utilize this phenomenon was variolation – the deliberate infection of children with material from the pustules of a person with a mild form of smallpox to protect against more virulent forms of the disease. This was a commonplace practice in Turkey and was observed by Lady Mary Wortley Montagu (1689–1762), the wife of a British Consul in that country, and introduced by her into the UK in the early eighteenth century. After initial safety studies in convicted criminals (who, it is to be hoped, gave full written informed consent), variolation was widely applied, as outbreaks of smallpox in those days caused numerous deaths, but it was not free of risk, including a low level of fatality. Accordingly, safer methods of immunization were sought.

There was at that time a folklore tale that milkmaids frequently caught cowpox, a benign and self-limiting infection of the skin of the hand, and this protected them against smallpox. In 1796, an English country doctor, Edward Jenner (1749–1823), inoculated an 8-year-old boy with material from a pustule of a milkmaid with cowpox. Six weeks later, after the boy had developed a pustule, Jenner inoculated him with material from a case of virulent smallpox and, fortunately, the lad remained well. Although such an experiment might cause raised eyebrows at an ethics committee today, it firmly established the practice of vaccination (from the Latin *vacca* – a cow), which eventually led to the conquest of smallpox and saved millions of lives.

Further developments in the field of vaccination had to await the experimental confirmation of the germ theory of disease by the French chemist Louis Pasteur (1822–1896) and techniques for isolating the causative organisms of infectious diseases. Pasteur found that old, 'stale' cultures of the causative organism of chicken cholera did not cause the disease when injected into healthy birds. He then found that these birds did not develop the disease when injected with fresh virulent cultures that caused disease in control birds. Inspired by this success, Pasteur developed several techniques for weakening (**attenuating**) the virulence of microorganisms and, using these techniques, he developed an anthrax vaccine in 1881. Subsequently, although he could not isolate the causative organism, he developed a rabies vaccine from dried spinal cords of rabbits infected with rabid material.

Other workers took up the challenge of developing new vaccines, and several were soon made available, some living attenuated, some killed and some, as in the case of diphtheria, prepared from inactivated toxins (toxoids) extracted from bacteria. Thus, Koch's discovery of the tubercle bacillus in 1882 came at the time when the science of vaccine development was becoming well established and many workers sought to produce a tuberculosis vaccine. Early studies led to the conclusion that, in order to afford protection, a vaccine prepared from the tubercle bacillus would have to be a living attenuated one rather than a killed one, as it would have to induce 'a limited tuberculous process'. This assertion might now be challenged, but it became the 'received wisdom' of those days. Indeed, several workers produced strains of *Mycobacterium tuberculosis* that were attenuated in experimental animals, and two are still available from culture collections, but none was used in clinical trials. Some workers attempted to use other species of mycobacteria, and the 'turtle tubercle bacillus' (*M. chelonae*), isolated from a turtle at the Berlin Zoo that was found to have a tuberculosis-like disease, was investigated sporadically between 1903 and 1933 as a vaccine and immunotherapeutic agent for human tuberculosis, though with conflicting results.

Eventually, by coincidental analogy with the use of the cowpox virus to protect against smallpox, the tuberculosis vaccine was developed from the bovine tubercle bacillus *M. bovis*. The choice of this organism was, at least in part, influenced by an error promulgated by Koch, who was following up the work of Theobald Smith (1859–1934) showing that the human and bovine tubercle bacilli displayed small but constant differences (see Chapter 2). Koch's studies led him to the false conclusion that *M. bovis* was of very low virulence in humans and no threat to human health, so that control measures in cattle were unnecessary. This conclusion was presented at the British Congress on Tuberculosis in 1901 and it met with vigorous condemnation by several eminent veterinary surgeons, who, on the basis of extensive observations, held a firmly opposing view.

As a direct result of the furore at this congress, the Royal Commission on Tuberculosis – the forerunner of the British Medical Research Council – was established. The excellent and extensive work of the Royal Commission, completed in 1911, fully justified the fears of these veterinary surgeons and firmly proved that tuberculous cattle posed a serious health threat to the human population.[1] Nevertheless, the statement by such a revered authority as Koch had made a lasting impact. In addition, there was a rather dubious concept at that time, known as 'Marfan's law', that self-limiting tuberculous cervical lymphadenitis (scrofula) in children caused by *M. bovis* in milk protected them against the more serious pulmonary tuberculosis later in life.

THE DEVELOPMENT OF BACILLE CALMETTE–GUÉRIN

Accordingly, two French scientists, Albert Calmette and Camille Guérin, working at the Institut Pasteur in Lille, began the very long process of attenuating a strain of *M. bovis* isolated from cows' milk so as to render it a safe vaccine for human use. They achieved this by making a total of 230 serial subcultures of their strain, on potato slices dipped in a mixture of glycerol and bile, between the years 1907 and 1920. (We will, unfortunately, never know how this bizarre process of attenuation worked, as the starting strain has been lost.) Eventually, in 1921, after conducting extensive animal experiments to ensure that it was irreversibly attenuated, the vaccine was administered by mouth to neonates born to mothers with active tuberculosis and therefore at a very great risk of developing the disease. The Bacille Calmette–Guérin (BCG) vaccine appeared to afford 90 per cent protection in these infants. (In this context, it is important to remember that this vaccine was intended as a substitute for natural infection of young children by *M. bovis* in milk and was therefore given by mouth at a very young age.) News of the success of this clinical trial spread and, despite the strongly expressed fears of many scientists that the vaccine could revert to virulence, subcultures were distributed to other countries where they were cultivated in local laboratories and administered to infants. This rather haphazard practice continued until 1930 when, owing to a tragic labelling accident, 251 infants in the north German city of Lübeck were accidentally given a virulent strain of *M. tuberculosis* and 72 died of tuberculosis over the next few months. Calmette never recovered from the shock, and Guérin reported that he died a few years later of a broken heart.

As a result of this disaster, BCG was subsequently manufactured under tightly controlled conditions for intradermal rather than oral administration. By that time, however, there were many 'daughter strains' of BCG worldwide, which, owing to different manufacturing procedures, vary slightly in their bacteriological properties.

In 1928, the League of Nations gave its approval to BCG, and its use spread across the world. There were, however, very few data on the protective efficacy of BCG at that time, and several major controlled evaluation studies, the first commencing in 1935, were therefore set up in a number of countries. When the results of these were compared, it was apparent that the observed protection given by BCG in different studies varied greatly, from around 78 per cent protection in the UK, north-western USA and Uganda to hardly any protection in Florida, Burma and South India. Some examples of the variation in demonstrated efficacy are shown in Table 6.1. Many explanations were advanced, but many doubts remained. In an attempt to settle the matter once and for all, the World Health Organization

TABLE 6.1 Protection afforded by BCG vaccination in nine major trials

Country	Year of commencement of trial	Age range at time of vaccination	Protection afforded (%)
North America	1935	0–20 years	80
Chicago, USA	1937	3 months	75
Great Britain	1950	14–15 years	78
Puerto Rico	1949	1–18 years	31
South India	1950	All ages	31
Georgia, USA	1950	5 years	14
Illinois, USA	1948	Young adults	0
South India[a]	1968	All ages	0
Malawi	1978	All ages	0

[a]No protection at 7.5-year follow-up but some protection at 15-year follow-up in those vaccinated in infancy.

(WHO) set up an enormous and well-controlled study, involving people of all ages up to 20 years, in the Chingleput region of South India. To universal consternation, a follow-up after 7.5 years revealed no protection at all; indeed, the vaccinated people seemed slightly more prone to active tuberculosis than the unvaccinated controls.[2] However, a 15-year follow-up did show that those who had been vaccinated in infancy had a moderate level of protection against both tuberculosis and leprosy. In view of this, the WHO sponsored several studies, which confirmed the efficacy of neonatal BCG vaccination even in regions in which vaccination of older children or young adults gave little protection.

In a critical analytical review of many studies (a process known as a **meta-analysis**), the average protection, though with very large variations between studies, was 50 per cent, but average protection against tuberculous meningitis and disseminated disease in children was 64 and 78 per cent respectively.[3] This confirmed the prevalent view that the principal role of BCG vaccination is the protection of children against these serious forms of the disease.

The Chingleput study, predictably, led to extensive head scratching, and several explanations, of widely differing credibility and rationality, emerged. One explanation that elicited considerable interest is that prior exposure to populations of environmental mycobacteria (EM) has profound effects on immune responses following infection by the tubercle bacillus.[4] One school of thought argued that, in some regions, prior exposure to EM would generate so much protective immunity that BCG vaccination would add very little and no efficacy would therefore be demonstrable in clinical trials. Another school maintained that, under some circumstances, exposure to EM generates immune responses that block the action of BCG or cause it to induce tissue necrotizing immunopathology rather than protective immunity.[5] This hypothesis would explain why, in the Chingleput study and in a subsequent study in Malawi, BCG given to older people appeared to predispose slightly to tuberculosis rather than to give protection. BGG has therefore been described as a 'two-edged sword', as it appears to boost both protective and adverse immune responses, which in turn may reflect the involvement of the two subsets of T helper (Th) cells – Th1 and Th2 – as described in the previous chapter. In this context, neonatal BCG vaccination, which (as described above) invariably gives good protection, is known to induce Th1 T cell-mediated immune reactivity.[6]

HOW DOES BCG PROTECT AGAINST TUBERCULOSIS?

The simple answer is – we do not know! Many vaccines are highly species or even strain specific and their 'protective antigens' have been well characterized and in some cases used to prepare subunit vaccines. A classical example is the inactivated toxin (toxoid) from the diphtheria bacillus. BCG is different – no definite mycobacterial 'protective antigens' have been identified and the protection afforded by this vaccine is certainly not species specific. Thus, in some regions, BCG protects as well, or even better, against leprosy, and the only antigens shared between *M. tuberculosis* and *M. leprae* are also shared by all other mycobacteria and, to a large extent, by many other bacteria. Indeed, BCG also protects children against lymphadenitis due to various species of environmental mycobacteria.

There are, however, a number of theories about how BCG gives protection. One is that it does not induce immune responses specifically against pathogenic mycobacteria but has a much broader effect on the maturation of T cell-mediated immunity when given early in life. This possibility is supported by intriguing observations that BCG vaccination of neonates and infants has beneficial effects on overall health in addition to protection against tuberculosis.[7] In addition, several surveys have strongly indicated that BCG vaccination significantly reduces the risk of children and young adults developing leukaemia, melanoma and possibly other cancers.[8] It has been suggested that, by non-specifically stimulating cell-mediated immunity, BCG enables the maturing immune system to hunt and destroy embryonic cell remnants from which such cancers of childhood may arise.[9]

Although protection usually implies prevention of a disease, there is evidence from a study in the Gambia that prior BCG vaccination may improve the prognosis and response to therapy in those who develop tuberculosis. Thus, 35 of 200 patients with no BCG scar died during the course of chemotherapy but none of 85 with BCG scars died.[10] Other factors that may have affected survival were sought but not found, so this effect of BCG seems genuine, although further confirmatory studies are required in other regions.

HOW LONG DOES PROTECTION BY BCG LAST?

Again, this is a difficult question to answer. Apart from the actual development of active disease, there is no good way of assessing protection. As mentioned above, tuberculin reactivity cannot be used reliably for this purpose. A major controlled trial of BCG in the UK was followed for 15 years and showed a gradual decline in protection, with no protection at 15 years.[11] Some other trials were likewise followed up but they showed more variable and usually statistically insignificant trends, possibly as several showed low initial levels of protection. It is possible that, as environmental factors such as repeated exposure to environmental mycobacteria affect the initial protective efficacy of BCG, they could also affect the duration of such protection.

WHO IS, AND WHO IS NOT, PROTECTED BY BCG VACCINATION?

In order to understand who is protected by BCG, it is necessary to be clear what we mean when we say that BCG affords a certain level of protection. It is also necessary to review a few aspects of the epidemiology and immunology of tuberculosis that have been discussed in previous chapters.

If a clinical trial revealed that, for example, BCG afforded 75 per cent protection against tuberculosis, it does not mean that 75 per cent of the vaccinated population were given protective immunity. Instead, it means that three-quarters of people expected to develop active tuberculosis did not do so. Thus, if a population of 100 000 is vaccinated and another of the same number acts as the control group, and if 250 cases of tuberculosis are observed over the subsequent 10 years in the vaccinated group compared to 1000 in the control group, then the protection would have been 75 per cent.

As their immune systems are immature, neonates and infants are at high risk of developing tuberculosis, especially serious disseminated forms such as tuberculous meningitis, after infection. This enhanced risk is no longer evident by around the age of 5 years owing to maturation of the immune system and, until the onset of puberty, children are then relatively well protected – the **safe school age**. From puberty onwards, the risk of developing tuberculosis following infection is similar to that in adults.

Accordingly, one would expect to see the greatest expression of protection of BCG when given to very young children with immature immune systems and a high risk of progression of infection to disease, especially as there is evidence that an important effect of BCG is to stimulate the maturation of the immune system. This is, in fact, what has been seen in the major BCG trials.

If, after the initial few years of high susceptibility to disease, a child or young adult is infected, the primary complex usually resolves. As described in Chapter 1, around 95 per cent of infected people successfully overcome their primary infection and, of these, only a minority (some 5 per cent) subsequently develop post-primary disease. Thus, 90 per cent of people do not develop tuberculosis following infection, indicating that such infection induces highly effective immunity in most people. Indeed, the immunity induced by 'natural' infection appears to be more powerful and lasting than that induced by BCG vaccination.

Despite this high level of long-lasting protective immunity, tubercle bacilli are able to persist in the lung tissues in a poorly understood form for years or decades. If the naturally induced protective immunity is unable to prevent this persister state, it is difficult to see why BCG vaccination should do so. In fact, the observed very small impact of vaccination on the incidence of post-primary tuberculosis is a clear indication that it does not significantly do so.

The natural protective immunity after resolution of the primary complex wanes over time, explaining why some 5 per cent of such people develop post-primary tuberculosis years or decades later. It is known that the protective efficacy of BCG also wanes with time, with, for example, a drop from 78 per cent protection to no protection over 15 years in the British vaccination trials. Of course, 5 per cent of the world's infected population (a third of the entire human population) is a huge number of people, explaining why tuberculosis is a global emergency, but it is asking a very great deal of a vaccine, which, by inducing a 'limited tuberculous process' merely mimics natural infection, to raise the protection induced by natural infection by *M. tuberculosis* from around 95 per cent to approaching 100 per cent and to maintain this for decades.

It might be argued that, as post-primary tuberculosis appears to be the result of a waning of the protective immunity induced by the resolving primary infection, BCG vaccination or re-vaccination given later in life to previously infected people would boost such waning immunity. Many such infected people would be tuberculin positive and therefore be unsuitable for vaccination, as it could cause severe hypersensitivity reactions. It is arguable that those becoming tuberculin negative might benefit from vaccination or re-vaccination, even though there is no evidence that a loss of tuberculin reactivity indicates a waning of protective immunity. There are, however, several reasons why vaccination or re-vaccination would not be of benefit to such people. If immune responses are waning due to old age or to various apparent or unapparent conditions that compromise immunity (such as dietary and genetic factors), vaccination might not have any beneficial effect. More worrying is the finding that BCG vaccination of adults was ineffective in clinical trials in several regions where tuberculosis is rife. Whatever the explanation, BCG given to older people would not be expected to have an impact in such regions.

In countries with a very low incidence of the disease, there will be many older people who have never been infected and some of these will never have received BCG. These people might, in principle, benefit from vaccination, although even if it could be shown to be effective, very many people would have to be vaccinated in order to prevent a single case of the disease, especially as the great majority of those who actually became infected would not develop overt disease. Exceptions would be adults anticipating exposure to risk through occupation or travel.

A major problem, however, is that there have been no extensive controlled trials of BCG vaccination in older people and there are therefore no firm data on which to base decision making, for the protection of either communities or individuals.

In summary, BCG protects the young child, uninfected at the time of vaccination, from primary tuberculosis, including the serious forms such as tuberculous meningitis. In some regions, it also protects older children and young adults against primary tuberculosis. In other regions this is not the case, and vaccination may even slightly predispose to the disease. Vaccination of those already infected does not protect them against developing post-primary tuberculosis, and may induce local hypersensitivity reactions.

WHO SHOULD RECEIVE BCG VACCINE?

From the foregoing, those in greatest need of vaccination are infants at risk of developing serious forms of primary tuberculosis. In regions where infants are at a very low risk, as in rural parts of the UK, vaccination may be delayed until the child is older. The argument in the UK is that tuberculosis is not a common disease and that children under the age of 12 are infrequently exposed to it. Also, there is clear evidence from a major BCG trial and more recent confirmatory studies that, in contrast to some other parts of the globe, vaccination at this age gives a high level of protection in the UK.[11,12] If, however, the child is at high risk of infection, as is the case in certain districts and communities, BCG should be given neonatally according to local Health Authority policies.

As mentioned above, vaccination or re-vaccination of older people is not generally recommended, as there is limited evidence that it would be of benefit.[13] On the other hand, a comparison of the incidence of tuberculosis in adult tuberculin-negative immigrants from South Asia who were vaccinated on entry to the UK with that in unvaccinated people of the same age and origin suggested that BCG gave a high level of protection. Accordingly, vaccination is recommended in this high-risk group.[14] In addition, vaccination is recommended for previously unvaccinated and tuberculin-negative people who anticipate exposure to risk through occupation or travel. Those who are not sure if they have had BCG vaccination in the past should only be vaccinated if they are tuberculin negative and have no characteristic BCG scar. Health authorities in some countries issue guidelines to the use of BCG in various groups of people, and these should be adhered to.[13,15,16]

In countries where tuberculosis is very uncommon, such as the USA, BCG is not routinely given to children unless they are at high risk of infection, as it is considered preferable to use the tuberculin test to identify the relatively few infected people and to give them preventive therapy, as explained in Chapter 12. In the USA, this policy has been modified to permit vaccination of those in high-risk situations, particularly those, including children and nurses, exposed to multidrug-resistant tuberculosis.[15,16] High-risk children are defined as those who are exposed continually to an untreated or ineffectively treated patient who has infectious pulmonary tuberculosis and cannot be separated from that infectious patient or, in the case of drug-susceptible disease, cannot be given long-term preventive therapy. High-risk health professionals are those working in facilities in which a high percentage of the tuberculosis patients are infected with strains resistant to both isoniazid and rifampicin and in which comprehensive tuberculosis infection-control precautions have been implemented and have not been successful.[16]

IS POST-VACCINATION TUBERCULIN TESTING INDICATED?

The use of post-vaccination tuberculin testing to assess the immune status of vaccinated persons is controversial. As mentioned above, no relationship between tuberculin reactivity and protective immunity has been reliably demonstrated. Tuberculin testing soon after BCG as an indication that the vaccine has 'taken' is not required. A scar is adequate indication of successful vaccination. The authors have seen a biomedical scientist who had many unsightly keloid scars on her upper arm as a result of repeated BCG vaccinations in an unsuccessful and unnecessary attempt to induce tuberculin positivity. In this context, a minority of people have a genetically determined failure to develop indurated reactions to tuberculin after natural infection or BCG vaccination, although biopsies of the test site reveal intense cellular activity in the dermis.

DOES RE-VACCINATION CONFER ADDITIONAL PROTECTION?

Re-vaccination, sometimes repeated, is practised in some countries, but there is no convincing evidence that it is of benefit. It is probable that, as the protective effect of vaccination varies considerably from region to region, the effect of re-vaccination may likewise vary. Unfortunately, there is very little firm information on which to base decision making. In the opinion of the WHO, re-vaccination is of little or no benefit,[17] and this is supported by a large study in Hong Kong.[18] The potential benefit of re-vaccination at school age is, however, currently being investigated in a very large randomized study in Brazil, which commenced in 1996.[19]

HOW IS BCG GIVEN?

Although originally developed as a vaccine for oral administration – and almost certainly effective when given by this route – BCG is now always given intradermally. This is done either by intradermal (intracutaneous) injection or by use of a multipuncture device.

In the former method, the freeze-dried BCG is suspended in the diluent fluid supplied with the vaccine according to the manufacturer's instructions, mixed well and drawn into a 1 mL tuberculin syringe. A 0.1 mL amount, or 0.05 mL for neonates, of the suspension is injected into the dermal layer of the skin overlying the insertion of the deltoid muscle in the upper arm. It is important that nurses are properly trained to give injections into the dermis – a procedure resulting in a distinct skin bleb, around 8 mm across, with minute pitting like the skin of an orange – rather than into the subcutaneous tissues. The latter is more likely to lead to abscess formation. The skin over the insertion of the deltoid muscle is the preferred site: vaccinations given higher on the shoulder are more likely to lead to raised and unsightly keloid scarring and the use of a standard site facilitates subsequent examination for a vaccination scar, should the need arise. Requests to give the vaccination in other sites for cosmetic or other reasons should be firmly resisted as, if abscesses or other complications were to occur, a claim for compensation would be indefensible.

In some countries, the recommended alternative in neonates, in whom the dermis is thin and who have a distinct propensity for wriggling, is the multipuncture method. In this, the BCG is applied to the skin as a paste and the prongs of the multipuncture device are pushed into the skin through the paste. This ensures that the vaccine is carried into the dermis to a fixed depth. Although the procedure looks rather alarming at first, it causes little discomfort and, in most cases, no residual scarring. It is important to use the correct vaccine for the selected method. Preparations for multipuncture application contain more bacilli than those for intradermal injection. Complications have resulted from accidental use of the wrong preparation.

Although no formal comparisons of protective efficacy between multipuncture application and intradermal injection have been made, both techniques have been used in trials showing good protection (and also in those showing poor protection). Thus there is limited and indirect evidence that the protection conferred by the two methods is of a similar order. In a study in the UK, multipuncture vaccination with a device bearing 18 or 20 needles induced the same degree of tuberculin reactivity as the standard intradermal vaccination in children aged under 2 years.[20] Older children required two applications of the instrument for the same effect, although it must be emphasized that, as discussed above, there is no evidence of a correlation between tuberculin reactivity and protection conferred. Nevertheless, for this reason, multipuncture vaccination is only licensed for use with children under the age of 2 years in the UK.

DO MASS BCG VACCINATION CAMPAIGNS CONTRIBUTE SIGNIFICANTLY TO GLOBAL TUBERCULOSIS CONTROL?

A frequently asked question is whether money and efforts would be better invested in mass BCG vaccination programmes than in the detection and treatment of infectious patients. As discussed above, BCG generally affords good protection against the serious extrapulmonary forms of primary tuberculosis in children, but such disease is usually not infectious. By contrast, it does very little to prevent infectious post-primary tuberculosis and, therefore, to block the transmission of the disease in the community. Notwithstanding, anyone who has seen a child rendered blind and paralysed by tuberculous meningitis could not fail to become a firm advocate for vaccination, even though it has little to offer in the overall global prevention of the spread of tuberculosis.

BCG VACCINATION IN THE ERA OF HIV INFECTION

There is no information on to what extent, if any, BCG vaccination prevents or delays the development of active tuberculosis in those infected with the human immunodeficiency virus (HIV). Logically, as HIV infection leads to suppression of the immune responses that normally prevent the progression of infection by the tubercle bacillus to active disease in most infected people, it would also suppress any protective immunity induced by BCG vaccination.

When considering vaccination strategies in regions where HIV infection is common, it must be remembered that BCG is a living vaccine and that, though attenuated, it has the potential to cause disease, even fatal disseminated disease, in immunosuppressed individuals (see below). This leads to an ethical dilemma. Nobody would want to inflict a potentially fatal condition on infants in attempting to protect them against such a condition. On the other hand, infants are at risk of developing serious forms of tuberculosis following infection and there is a duty to offer them protection, especially where the risk of infection is high. In view of this, the WHO recommendation is that, although BCG should never be given to people known to be infected with HIV, routine immunization of infants should continue in areas with a high incidence of tuberculosis and HIV infection.[21] In other countries, official advice may vary. In the UK, for example, it is advised that BCG should not be given to infants born to mothers known or suspected to be infected with HIV, unless the infants are subsequently confirmed to be uninfected.[22]

HOW SAFE IS BCG?

BCG is very safe. Most problems and complications are the result of faulty technique and a failure to follow national guidelines, such as those periodically updated in the UK and the USA.[13,15] In brief, BCG should only be given to those who are tuberculin negative (Heaf grades 0 and 1 and Mantoux responses of 0–4 mm), although infants under 3 months of age may be vaccinated without prior tuberculin testing. Contraindications include malignancy, steroid therapy, fever, pregnancy (even though no harmful effects on the fetus have been reported), generalized septic skin conditions and immunosuppressive disorders. Children prone to atopic dermatitis should be vaccinated when that condition is in remission.

A number of complications of BCG vaccination have been described and are summarized, together with their management, in Table 6.2.[23] The most frequently seen ones are hypersensitivity reactions and abscesses at the injection site and axillary lymphadenopathy. Outbreaks of complications have followed the accidental intracutaneous injection of vaccine

TABLE 6.2 The principal complications of BCG vaccination and their treatment

Complication	Treatment
Local hypersensitivity reaction	None; dry dressing, steroid ointment as 'placebo'
Abscess or ulcer at vaccination site	Drainage or needle aspiration if required, topical or systemic isoniazid or erythromycin
Axillary lymphadenopathy	None, or surgery for excessive enlargement, chronic suppuration or sinus formation
Distant lesion, such as osteitis	Antituberculosis therapy
Disseminated 'BCG-osis'	Antituberculosis therapy

for multipuncture use, as the latter contains many more bacilli. On occasions, health workers with inadequate experience of BCG vaccination, usually doctors giving 'one-off' vaccinations, have injected the entire 10-dose ampoule of BCG intramuscularly! More serious complications, such as osteitis, are extremely rare.

A very small minority of vaccinated children, fewer than one in a million, develop disseminated **BCG-osis** due to congenital immune defects.[24] Children who are infected with HIV are at an increased risk of developing infective complications after BCG vaccination and, although most of the cases reported to date have been relatively mild,[25] the occurrence of disseminated BCG-osis is a possibility.

Large local hypersensitivity reactions develop within a day or two and usually resolve spontaneously, although severe reactions may ulcerate and become secondarily infected. Steroid ointments are sometimes prescribed, more as a placebo to calm parental anxiety, as there is no published evidence that they are effective. Abscesses develop between 1 and 5 months after vaccination. If available, bacteriological investigations show whether BCG or another bacterium such as *Staphylococcus aureus* is responsible. Several treatments have been tried for BCG abscesses, including aspiration, topical or systemic isoniazid and systemic erythromycin. Enlarged axillary lymph nodes do not respond to antimicrobial therapy but often resolve spontaneously. Surgery is advocated for grossly enlarged and suppurating nodes or chronically discharging sinuses.

Post-vaccination osteitis is a rare complication, but clusters of cases have been seen in some countries where certain strains of vaccine were used. Also, it is more likely to occur when the vaccine is given in the thigh rather than the recommended site on the arm. Osteitis and other serious infective complications are treated as for tuberculosis (as described in Chapter 12), except that, in common with *M. bovis*, BCG is naturally resistant to pyrazinamide.

ARE THERE HOPES FOR AN IMPROVED VACCINE?

Much research effort is being put into developing novel vaccines, and the recently achieved complete sequencing of the genomes of both *M. tuberculosis* and *Homo sapiens* may well facilitate useful advances. The ideal vaccine will be a non-viable one so that it can be given

TABLE 6.3 Alternative immunizing strategies against tuberculosis currently being investigated

Standard BCG	Revision of dose and timing of vaccination Alternative routes of delivery – oral and intranasal
Modified BCG	'Engineered' BCG with several copies of genes coding for protective antigens
Modified *M. tuberculosis*	Strains with virulence-determining genes deleted or with mutations that permit only limited replication in tissues
Alternative carriers	'Engineered' viruses, especially smallpox vaccine, expressing protective mycobacterial antigens
Non-viable subunit vaccines	Isolated antigens, or mixtures of antigens, with or without adjuvants
Free or 'naked' DNA	Injected free DNA enters antigen-presenting cells where it codes for antigenic protein
Immunoregulatory vaccines	BCG 'engineered' to express cytokines, or mixed with adjuvants that induce Th1-mediated immune reactions
Prime and boost strategies	One vaccine, usually a DNA vaccine, which primes for an immune response, followed by a more complete vaccine, usually BCG, to boost the response

safely to immunosuppressed people and it will prevent those already infected by the tubercle bacillus from developing infectious forms of the disease. This is an enormous challenge, but a few potentially useful approaches are being explored.[26] The principal novel approaches to vaccination against tuberculosis are summarized in Table 6.3. A major problem is that there is no experimental animal model that closely mimics human tuberculosis. Thus any new candidate vaccine will have to be evaluated in the human population and this will be a very difficult and time-consuming task.

Summary

Although we have been using BCG for 80 years, many aspects are still shrouded in mystery. Numerous questions surround its mode of action, its efficacy and the reasons for its geographical variation in efficacy. An undoubted beneficial effect of BCG vaccination is the protection of children against primary tuberculosis, including serious extrapulmonary forms such as tuberculous meningitis – an effect that fully justifies its continued widespread use. By contrast, it is ineffective in preventing cases of post-primary tuberculosis later in life, which are responsible for the transmission of the disease in the community. For this reason, BCG vaccination will contribute relatively little to the eventual eradication of the disease. Much research is required to develop more effective vaccination strategies, although this is a tough challenge.

Prologue to the next chapter

As we have not been able to develop vaccination strategies that have facilitated the eradication of tuberculosis, the control of this disease will, for the foreseeable future, be based on therapy designed to render the patients rapidly non-infectious and then to cure them completely so the disease does not relapse. Before they can be treated, their disease must be diagnosed, but this is no easy matter. Therefore, before looking at the clinical features and care of patients with tuberculosis, the next chapter looks at the various techniques that are used to diagnose the very variable forms of the disease seen in clinical practice.

REFERENCES

1. Francis J. The work of the British Royal Commission on Tuberculosis, 1901–1911. *Tubercle* 1959; **40**: 124–32.
2. Tuberculosis Research Centre (ICMR), Chennai. Fifteen year follow up of trial of BCG vaccines in south India for tuberculosis prevention. *Indian J Med Res* 1999; **110**: 56–69.
3. Colditz GA, Brewer TF, Berkey CS et al. Efficacy of BCG vaccine in the prevention of tuberculosis: meta-analysis of the published literature. *J Am Med Assoc* 1994; **271**: 698–702.
4. Fine PEM. Variation in protection by BCG: implications of and for heterologous immunity. *Lancet* 1995; **346**: 1339–45.
5. Stanford JL, Shield MJ, Rook GAW. How environmental mycobacteria may predetermine the protective efficacy of BCG. *Tubercle* 1981; **62**: 55–62.
6. Marchent A, Goetghebuer T, Ota MO et al. Newborns develop a Th1-type immune response to *Mycobacterium bovis* bacillus Calmette–Guérin vaccination. *J Immunol* 1999; **163**: 2249–55.

7. Kristensen I, Aaby P, Jensen H. Routine vaccinations and child survival: follow up study in Guinea-Bissau, West Africa. *BMJ* 2000; **321**: 1435–9.
8. Grange JM, Stanford JL, Stanford CA, Kölmel KF. Prospects for vaccination strategies to reduce the risk of leukaemia and melanoma. *J R Soc Med* 2003; **96**: 389–92.
9. Crispin RG, Rosenthal SR. BCG vaccination and cancer mortality. *Cancer Immunol Immunother* 1976; **1**: 139–42.
10. Corah T, Byass P, Jaffar S et al. Prior BCG vaccination improves survival of Gambian patients treated for pulmonary tuberculosis. *Trop Med Int Health* 2000; **5**: 413–17.
11. Hart PD, Sutherland I. BCG and vole bacillus vaccines in the prevention of tuberculosis in adolescence and early adult life. *BMJ* 1977; **2**: 293–5.
12. Springett V, Sutherland I. A re-examination of the variations in the efficacy of BCG vaccination against tuberculosis in clinical trials. *Tuber Lung Dis* 1994; **75**: 227–33.
13. Department of Health. *Immunisation against infectious disease*. London: HM Stationery Office, 1996. Also available online via <http://www.dh.gov.uk/>
14. Chaloner JH, Ormerod LP. Assessment of the impact of BCG vaccination on tuberculosis incidence in South Asian adult immigrants. *Commun Dis Public Health* 2002; **5**: 338–40.
15. Centers for Disease Control and Prevention. The role of BCG vaccine in the control of tuberculosis in the United States: a joint statement by the Advisory Council for the Elimination of Tuberculosis and the Advisory Committee on Immunization Practices. *MMWR* 1996; **45**(RR-4): 1–18. Also available online at <http://www.cdc.gov/mmwr/PDF/RR/RR4504.pdf>
16. National Center for HIV, STD and TB Prevention. Division of Tuberculosis Elimination. BCG vaccination. In *Core curriculum on tuberculosis*. Atlanta GA: Centers for Disease Control, 2002.
17. World Health Organization. Global Tuberculosis Programme and Global Programme on Vaccines. Statement on BCG revaccination for prevention of tuberculosis. *Wkly Epidemiol Rec* 1995; **70**: 229–31.
18. Leung CC, Tam CM, Chan SL et al. Efficacy of the BCG revaccination program in a cohort given BCG vaccination at birth in Hong Kong. *Int J Tuberc Lung Dis* 2001; **5**: 717–23.
19. Barreto ML, Rodrigues LC, Cunha SS et al. Design of the Brazilian BCG-REVAC trial against tuberculosis. A large, simple randomized community trial to evaluate the impact on tuberculosis of BCG revaccination at school age. *Control Clin Trials* 2002; **23**: 540–53.
20. Al Jarad N, Empey DW, Duckworth G. Administration of BCG vaccination using the multipuncture method in schoolchildren: a comparison with the intradermal method. *Thorax* 1999; **54**: 762–4.
21. World Health Organization. HIV and routine childhood immunization. *Wkly Epidemiol Rec* 1987; **62**: 297–9.
22. Joint Tuberculosis Committee of the British Thoracic Society. Control and prevention of tuberculosis in the United Kingdom: Code of Practice 2000. *Thorax* 2000; **53**: 887–901.
23. Grange JM. Complications of Bacille Calmette–Guérin (BCG) vaccination and immunotherapy and their management. *Commun Dis Public Health* 1998; **1**: 84–8.
24. Talbot EA, Perkins MD, Silva SFM, Frothingham R. Disseminated Bacille Calmette–Guérin disease after vaccination: case report and review. *Clin Infect Dis* 1997; **24**: 1139–46.

25. O'Brien KL, Ruff AJ, Louis MA et al. Bacillus Calmette–Guérin complications in children born to HIV-1-infected women with a review of the literature. *Pediatrics* 1995; **95**: 414–18.
26. Doherty M, Andersen P. Tuberculosis vaccines: developmental work and the future. *Curr Opin Pulm Med* 2000; **6**: 203–8.

FURTHER READING

Malin AS, Young DB. Designing a vaccine for tuberculosis. Unraveling the tuberculosis genome – can we build a better BCG? *BMJ* 1996; **312**: 1495.

Rieder H. BCG vaccination. In Davies PDO (ed.), *Clinical tuberculosis*, 3rd edn. London: Arnold, 2003, 337–53.

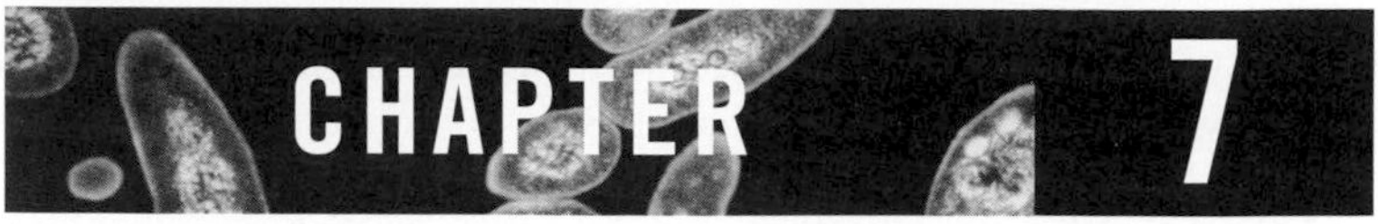

Diagnosis of tuberculosis and other mycobacterial diseases

Introduction

If you think diagnosing tuberculosis is easy – think again! The diagnosis of this disease is fraught with difficulties that present many obstacles to its effective control. There are no clearly recognizable signs and symptoms of tuberculosis that distinguish it with certainty from other diseases, and a bacteriological confirmation of a diagnosis is not always possible. Many patients present with vague illness or respiratory symptoms that could have many other causes. In regions where tuberculosis is now a rarity, diagnosis in many patients is delayed and, tragically, is sometimes not made until after the patient has died.

Learning outcomes

After studying and reflecting on the material in this chapter, you will be able to:

- discuss the need to evaluate critically a diagnostic test in respect to its sensitivity, specificity and predictive value,
- describe the role of the laboratory and the principal bacteriological investigations available for the diagnosis of tuberculosis,
- explain why sputum microscopy is of central importance in tuberculosis control programmes,
- describe why clinical examinations, including history taking and radiology, have a key place in diagnosis,
- outline the particular diagnostic challenge posed by childhood tuberculosis.

Tuberculosis is diagnosed, like many other illnesses, by a combination of clinical examinations and tests. Broadly speaking, an examination involves collection of many bits of information by means of history taking, conducting a physical examination and looking at radiographs (X-rays). The data thus obtained are then sifted by mental processes based on experience to give an idea of the likely diagnosis. In some cases, decision making is based on the use of formal flow charts or algorithms, as have been developed for aiding the diagnosis of tuberculosis in children (see Chapter 8).

Tests, by contrast, are usually single investigations giving a 'yes or no' type of answer. In order to know how much reliance can be put on a result, tests are evaluated to determine their **sensitivity** and **specificity**. Sensitivity is the measure of the ability of a test to detect a characteristic of a disease when it is present. Thus, for example, a test of 100 per cent sensitivity for detecting tubercle bacilli would be positive for all specimens containing them. Specificity is the measure of the ability of the test to distinguish between those with and those without the disease. Use of a test of low specificity would result in many patients with other conditions being mis-classified as having tuberculosis and receiving inappropriate treatment. Put another way, a test of low sensitivity would give many 'false-negative' results, whereas a test of low specificity would give many 'false-positive' results. The actual usefulness of a test depends very much on the circumstances in which it is used. A test of 95 per cent specificity looks quite good on paper, as only one in 20 patients without tuberculosis would be misdiagnosed as having the disease, but, if the test was applied routinely to all patients with a cough or fever in a region with a low incidence of tuberculosis, one could well have many more misdiagnosed patients than correctly diagnosed ones. A statistical method based on Bayes' theorem can be used to calculate the predictive value of a positive or negative result in a given situation.[1] It is very important that all new tests are thoroughly evaluated for their sensitivity, specificity and predictive values. There have, for example, been hundreds of descriptions of various 'blood tests' for tuberculosis, mostly based on antibody detection, but very few have been properly evaluated and even fewer have been introduced into clinical practice.

BACTERIOLOGICAL DIAGNOSIS OF TUBERCULOSIS

The only certain way of diagnosing tuberculosis is by finding the tubercle bacillus, but this is not always straightforward. Adult patients with post-primary tuberculosis and cavities in their lungs will often have enough tubercle bacilli in their sputum to be seen on microscopical examination. Indeed, as the microscopical detection of such bacilli is a clear indication of infectiousness, this investigation is the principal one used in tuberculosis control programmes. Patients with tuberculosis of the lungs but without cavities, especially children, do not usually have enough tubercle bacilli in their sputum, if they produce sputum at all, for them to be detected microscopically. These, and patients who have tuberculosis in organs other than the lung, require special approaches to diagnosis.

By far the most common specimen submitted from patients with tuberculosis is sputum, and the most frequent test is microscopical examination of sputum smears after staining for acid-fast bacilli (AFB).[2,3] It is an axiom of clinical microbiology that 'no test is better than the specimen received'. The nurse therefore has a key role in ensuring that adequate specimens are taken, that the patient is actually producing sputum and not just saliva, and that the patient is carefully instructed as to what is required. Unfortunately, the word 'spit' is often used as a slang word for sputum, even by qualified health workers. It is also essential that sputum is collected directly into sterile containers. (In some centres, sputum used to be collected in metal pots that had been simply rinsed under a hot tap and was then decanted into sterile containers. This led to diagnostic confusion, as hot-water taps may be contaminated by environmental mycobacteria, especially *Mycobacterium xenopi*, which thrives at high temperatures.) Finally, the nurse should ensure that specimens are labelled properly and accompanied by a request form correctly filled in, that their containers are not contaminated on the outside by sputum and that they are transferred to the laboratory with a minimum of delay.

The number of AFB in samples of sputum from a patient will vary greatly, even from hour to hour. Ideally, therefore, several samples should be taken, as these increase the chance of detection of the bacilli. When possible, the patient should produce one specimen of sputum on his or her first visit to the clinic and then be given an appropriate sterile container in which to collect sputum produced during the first hour or two after rising the following morning. The patient should bring this morning sputum to the clinic, when a third specimen will be collected. Although examination of three specimens is better than just one, it does require the availability of technical staff to do the extra examinations and nurses or public health workers to locate those patients who do not return on the second day. According to an International Union Against Tuberculosis and Lung Disease technical guide,[2] of the patients eventually found to be sputum positive, 80 per cent are diagnosed on the first spot specimen, an additional 15 per cent on the morning specimen and 5 per cent more on the third specimen. Another report based on an extensive study in Ethiopia gives the analogous percentages for the three specimens as, respectively, 91.6, 7.4 and 1, indicating that there is limited benefit in examining the third specimen.[4]

In the laboratory, purulent portions of the sputum sample will be spread as a smear on a glass microscope slide, allowed to dry, 'fixed' by heating and then stained by the Ziehl–Neelsen (ZN) method based on the characteristic acid-fast staining property of mycobacteria. The smear is then examined for AFB under high-power microscopy. It must be remembered that a very small amount of sputum covers a very large area when smeared on a slide and examined at a magnification of around 1000 times. Thus it has been calculated that, for there to be a reasonable chance of seeing any AFB, there must be between 5000 and 10 000 of them in every millilitre of sputum. Therefore, microscopical examination cannot be hurried and 100 high-power fields should be examined – a process taking 5–10 minutes for each slide.

Fluorescence microscopy, based on the same principle as the ZN method but utilizing a fluorescent stain rather than a red one, is much less tiring for the technical staff. The slides are examined at low power and, if a fluorescing spot is seen against the black background, it is examined under high power to see if it is a bacterium. The equipment is expensive, however, and requires more skilled maintenance than the standard light microscope, but fluorescence microscopy is justified in resource-poor settings on account of its greater sensitivity and cost effectiveness.[5]

It is obvious, therefore, that the accuracy of diagnosis by microscopy depends greatly on the quality of the specimen, the care with which smears are made and the time and concentration given to their microscopical examination. The fact is that examining a large batch of stained slides for AFB can be very dull and tedious work, especially when most or all of the slides are negative. Without good motivation and support, technical staff may 'cut corners'. It has been recommended that no microscopist should prepare and examine more than 25 sputum smears each day and that this activity should be only one aspect of varied and intellectually stimulating work within a good career structure. Unfortunately, this ideal is not met in many working environments.

Microscopy does not distinguish between tubercle bacilli and other species of mycobacteria. The report will therefore just state 'acid-fast bacilli seen'. In some services, an indication of the number of AFB seen will be given even though, as stated above, the number may vary considerably from specimen to specimen from the same patient, even when taken just a few hours apart. One reported scheme, recommended by the International Union Against Tuberculosis and Lung Disease, is shown in Table 7.1, although this is not the only scheme in use.[2] The presence of a very small number of bacilli – one to three in 100 high-power fields – is of doubtful significance. These may be environmental mycobacteria, staining artefacts or accidental 'carry over' from one specimen to the next. Fresh specimens should be requested and examined.

TABLE 7.1 System for reporting sputum smears as recommended by the International Union Against Tuberculosis and Lung Disease

Counts of AFB	Reporting
No AFB seen in 100 high-power fields	Negative
1–9 AFB seen in 100 high-power fields	Actual numbers
10–99 AFB seen in 100 high-power fields	+
1–10 AFB seen per field in at least 50 fields	++
More than 10 AFB seen per field in at least 20 fields	+++

AFB, acid-fast bacilli.

Some centres have facilities for more sophisticated laboratory examinations, especially cultivation of tubercle bacilli.[3] Cultivation is more sensitive than smear microscopy but requires experienced staff, takes time to set up and the incubation period is long. Positive results may not be available for several weeks after the specimen is received. Cultivation detects those patients who have active tuberculosis but relatively few AFB in their sputum – the so-called smear-negative, culture-positive patients. Ideally, such patients should be detected and treated, but in many regions priority must be given to the detection and treatment of the more infectious, smear-positive, patients. Cultivation is, however, essential for distinguishing between tubercle bacilli and environmental mycobacteria and for obtaining bacteria for performing standard drug susceptibility tests.

Other techniques for obtaining specimens for bacteriological examination are used in some centres. Laryngeal swabbing is used in patients who do not produce sputum and collects secretions coming from the lung on the ciliary escalator before they are swallowed. It is essential that it is only performed by those trained to visualize the larynx; 'blind' swabbing of the larynx is useless. The operator is at risk of infection and must therefore wear a mask and visor, as the procedure invariably induces a bout of violent coughing.

The stomachs of children may be aspirated to harvest any AFB swallowed during the night, although this procedure is unpleasant for the child and the diagnostic yield is low. It is essential that the acidic gastric contents are neutralized or that the specimen is transferred straightaway to the laboratory. In one study, induction of sputum by the use of inhaled nebulized bronchodilators and 5 per cent saline together with physiotherapy in children both with and without human immunodeficiency virus (HIV) infection, even very young ones (aged 3–20 months), who did not otherwise produce adequate specimens, was shown to be effective and slightly more sensitive than gastric lavage.[6] Sputum induction, which is also useful in adults who do not produce sputum, should be done well away from other patients, in facilities for respiratory isolation where these are available,[7] or even in the open air. There have been outbreaks of tuberculosis in units caring for patients with HIV disease after inducing sputum in multi-bed wards.

Fibreoptic bronchoscopy is a safe procedure in adults by which bacilli and material for histological examination may be obtained by bronchial washing, brushing or biopsy, and is used to an increasing extent. If used in children, great care and considerable expertise are required in order to prevent injury. It is important that bronchoscopes are adequately cleaned and disinfected between patients by using approved equipment to prevent accidental infection of subsequent patients and cross-contamination of sputum specimens.[8]

Renal tuberculosis is diagnosed by bacteriological examination of urine. The best examination is culture, as AFB seen by microscopy in centrifuged deposits may be environmental mycobacteria that have contaminated the lower urethra. Examination of cerebrospinal fluid by very careful and prolonged microscopy is essential for the diagnosis of tuberculous meningitis, and this examination must be considered an emergency one. Other fluids submitted for bacteriological examination include pleural, pericardial and peritoneal exudates. For culture, some of the aspirated fluid may be added directly to an equal quantity of a suitable liquid medium at the bedside. Open biopsies or fine-needle aspirates of tissues are also examined, by acid-fast staining of histological sections or smears and by culture.

METHODS FOR CULTIVATING MYCOBACTERIA

In most centres worldwide, mycobacteria are isolated on simple culture media.[4] The most commonly used is Löwenstein–Jensen medium which, in essence, is made from heat-coagulated eggs, supplemented by some mineral salts and glycerol. A green dye (malachite green) is added, as this suppresses the growth of certain contaminating bacteria and provides a green background against which the off-white colonies of *M. tuberculosis* are more clearly seen. A very similar medium, containing sodium pyruvate instead of glycerol, is used for the isolation of *M. bovis*, which grows poorly or not at all on media containing glycerol. Most of the environmental mycobacteria causing human disease also grow on egg-based media. Liquid media are used in the automated culture systems described below and for certain special purposes.

The problem with cultivation of mycobacteria is the very slow growth rate of members of the *M. tuberculosis* complex and most other species causing human disease. Even the rapidly growing species may, paradoxically, take a long time to grow on first isolation from clinical specimens. Results of culture may therefore not be available for a month or more after receipt of the specimen. Identification takes even longer. Many centres use a set of simple tests to differentiate between members of the *M. tuberculosis* complex and environmental mycobacteria; some divide the former into its various species, but identification of environmental mycobacteria is usually undertaken in central reference laboratories. Some laboratories offer a more rapid identification by means of the various molecular techniques described below and a few use sophisticated equipment, such as mass spectroscopes, for this same purpose.

Tuberculosis laboratories are divided into three categories or levels according to their function, as shown in Box 7.1.

As mycobacteria grow very slowly, it is important that specimens should not contain other viable microorganisms that would grow more rapidly and contaminate the culture medium. Inevitably, many specimens, especially sputum and urine, will contain many other microorganisms. Contamination may be avoided by supplementing the culture medium with a 'cocktail' of antimicrobial agents that kill virtually all microorganisms other than mycobacteria. More usually, though, use is made of the relatively greater resistance of mycobacteria to killing by acids and alkalis. 'Hard' methods, such as treatment with 4 per

BOX 7.1 The three levels of tuberculosis laboratories

Level 1	Usually single rooms or part of a general laboratory in a primary healthcare setting Activities are restricted to collection of specimens and their dispatch to a higher level laboratory
Level 2	Usually in district hospitals and part of a general microbiology laboratory Activities include microscopical examination of specimens for acid-fast bacilli and, in some cases, setting up cultures, which are usually sent to level 3 laboratories for incubation
Level 3	These are more specialized and centralized facilities, which, in addition to doing the tasks of level 1 and 2 laboratories, identify isolated mycobacteria and do drug susceptibility tests More centralized reference laboratories do more detailed examinations (such as identification of environmental mycobacteria), organize quality control, undertake training and participate in research activities

cent sodium hydroxide (caustic soda), are used for specimens such as sputum that are likely to be heavily contaminated, and 'soft' methods are suitable for cleaner materials. The former will kill many mycobacteria as well as contaminants and thus give a reduced isolation rate, but this is a price to be paid for avoiding many contaminated cultures and incurring the wrath of the physicians submitting the specimens.

RAPID BACTERIOLOGICAL METHODS

As sputum smear microscopy is rapid but relatively insensitive and culture, though more sensitive and specific, is very slow, considerable research effort has been put into developing tests with the triple merits of sensitivity, specificity and speed. These include automated culture systems and molecular methods.[9–11]

Automated culture systems

These are of two main types: **radiometric** and **non-radiometric**. In the radiometric systems, specimens are inoculated into liquid media containing a 'cocktail' of agents to prevent the growth of microorganisms other than mycobacteria, and a radiolabelled substrate (palmitic acid) that the mycobacteria are able to utilize for growth. Bacterial growth is indicated by the release of radioactive carbon dioxide from the substrate into the air spaces in the top of the bottles, which is automatically sampled through needles inserted through the caps of the bottles and counted for radioactivity. Growth is usually detectable between 2 and 10 days after inoculating the media, and the system may be used, with appropriate modified media, to differentiate the *M. tuberculosis* complex from other mycobacteria and to perform rapid drug susceptibility tests.

The disadvantage of this system is the need to dispose of radioactive waste, which, owing to increasingly strict legislation, poses serious difficulties in many countries. Accordingly, various non-radiometric systems have been developed and are based on changes in the colour of dyes or the activation of fluorescent substances on, respectively, the liberation of carbon dioxide and the consumption of oxygen. These systems are comparable in performance to the radiometric systems.

Molecular technology

Great interest has been shown in recent years in the detection of specific nucleic acids, DNA or RNA, of tubercle bacilli and other mycobacteria in clinical specimens. These methods are based on the unique structure of nucleic acid, which consists of very long molecular chains with the genetic code written, in the case of DNA, in a 'language' of four bases, A, T, C and G. The famous 'double helix' consists of complementary strands, where A in one strand is linked to T in the other, with C and G being similarly linked. In a dividing cell, the double helix separates into its two strands, after which the corresponding complementary strands are synthesized, giving two new double helices. In the test tube, a double helix can be separated by heat. On cooling, separated strands will only recombine to form a double helix if the sequences of the bases in the two single strands are complementary. Thus, if a single strand of DNA with a base sequence complementary to, for example, a species-specific part of the genome of *M. tuberculosis*, is added to DNA extracted from a cultivated strain of this species and separated into single strands by heating, binding or hybridization to the added **DNA probe** will occur and can be detected by several methods. Several DNA probes specific for commonly encountered mycobacteria are commercially available but, as they are not sensitive enough to detect mycobacterial DNA in clinical specimens, they are only suitable for the identification of cultivated mycobacteria.

Fortunately, the problem of sensitivity has been largely overcome, as the replication of DNA that occurs in living cells can also be carried out in the test tube. A clinical specimen is added, after treatment to liberate DNA from bacterial cells, to a tube containing a DNA polymerase enzyme which catalyses the synthesis of new strands of DNA, the bases or 'building blocks' A, T, C and G, and so-called primers, which are short sequences of DNA specific for selected short sequences on the two complementary strands of DNA in the organism being sought. The mixture is heated to separate any double helices and then cooled so that if the specific primers bind to their respective single strands, corresponding new strands of DNA are synthesized, starting at the points where the primers are bound and thus yielding two double helices. The mixture is re-heated (a heat-resistant DNA polymerase is used so that addition of new enzyme is unnecessary) and the process is repeated, yielding four double helices from part of the original one. The entire bacterial chromosome is not replicated in this process, just the part determined by the distance separating the primer-binding sites on the complementary DNA strands. Each heating and cooling cycle lasts for about 2 minutes, so that over a 2-hour period, millions of new helices of DNA of identical length are generated and are easily detected. In view of the almost explosive doubling rate of DNA synthesis, the method is known as the **polymerase chain reaction** (PCR).

The choice of primers is important. Depending on their specificity, primers may, for example, be selected to permit detection of any mycobacterium, a member of the *M. tuberculosis* complex or, more specifically, *M. tuberculosis* or *M. bovis*.[12] Various modifications of the PCR are commercially available and PCR-related techniques are used, without the need for isolating the organisms by culture, to 'fingerprint' tubercle bacilli for epidemiological purposes and to determine, with around 95 per cent accuracy, whether strains are resistant to rifampicin. Elucidation of the genetic basis of drug resistance is paving the way for a range of novel rapid tests for such resistance.[13] In an ideal world, a physician could know within a day whether a patient has tuberculosis, within 2 days whether the patient is likely to respond to standard therapy and, in some circumstances, could have information on the possible source of the infection.

Unfortunately, it is not an ideal world, and nucleic acid-based methods have met with various problems. The PCR can be made very specific and it should be extremely sensitive. In practice, it is usually positive in patients who are sputum-smear positive but, probably due to the presence of inhibitory substances in sputum, sensitivity is significantly lower, around 48–53 per cent, in those who are smear negative but culture positive. This somewhat defeats the object of the test, but sensitivity is greatly improved by inoculating specimens on solid media for a day or two. This may permit some bacillary replication and, possibly, allow inhibitory substances to diffuse out of the specimen.[14] There is, however, a high commercial and humanitarian incentive to develop more rapid, sensitive and specific diagnostic tests for tuberculosis, and continuing developments and improvements are thus likely to occur. Another problem is that of cost, but, like the cost of drugs, this could be considerably reduced with international support and aid.

DNA 'fingerprinting'

In addition to diagnosis, the tuberculosis laboratory may assist epidemiological investigations by dividing isolates of tubercle bacilli into many types according to differences in their DNA structure, as briefly outlined in Chapter 2. Application of these techniques enables the spread of disease in mini-epidemics to be investigated, the distinction between endogenous reactivation and re-infection to be made and laboratory cross-contamination to be detected.[15]

RADIOLOGICAL EXAMINATIONS

Radiology, particularly of the chest, is used widely for the diagnosis of tuberculosis.[16] This has traditionally involved the use of full-size chest radiographs, miniature chest radiographs and fluoroscopy. In fluoroscopy, the image is shown on a fluorescent screen rather than a photographic plate but it exposes the investigator to unacceptably high levels of radiation and is of very limited diagnostic value. Accordingly, the World Health Organization (WHO) has advised that this technique should be universally abandoned. Miniature X-ray has been used in mass screening but it is not cost-effective and is now rarely used routinely. Radiology with the use of full-size radiographs is sensitive as it allows even very small pulmonary lesions to be seen. It is not specific, however, and even experienced radiologists often have difficulty in determining whether lesions are caused by tuberculosis or by one of the many other causes of lung disease, especially in HIV-infected people.[17] Even large pulmonary cavities are not necessarily indicative of tuberculosis, as a very similar appearance may be seen in lung cancer. Accordingly, radiology may be of great help, but other investigations are required to confirm the diagnosis.

Radiology is also used for the diagnosis of tuberculosis in sites other than the lung, especially the bones, joints, kidney and renal tract, but, as in the case of the lung, radiological appearances are not specific and other confirmatory investigations are required. In some centres, computerized tomography (CT) and magnetic resonance imaging (MRI) have proved very useful for imaging tuberculous lesions, particularly those in the brain and spine.

TUBERCULIN TESTING

As described in Chapter 5, a positive tuberculin test indicates that a person is reacting immunologically to mycobacterial antigens. This reactivity may result from latent infection by the tubercle bacillus, active tuberculosis, prior vaccination with Bacille Calmette–Guérin (BCG) or, in some cases, infection by or disease due to environmental mycobacteria. The test is therefore by no means diagnostic for active tuberculosis. In regions with a high incidence of infection, many adolescents and adults will have converted to tuberculin positivity. On the other hand, in regions with a very low risk of infection and where people are not vaccinated with BCG, such as many parts of the USA, a positive tuberculin test in targeted populations can be taken as a fairly reliable indication of infection by the tubercle bacillus and the need for preventive therapy.[18] Also, strong tuberculin reactions in young children are indicative of recent infection or overt disease and the need for therapy.

In some regions, small tuberculin reactions are due to sensitization by mycobacteria in the environment. Thus the 'cut-off' point of size or intensity of the tuberculin reaction that distinguishes between such sensitization and possible active tuberculosis will differ from region to region and will need to be established locally. Conversely, a negative tuberculin test does not mean that the patient does not have active tuberculosis. The immune responses of a patient with advanced untreated tuberculosis, or whose disease is associated with severe immunosuppression due to HIV infection or other causes, may be too weak to give the reaction – a condition known as **anergy**. Also, acute infections, particularly measles in children, may temporarily suppress the tuberculin response. In addition, a few people of a particular genetic type fail to react to tuberculin, even though they have been sensitized by infection or BCG vaccination, or have active tuberculosis.

Originally, tuberculin testing was done by applying a drop of concentrated Old Tuberculin on the skin and making a scratch through it. More quantitative methods are now in use – the **Mantoux** and **Heaf tests** and, occasionally, the **tine test**. In addition, as non-specific reactions were commonly caused by the use of Old Tuberculin, the reagent is now partly purified by precipitation of the protein antigens and the resulting product is termed **Purified Protein Derivative** (PPD).

Preparations of PPD are standardized before use and their strength is stated in International Units (IU). Batches of PPD vary slightly qualitatively and are thus usually made up in large amounts so as to avoid batch-to-batch variation. One gigantic batch, termed RT23, was prepared at the State Serum Institute, Copenhagen, and is used internationally in epidemiological studies, but it is rather expensive for routine use.

In the Mantoux method, a tuberculin syringe is used to inject a specified amount of PPD, usually 0.1 mL (or 0.05 mL in infants), into the dermal layer of the skin, usually on the forearm. The routinely used strength of PPD varies from country to country and is usually 1 IU, 2 IU or 5 IU. The test is read after 2–3 days by measuring the transverse diameter of the induration that can be felt. Redness (**erythema**) of the skin spreading beyond the induration should not be read. One way of reading the induration is to slide a ball-point pen along the skin from a few centimetres outside the test site until it 'catches' on the distinct edge of the induration and to make a mark with the pen at that point.

The great advantage of the Mantoux method is that it gives a quantitative result expressed as the diameter of the induration, which is of importance in epidemiological surveys and for research purposes.[19] For routine diagnosis, an induration of 10 mm or more in adults and in children who have not had BCG, and 15 mm or more in BCG-vaccinated children, is strongly indicative of active tuberculosis, although interpretation should be based on local guidelines where these are available. As mentioned above, local interpretations should take into account the extent of sensitization by environmental mycobacteria, as this varies from region to region, as illustrated in Figure 7.1.[20] A distinction between sensitization by *M. tuberculosis* and by environmental mycobacteria may be made by testing with tuberculin and, at the same time, also with an analogous reagent prepared from *M. avium*. This procedure has long been used in cattle and has recently been evaluated in humans.[21]

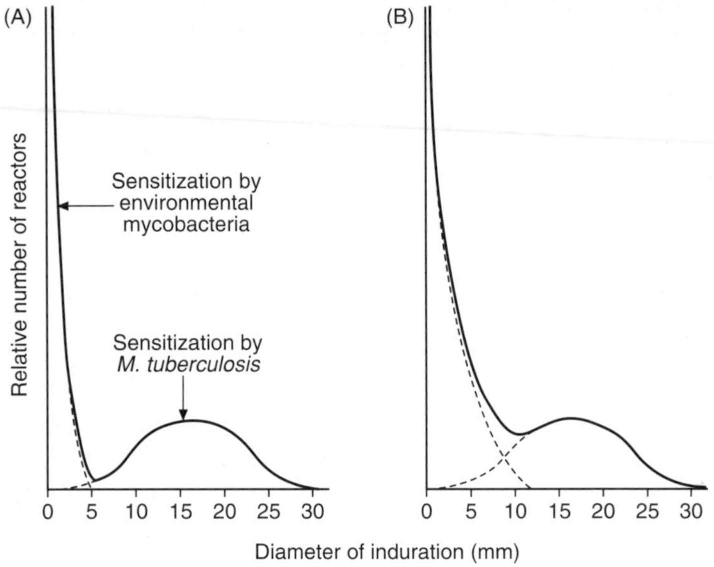

FIGURE 7.1 *Distribution of induration sizes of the Mantoux tuberculin test: (A) in region with low level of sensitization by environmental mycobacteria; (B) in region with high level of sensitization by environmental mycobacteria. A cut-off point of 5 mm in region A will clearly differentiate infection by* M. tuberculosis*, but in region B, many such reactions will be due to sensitization by environmental mycobacteria.*

The disadvantage of the Mantoux method is that, as in the case of BCG vaccination, experience in giving intradermal injections is required. This requirement is avoided in the Heaf method, which employs a spring-loaded 'gun' which drives six needles to a set depth into the dermis, usually 2 mm but 1 mm in young children, through a drop of concentrated PPD (100 000 IU/mL) placed on the skin. The Heaf test is read after 2–3 days and, rather than measuring the diameter of the reaction, it is graded I to IV, as shown in Table 7.2. Although not as quantitative as the Mantoux method, Heaf reactions of grade II or

TABLE 7.2 The grades of tuberculin reactivity in the Heaf test

Grade 0	No reaction
Grade I	At least four discrete papules
Grade II	Confluent papules forming a ring
Grade III	An entire disc of induration
Grade IV	A disc of induration greater than 10 mm in diameter or vesicles in the indurated skin

stronger are suggestive of tuberculosis. One disadvantage of the Heaf test is that the guns must be properly sterilized between use to prevent transmission of hepatitis, HIV and other viruses. The older practice of dipping the head of the gun in spirit and flaming it between uses is no longer acceptable. Detachable, sterilizable heads for the guns are now available.

The tine test resembles the Heaf test in principle. It consists of a small hand-held device with four prongs (tines) coated with dried PPD and is supplied pre-sterilized in an individual sealed package for single use only. The device is taken out of its package, pushed firmly into the dermis and discarded in a container suitable for medical 'sharps'. It is important to hold it in place for several seconds after insertion into the skin so that the dried PPD has time to dissolve in the tissue fluids. It is principally used for 'one-off' tests but is not regarded as being as sensitive as the other two techniques.

Booster effect

If a tuberculin test is repeated after an initial test giving a negative or weak reaction, a stronger reaction may be observed. This is thought to be due to the tuberculin in the initial test recalling immunological memory of prior sensitization by mycobacterial antigens, whether as the result of infection, BCG vaccination or contact with environmental mycobacteria. The phenomenon is usually seen when re-testing is done between 1 and 5 weeks after the initial test. In one study in the UK, a booster effect was clearly demonstrated when the second test was performed 1 week after the initial one.[22] However, the effect is uncommon after 8 weeks, and is only very occasionally observed a year or more later. It could, therefore, lead to a small minority of people being misclassified as tuberculin converters if they are tuberculin tested regularly.[23]

CLINICAL DIAGNOSIS

In view of the problems and shortcomings of bacterial and radiological examinations and the inherent problems of tuberculin testing, diagnosis must often be made on the basis of clinical features. Unfortunately, the clinical signs and symptoms of tuberculosis are very similar to those of a range of other conditions, especially in children and in cases of extrapulmonary tuberculosis, in which bacteriological diagnosis is often difficult.

The usual features suggesting tuberculosis of the lung in adults are a cough, particularly if it is of over 3 weeks' duration (most patients with acute lung infections get better within 3 weeks), and production of sputum which may contain blood. There may be breathlessness and chest pain. More general symptoms include loss of appetite, tiredness, weight loss, fever and night sweats. Chest signs, such as wheezing, crepitations and dullness on percussion, may be detected by clinical examination, although the signs are often much less than would be suggested by the extent of disease apparent on chest X-ray.

The clinical features of tuberculosis in HIV-infected people are often bizarre and not easily differentiated from those of other HIV-related conditions. Cavity formation is reduced as a result of immunosuppression, so there is a lower likelihood of finding AFB in sputum. The skin test may be weak or negative and chest X-rays may reveal non-specific shadowing.

More details on clinical features of diagnostic usefulness are given in the following three chapters. The particular problems encountered in the diagnosis of tuberculosis in infants and children are discussed in Chapter 8.

OTHER INVESTIGATIONS

Haematological features, especially a mild anaemia, a high erythrocyte sedimentation rate (ESR) and an elevated lymphocyte count, may suggest or support a diagnosis of tuberculosis. More sophisticated biochemical and haematological tests are no more informative than these simple routine ones. Numerous attempts have been made to develop serological tests for tuberculosis and a few are available commercially, but, in general, they have not been adopted in routine clinical practice. A recently described test for the detection of T cells binding to an antigen specific for *M. tuberculosis* differentiates those latently infected by this organism from those sensitized by BCG or environmental mycobacteria and could be used to delineate those suitable for preventive therapy in low-incidence regions.[24]

Summary

The diagnosis of tuberculosis is not easy, particularly in children and in adults who do not produce sputum or when any sputum that is produced is microscopically negative. The laboratory has a key role in the diagnosis of tuberculosis. The priority in control programmes is the detection of infectious patients, and sputum microscopy is therefore of prime importance. Some laboratories are able to cultivate mycobacteria and some use more rapid automated equipment for this purpose. Interest has focused recently on molecular methods for the detection and identification of mycobacteria in clinical specimens. These are very specific, but problems of sensitivity need to be solved. History taking, physical examination, radiology and, subject to careful interpretation, tuberculin testing also play a major part in the diagnosis of tuberculosis.

Prologue to the next chapter

Having considered how tuberculosis is diagnosed, it is now time to move on to the clinical features of the disease, and this will be the theme of the next three chapters. It has been said that if one knows tuberculosis, one knows all of medicine. Certainly, tuberculosis can involve any tissue or organ and may mimic almost all other conditions. Among the many epithets that the disease has acquired over the ages, one is *Morbus percorpus* – the disease affecting the entire body. An awareness of the great diversity of forms that this disease takes – a diversity enhanced in recent decades by the HIV/acquired immunodeficiency syndrome (AIDS) pandemic – enables the healthcare worker to 'think tuberculosis'. Sadly, for many people, the problem is not so much that they have tuberculosis, but that their doctors do not realize that they have it.

REFERENCES

1. Grange JM, Laszlo A. Serodiagnostic tests for tuberculosis: a need for assessment of their predictive accuracy and acceptability. *Bull World Health Organ* 1990; **68**: 571–6.
2. International Union Against Tuberculosis and Lung Disease (IUATLD). *Technical guide. Sputum examination for tuberculosis by direct microscopy in low income countries*, 5th edn. Paris: IUATLD, 2000.

3. Collins CH, Grange JM, Yates MD. *Tuberculosis bacteriology. Organization and practice*, 2nd edn. Oxford: Butterworth Heinemann, 1997.
4. Yassin MA, Cuevas LE. How many sputum smears are necessary for case finding in pulmonary tuberculosis? *Trop Med Int Health* 2003; **8**: 927–32.
5. Kivihya-Ndugga LE, van Cleeff MR, Githui WA et al. A comprehensive comparison of Ziehl–Neelsen and fluorescence microscopy for the diagnosis of tuberculosis in a resource-poor urban setting. *Int J Tuberc Lung Dis* 2003; **7**: 1163–71.
6. Zar HJ, Tannenbaum E, Apolles P et al. Sputum induction for the diagnosis of pulmonary tuberculosis in infants and young children in an urban setting in South Africa. *Arch Dis Child* 2000; **82**: 305–8.
7. McWilliams T, Wells AU, Harrison AC et al. Induced sputum and bronchoscopy in the diagnosis of pulmonary tuberculosis. *Thorax* 2002; **57**: 1010–14.
8. Larson JL, Lambert L, Stricof RL et al. Potential nosocomial exposure to *Mycobacterium tuberculosis* from a bronchoscope. *Infect Control Hosp Epidemiol* 2003; **24**: 825–30.
9. Woods GL. The mycobacteriology laboratory and new diagnostic techniques. *Infect Dis Clin North Am* 2002; **16**: 127–44.
10. Caws M, Drobniewski FA. Molecular techniques in the diagnosis of *Mycobacterium tuberculosis* and the detection of drug resistance. *Ann N Y Acad Sci* 2001; **953**: 138–45.
11. Drobniewski FA, Caws M, Gibson A, Young D. Modern laboratory diagnosis of tuberculosis. *Lancet Infect Dis* 2003; **3**: 141–7.
12. Cobos-Marin L, Montes-Vargas J, Riviera-Gutierrez S et al. A novel multiplex PCR for the rapid identification of *Mycobacterium bovis* in clinical isolates of both veterinary and human origin. *Epidemiol Infect* 2003; **130**: 485–90.
13. Marttila H.J, Soini H. Molecular detection of resistance to antituberculous therapy. *Clin Lab Med* 2003; **23**: 823–41.
14. Fernstrom MC, Dahlgren L, Ranby M et al. Increased sensitivity of *Mycobacterium tuberculosis* Cobas Amplicor PCR following brief incubation of tissue samples on Löwenstein–Jensen substrate. *Acta Pathol Microbiol Immunol Scand* 2003; **111**: 1114–16.
15. Sonnenberg P, Godfreey-Fausset P. The use of DNA fingerprinting to study tuberculosis. In Davies PDO (ed.), *Clinical tuberculosis*, 3rd edn. London: Arnold, 2003, 60–73.
16. Van Dyck P, Vanhoenacker FM, Van den Brande P, De Schepper AM. Imaging of pulmonary tuberculosis. *Eur Radiol* 2003; **13**: 1771–85.
17. Tshibwabwa-Tumba E, Mwinga A, Pobee JOM et al. Radiological features of pulmonary tuberculosis in 963 HIV-infected adults at three central African hospitals. *Clin Radiol* 1997; **52**: 837–41.
18. American Thoracic Society. Targeted tuberculin testing and treatment of latent tuberculosis infection. *Am J Respir Crit Care Med* 2000; **161**: 5221–47.
19. Fourie B. The tuberculin skin test, with special reference to the application and interpretation of the Mantoux intradermal method. In Donald PR, Fourie B, Grange JM (eds), *Tuberculosis in childhood*. Pretoria: JL van Schaik, 1999, 119–31.
20. Fitzgerald JM, Menzies D. Interpretation of the tuberculin test. In Davies PDO (ed.), *Clinical tuberculosis*, 3rd edn. London: Arnold, 2003, 323–36.
21. Hersh AL, Tosteson AN, von Reyn CF. Dual skin testing for latent tuberculosis infection. A decision analysis. *Am J Prev Med* 2003; **24**: 254–9.
22. Singh D, Sutton C, Woodcock A. Repeat tuberculin testing in BCG-vaccinated subjects in the United Kingdom. *Am J Respir Crit Care Med* 2001; **164**: 962–4.

23. Menzies D. Interpretation of repeated tuberculin tests. Boosting, conversion, and reversion. *Am J Respir Crit Care Med* 1999; **159**: 15–21.
24. Ewer K, Deeks J, Alvarez L et al. Comparison of T-cell-based assay with tuberculin skin test for diagnosis of *Mycobacterium tuberculosis* infection in a school tuberculosis outbreak. *Lancet* 2003; **361**: 1168–73.

FURTHER READING

Collins CH, Grange JM, Yates MD. *Tuberculosis bacteriology. Organization and practice*, 2nd edn. Oxford: Butterworth Heinemann, 1997.

Fitzgerald JM, Menzies D. Interpretation of the tuberculin test. In Davies PDO (ed.), *Clinical tuberculosis*, 3rd edn. London: Arnold, 2003, 323–36.

International Union Against Tuberculosis and Lung Disease (IUATLD). *Technical guide. Sputum examination for tuberculosis by direct microscopy in low income countries*, 5th edn. Paris: IUATLD, 2000.

CHAPTER 8

Pulmonary tuberculosis

Introduction

As tuberculosis is principally spread by the respiratory route, most cases of the disease affect the lung. In a significant number of cases, however, the disease spreads beyond the confines of the lung and the closely related pleurae to other tissues and organs. The nomenclature of tuberculosis within and outside the lung is confusing. Expressions used in the literature include pulmonary and extrapulmonary (or non-pulmonary), respiratory and non-respiratory, and intrathoracic and extrathoracic tuberculosis. In the USA, the term pulmonary tuberculosis refers to disease confined to the lung tissues, whereas in the UK it includes disease of the pleurae. This distinction is important, as, by the USA definition, pleural tuberculosis is the commonest form of extrapulmonary tuberculosis. The terms pulmonary and extrapulmonary tuberculosis are used in this book, with the former including pleural manifestations of the disease. Some patients will, of course, have both forms of the disease.

Learning outcomes

After studying and reflecting on the material in this chapter, you will be able to:

- describe the differences between primary and post-primary tuberculosis,
- in the case of post-primary tuberculosis, appreciate the difference between endogenous reactivation of disease and exogenous re-infection,
- describe the evolution of the primary pulmonary complex following infection,
- describe the differences between tuberculosis as it usually presents in childhood and adult life,
- describe the evolution of the post-primary pulmonary lesion and how this enables the disease to become infectious,
- appreciate the serious problems encountered in making a correct diagnosis of pulmonary tuberculosis in children and adults.

Traditionally, tuberculosis is divided into childhood, or primary, and adult, or post-primary, forms. This division is not applicable in all situations, as, in regions where the incidence of the disease is low, primary infection may not occur until well into adult life. Also, there is a 'grey area' between the two types of the disease, with some patients progressing directly from the primary to the post-primary pattern of disease. In the past, when tuberculosis was prevalent in the industrialized nations, many people were infected, and developed primary tuberculosis, before puberty, which was of later onset than today. Nowadays, infection is more likely to occur around or after puberty, when direct progression to post-primary disease often occurs. Also, as described in Chapter 10, the increasing prevalence of people showing some form of immunosuppression, notably, but not exclusively, as a result of human immunodeficiency virus (HIV) infection, further blurs the clinical classification. Nevertheless, it is of practical help to consider the disease according to the age of those affected.

TUBERCULOSIS IN INFANTS AND CHILDREN

Children are prone to tuberculosis – including serious life-threatening forms – and the presentation and course of the disease differ in several important respects from the disease in adults.[1] Tuberculosis is one of the major diseases affecting children worldwide but, owing to the diagnostic difficulties discussed below, accurate information concerning its overall extent and distribution is not available.[2] Children may be born with active tuberculosis as a result of infection in the uterus from the mother (congenital tuberculosis), but this is a very rare occurrence.[3] The newborn infant is, however, very susceptible to development of the disease following exposure to a source case of infection, usually the mother or other close family contact. Children under the age of 3 years are particularly susceptible to serious forms of tuberculosis, including miliary disease and tuberculous meningitis, probably due to the immaturity of their immune systems.[4]

By contrast, children between the age of 3 years and puberty are relatively resistant to the disease and are said to be in the 'safe school age'. The reason for this is unknown, but endocrine factors are suspected. Adolescents are more susceptible and their disease may go

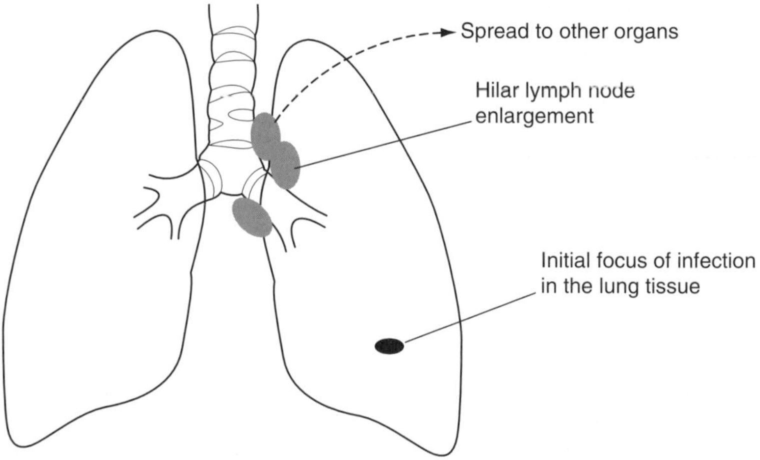

FIGURE 8.1 *The primary complex of pulmonary tuberculosis showing the lesion at the site of infection, enlarged hilar lymph nodes and distant spread.*

straight from the primary form to the post-primary or 'adult' form – so-called **progressive primary tuberculosis**. Gender differences in the incidence and response to the treatment of tuberculosis in various age groups have been described, but the data are conflicting and may reflect better access to health care for males in some societies rather than biological differences.[5]

The classic form of the disease seen in children is primary pulmonary tuberculosis, consisting of the focus of infection in the lung tissue and enlargement of the lymph nodes at the root or hilum of the lung (Fig. 8.1). This is known as the **primary complex** and is often, but not always, visible on chest radiographs. In most cases, this primary complex resolves, and fibrous scarring in the pulmonary component may later become calcified and thus remain visible on chest radiographs.

Self-limiting primary tuberculosis is often undetected clinically and the affected person may, at the most, have only mild and non-specific symptoms. During the primary process, conversion to tuberculin test positivity occurs – a process taking 3–8 weeks – and a minority, almost always children, develop certain 'allergic' phenomena, namely, **erythema nodosum**[6] and **phlyctenular conjunctivitis** (Box 8.1).[7]

BOX 8.1

Erythema nodosum is most often seen in children aged between 5 and 10 years and is commoner in girls, especially those with fair skin. It is characterized by firm, painful red patches or nodules, usually on the lower limbs, and sometimes by joint pain. It usually clears up within 2 weeks, although reddening of the skin may remain for several weeks. No specific treatment is indicated unless joint pain is severe, in which cases steroids may be given. Erythema nodosum also occurs in other conditions, including streptococcal infections, leprosy, systemic fungal infections, sarcoidosis, leukaemia and as a reaction to certain drugs.

Phlyctenular conjunctivitis is characterized by itching or pain, excessive production of tears and sensitivity to light and usually affects just one eye. Small grey nodules are seen near the edge of the cornea, and the adjacent area of the eye is reddened due to dilatation of blood vessels. The condition usually clears up within a few days, although it may recur. It is most common in children aged between 5 and 10 years, and affects more girls than boys. Although it usually occurs soon after primary infection, it occasionally occurs much later. It is also associated with staphylococcal infections and worm infestations, although it is usually less severe than when associated with tuberculosis.

In most cases, the primary complex resolves and there is no further problem, except in the small minority who develop post-primary tuberculosis years or decades later. However, around 5 per cent of those with primary complexes do become ill with tuberculosis, of either the lung or other parts of the body. The latter are described in the next chapter.

Physicians in the days before antituberculosis therapy was available noticed that the course of primary tuberculosis, particularly involvement of organs other than the lung, tended to follow a 'timetable' of events,[8,9] as shown in Table 8.1.

Within the lung, the primary focus of disease may enlarge. In some cases, chest X-rays reveal a struggle between the disease and immune defences so that the lesion shows several concentric rings of healing and calcification. Radiologically, such lesions have a 'laminated'

TABLE 8.1 The 'timetable' of primary tuberculosis

Stage	Duration	Features
1	3–8 weeks	The primary complex develops; conversion to tuberculin positivity occurs
2	About 3 months	Life-threatening forms of disease due to haematogenous dissemination occur, i.e. tuberculous meningitis and miliary tuberculosis
3	3–4 months	Tuberculous pleurisy may be the result of either haematogenous spread or direct spread from an enlarging primary focus
4	Up to 3 years	This stage lasts until the primary complex resolves. Extrapulmonary lesions that develop more slowly may appear, particularly in the bones and joints
5	Up to 12 years	Genito-urinary tuberculosis may occur as a late manifestation of primary tuberculosis

or 'onion-skinned' appearance. In other cases, the disease process fails to resolve and eventually develops the characteristic features of post-primary tuberculosis with cavity formation. In yet other cases, the lesion bursts into the pleural space surrounding the lung and a pleural effusion develops. This may be due either to a hypersensitivity reaction to antigens in the tubercle bacillus or to infection by the bacilli, or both. In children, problems arise from the enlarged lymph nodes at the root of the lung. In some cases, particularly in younger children, these lymph nodes may be so enlarged that they obstruct a major bronchus, leading to either hyper-inflation or collapse of a segment or lobe of the lung – a condition called **epituberculosis**. Alternatively, a diseased node may erode into a bronchial wall, allowing the disease process to spread within the bronchial tree – so-called **endobronchial tuberculosis**. The local manifestations of primary pulmonary tuberculosis are summarized in Figure 8.2. Diseased lymph nodes may also erode into the pericardial cavity, causing tuberculous pericarditis, as described in Chapter 9.

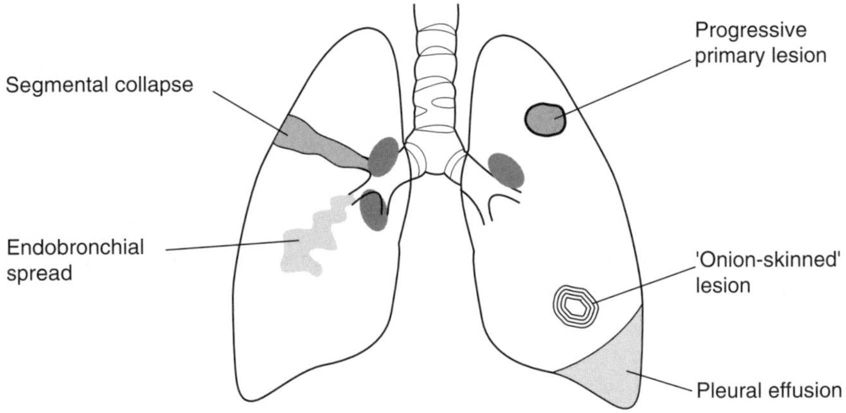

FIGURE 8.2 *The pulmonary complications of primary tuberculosis.*

DIAGNOSIS OF TUBERCULOSIS IN CHILDREN

As discussed in Chapter 7, diagnosis of tuberculosis in children is not easy. Most children with primary pulmonary lesions do not produce sputum and, even when they do, acid-fast bacilli are only occasionally seen. Specimens may be obtained for culture by early-morning gastric aspiration, but this is unpleasant for the child and confirms the diagnosis in less than half the cases. Sputum induction can be effectively and safely performed in young children and infants and there is evidence that this is more sensitive than gastric lavage for the isolation of *Mycobacterium tuberculosis*.[10] Clinical and radiological features are therefore important, though often vague, and it is very important to enquire whether a child suspected of having this disease is likely to have been exposed to infection, particularly from a close relative in the home. It is not uncommon for children with primary pulmonary tuberculosis to have normal chest X-rays, although in one study, computerized tomography (CT) revealed enlarged mediastinal lymph nodes in 9 of 15 such children.[11]

The younger the child, the more likely there are to be clinical signs, including coughing, wheezing, reduced chest expansion and crepitations on auscultation. In older children there may be no clinical signs, even when the disease in the lung is extensive.[12]

In view of the problems of obtaining bacteriological confirmation, diagnosis is usually based on radiological signs (when present), clinical signs and symptoms, including a failure to thrive, a positive tuberculin test conducted and interpreted according to national guidelines (a strongly positive tuberculin test is of greater diagnostic significance in a child than in an adult) and evidence of recent exposure to an infectious source case. Accordingly, it is not easy to distinguish between infection and active tuberculosis in children, and some children will not receive treatment while others will be treated unnecessarily.

Children are prone to develop extrapulmonary forms of primary tuberculosis, particularly forms involving the central nervous system, the lymph nodes, the bones and joints and the renal tract. Diagnosis of these forms requires considerable clinical experience and an awareness of the possibility of tuberculosis.

As discussed in Chapter 10, tuberculosis in HIV-infected children is particularly difficult to diagnose as it resembles several other infectious diseases, such as *Pneumocystis carinii* pneumonia, to which such children are prone. Also, the more generalized clinical features of childhood tuberculosis, such as prolonged cough, weight loss and a failure to gain weight, are caused by other HIV-related conditions and tuberculin tests are often negative.

In view of the diagnostic difficulties, there have been several studies aimed at developing scoring systems for determining whether children are likely to have active tuberculosis.[13] These include one conducted by the International Union Against Tuberculosis and Lung Disease, involving 879 children under the age of 15 years in 10 countries.[14] This study established that five clinical criteria – namely, history of contact with a case of tuberculosis, a positive skin test, persistent cough, low weight for age and an unexplained prolonged fever – gave positive predictive values which, depending on age and environment, ranged from 60 to 77 per cent. In regions with a low prevalence of tuberculosis, a history of household exposure to a source case and a positive skin test were of particular predictive value, whereas in high prevalence regions the other features – low body weight, prolonged fever and cough – were more reliable indicators of tuberculosis. This study was, however, conducted retrospectively on notified cases and did not address the growing problem of HIV-associated tuberculosis. By means of the above criteria, children may be divided into those who are suspect cases and those with probable tuberculosis, as shown in Box 8.2. Only those with acid-fast bacilli seen on microscopy of relevant specimens or isolation of *M. tuberculosis* on culture are regarded as having confirmed tuberculosis, but, as mentioned above, only a minority of children fall into this category.

Children who are clinically well but have an abnormal chest X-ray and a positive skin test and who are in close contact with an infectious adult should be regarded as having probable

BOX 8.2 Clinical features suggesting that children have suspected or probable tuberculosis

Features of suspected cases of tuberculosis

- Household exposure to an adult with infectious tuberculosis
- Failure to recover from a common infectious disease such as gastroenteritis, measles or whooping cough
- Failure to recover from an acute respiratory infection when given appropriate therapy
- Persistent wheeze and/or cough
- Failure to put on weight, or to recover from malnutrition, when given an adequate diet
- Intermittent or persistent fever and an enlarged liver or spleen
- Features suggestive of extrapulmonary tuberculosis, especially enlarged cervical lymph nodes, an abdominal mass, spinal tenderness or deformity, arthritis of a single joint and the features of meningitis (lethargy, loss of appetite, vomiting, irritability, convulsions and hemiplegia)

Features of probable cases of tuberculosis

- A positive tuberculin test, interpreted according to local guidelines; usually a Mantoux test with an induration of 10 mm or more, or 15 mm or more in those previously vaccinated with Bacille Calmette–Guérin (BCG)
- Chest X-rays showing lesions compatible with tuberculosis
- A histological appearance of biopsied lesions compatible with tuberculosis but without bacterial confirmation by microscopy or culture

tuberculosis. Those with abnormal chest X-rays but negative tuberculin tests should be treated for non-tuberculous chest infections and re-examined radiologically after 1 month. Suspected cases with normal chest X-rays and negative skin tests should likewise be re-assessed after 1 month. Seriously ill children who may have miliary disease or tuberculous meningitis and those with neurological signs associated with suspected spinal tuberculosis must be treated for tuberculosis in the absence of confirmatory evidence and their progress assessed during therapy.

A useful and concise consensus statement on the diagnosis of tuberculosis in children has been published by the Indian Academy of Pediatrics.[15] This statement lists and discusses the principal indicators of tuberculosis – fever, cough, loss of weight and appetite and a history of contact – and also discusses the values and limitations of available investigations and useful indicators of various forms of extrapulmonary tuberculosis.

POST-PRIMARY PULMONARY TUBERCULOSIS

The most common form of tuberculosis seen in clinical practice is post-primary disease of the lung in adolescents and adults. From the epidemiological point of view, this is the most important form of tuberculosis, as most patients at the time of diagnosis have cavities in the lung and are therefore highly likely to be infectious.[16] In most parts of the world, as explained in Chapter 13, a particular effort is made to find these patients. Thus, in many countries, other forms of tuberculosis are probably underdiagnosed.

As outlined in Chapter 5, it was widely assumed that post-primary tuberculosis was the result of endogenous reactivation of the primary infection after a period of latency. Accordingly, post-primary tuberculosis is sometimes referred to as reactivation tuberculosis. The introduction of techniques for 'fingerprinting' tubercle bacilli has shown that post-primary tuberculosis can also be due to exogenous re-infection with a new strain of the bacillus. Hence, the term reactivation tuberculosis is not always an accurate one.

For reasons that are not understood, post-primary tuberculosis preferentially affects the upper regions of the lung, irrespective of the site of the primary lesion (even if it was in the skin or intestine) or whether the disease is due to endogenous reactivation or exogenous re-infection.[17] Various explanations, such as higher oxygen levels in the upper parts of the lungs, have been proposed but none has been proven.

The usual symptoms of this form of tuberculosis are loss of appetite, weight loss, night sweats, low-grade fever, tiredness and general malaise. In advanced, untreated patients, the wasting and weight loss may be very severe. In most patients, symptoms develop gradually over several weeks or months, but some patients develop a more acute illness suggestive of pneumonia. Cough is a very common feature and most patients present with a persistent cough of over 3 weeks' duration and produce mucoid or purulent sputum that may contain blood. Some patients, including some with quite extensive disease, may be remarkably symptom free. Chest signs on physical examination are often much less evident than would be expected from the chest X-ray appearance and may be restricted to a few apical crackles or localized wheezing.

Chest X-rays characteristically show lesions in the upper zones of one or both lungs, some of which may show cavitation (Fig. 8.3). Solid, non-cavitating lesions resemble lung tumours, with which they may be confused diagnostically, and are termed tuberculomas. (In this context, some lung tumours and abscesses show central necrosis and may be confused with tuberculous cavities.) Smaller scattered lesions may be evident in the lower zones of one or both lungs and are the result of spread of disease from the open cavity through the bronchial tree.

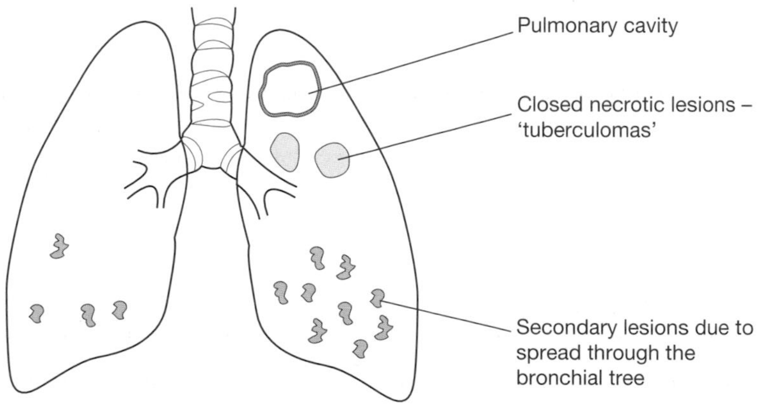

FIGURE 8.3 *Post-primary pulmonary tuberculosis, showing tuberculomas, cavity and secondary lesions due to intra-bronchial spread.*

The disease process may involve the pleural space, with the development of pleural effusions due either to direct bacterial invasion or to hypersensitivity reactions to mycobacterial antigens. The patient may present with dull chest pain and this condition, and progressive lung damage, leads to breathlessness and, in severe cases, to respiratory distress. If pleural effusions become infected by tubercle bacilli or secondary bacterial invaders, an **empyema** develops and the effusion becomes thick and purulent.[18] A cavity may rupture into the pleural space to form a bronchopleural fistula, which allows air to enter this space, a condition known as a **pneumothorax** or, if there is a purulent pleural effusion, to a **pyopneumothorax**. Very occasionally, an empyema ruptures into or through the chest wall to form, respectively, a **cold abscess** or sinus.

Bacilli may also occasionally lodge in the larynx, causing tuberculous laryngitis, which was a particularly painful and debilitating condition in the days before antituberculosis therapy was introduced. Bacilli may also be swallowed and give rise to gastrointestinal lesions, as described in the next chapter. In rare cases, bacilli may lodge in fissures at the angles of the mouth or track up the Eustachian tube and cause middle ear disease. On the other hand, unless the patient is immunosuppressed, spread of the disease to other organs and tissues by the lymphatics and bloodstream is much less often seen than in primary tuberculosis.

Adequate and appropriate therapy renders the disease quiescent, but healing of the lung may, in advanced cases, lead to scarring which, in turn, causes airway obstruction and respiratory failure. This is particularly seen in the elderly and in smokers. Tuberculous cavities that fail to close and heal may become infected with fungi of the *Aspergillus* group, which may lead to massive life-threatening haemoptysis or respiratory failure, and, if the patient is well enough, surgery may be undertaken to remove the fungally infected cavity.

DIAGNOSIS OF POST-PRIMARY PULMONARY TUBERCULOSIS

In contrast to primary pulmonary tuberculosis, sputum is produced in most cases and tubercle bacilli may usually be detected by microscopical examination, by culture or, where facilities exist, by use of one of the rapid molecular methods (see Chapter 7). If there is difficulty in obtaining sputum specimens, lesions may be sampled by bronchial brushing or biopsy through a flexible fibreoptic bronchoscope.[19] In this context, it is worthwhile examining material obtained at routine fibreoptic bronchoscopy, as unsuspected cases of tuberculosis will thereby be diagnosed.

Chest X-rays reveal the solid and cavitating lesions described above, and in old or recurrent cases there may be considerable scarring and distortion of the lung fields. Pleural effusions may be present and, in the case of bronchopleural fistulae, distinct fluid levels. None of these features is, however, specific to tuberculosis.

If a bacteriological diagnosis is not made, suspected pulmonary tuberculosis must be distinguished from a range of conditions, especially lung cancer, unresolved pneumonias, pulmonary infarct, parasitic infections of the lung and pulmonary fibrosis secondary to sarcoidosis or industrial dust disease. Lung cancers and abscesses, particularly those caused by *Staphylococcus aureus* or *Klebsiella pneumoniae*, may undergo central cavitation and resemble the cavitating lesions of tuberculosis.

In addition to tuberculosis, pleural effusions may be associated with bacterial and viral pneumonia, heart failure, cancer and pulmonary embolism. The general malaise, fever, night sweats and weight loss seen in tuberculosis are also features of acquired immunodeficiency syndrome (AIDS) and metastatic cancer.

Summary

The lung is the organ most frequently involved in tuberculosis, in both primary and post-primary disease. Both types of disease pose serious diagnostic problems, although in the latter, acid-fast bacilli are often seen on microscopical examination of smears of sputum. The lesions of primary tuberculosis are usually closed, whereas post-primary lesions often cavitate and permit the bacilli to enter the sputum and render the patient infectious. Clinical features, including a history of exposure to infection in the case of primary tuberculosis, are suggestive of the diagnosis. Radiological appearances and positive tuberculin tests may render the diagnosis probable, but only the demonstration of the causative organism by microscopy or culture confirms the diagnosis.

Prologue to the next chapter

In this chapter, the most common forms of tuberculosis – those affecting the lung and related structures – have been described. In a substantial minority of cases, however, the disease may spread beyond the lung and cause particularly serious forms of the disease. These challenging and important conditions are the subject of the next chapter.

REFERENCES

1. Milburn HJ. Primary tuberculosis. *Curr Opin Pulm Med* 2001; **7**: 133–41.
2. Walls T, Shingadia D. Global epidemiology of paediatric tuberculosis. *J Infect* 2004; **48**: 13–22.
3. Snider DE, Bloch AB. Congenital tuberculosis. *Tubercle* 1984; **65**: 81–2.
4. Maltezou HC, Spyridis P, Kafetzis DA. Tuberculosis during infancy. *Int J Tuberc Lung Dis* 2000; **4**: 414–19.
5. Diwan V, Thorson A, Winkvist A (eds). *Gender and tuberculosis*. Report from the Workshop at the Nordic School of Public Health, Göteborg, May 24–26, 1998. Göteborg: The Nordic School of Public Health, 1998.
6. Mert A, Ozaras R, Tabak F, Ozturk R. Primary tuberculosis cases presenting with erythema nodosum. *J Dermatol* 2004; **31**: 66–8.
7. Rohatgi J, Dhaliwal U. Phlyctenular eye disease: a reappraisal. *Jpn J Ophthalmol* 2000; **44**: 146–50.
8. Wallgren A. The timetable of tuberculosis. *Tubercle* 1948; **29**: 245–51.
9. Ustvedt HJ. The relationship between renal tuberculosis and primary infection. *Tubercle* 1947; **28**: 22–5.
10. Ip M, Chau PY, So S et al. The value of routine bronchial aspirate culture at fibreoptic bronchoscopy for the diagnosis of tuberculosis. *Tubercle* 1989; **79**: 281–5.
11. Delacourt C, Mani T M, Bonnerot V et al. Computed tomography with normal chest radiograph in tuberculous infection. *Arch Dis Child* 1993; **69**: 430–2.
12. Donald PR. Clinical manifestations of tuberculosis. In Donald PR, Fourie PB, Grange JM (eds), *Tuberculosis in childhood*. Pretoria: van Schaik, 1999, 61–99.
13. Hesseling AC, Schaaf HS, Gie RP et al. A critical review of diagnostic approaches used in the diagnosis of childhood tuberculosis. *Int J Tuberc Lung Dis* 2002; **6**: 1036–45.

14. Fourie PB, Becker PJ, Festenstein F et al. Procedures for developing a simple scoring method based on unsophisticated criteria for screening children for tuberculosis. *Int J Tuberc Lung Dis* 1998; **2**: 116–23.
15. Consensus Statement of IAP Working Group. Status report of diagnosis of childhood tuberculosis. *Ind Pediatrics* 2004; **41**: 146–55. Full text also available online: <www.indianpediatrics.net/feb2004/feb-146-155.htm>.
16. Rouillon A, Perdrizet S, Parrot R. Transmission of tubercle bacilli: the effects of chemotherapy. *Tubercle* 1976; **57**: 275–99.
17. Balasubramanian V, Wiegeshaus EH, Taylor BT, Smith DW. Pathogenesis of tuberculosis: pathway to apical localization. *Tuber Lung Dis* 1994; **75**: 168–78.
18. Epstein DM, Kline LR, Albelda SM, Miller WT. Tuberculous pleural effusions. *Chest* 1987; **91**: 106–9.
19. Willcox PA, Benatar SR, Potgeiter PD. Use of flexible fibreoptic bronchoscope in the diagnosis of sputum-negative pulmonary tuberculosis. *Thorax* 1982; **37**: 598–601.

FURTHER READING

Crofton J, Horne N, Miller F. *Clinical tuberculosis*, 2nd edn. London: Macmillan, 1999.

Davies PDO. Respiratory tuberculosis. In Davies PDO (ed.), *Clinical tuberculosis*, 3rd edn. London: Arnold, 2003, 107–24.

Davies PDO, Ormerod LP. *Case presentations in clinical tuberculosis*. London: Arnold, 1999.

Donald PR, Fourie PB, Grange JM. *Tuberculosis in childhood*. Pretoria: van Schaik, 1999.

Grange JM, Zumla A. Tuberculosis. In Cook G, Zumla A (eds), *Manson's tropical diseases*, 21st edn. London: WB Saunders, 2003, 995–1052.

Interactive tutorial on CD-ROM. *Tuberculosis*. Topics in International Health. London: Wellcome Trust, 1999. Available from CABI International, Wallingford, Oxon OX10 8DE, UK; <www.cabi.org>.

International Union Against Tuberculosis and Lung Disease. *Management of tuberculosis: a guide for low income countries*, 5th edn. Paris: IUATLD, 2000.

Zumla A, Rook G, Mwaba P, Lucas S. Tuberculosis. In James DG, Zumla A (eds), *The granulomatous disorders*. Cambridge: Cambridge University Press, 1999, 132–60.

CHAPTER 9

Extrapulmonary tuberculosis

Introduction

Tuberculosis outside the lung may result from infection by a route other than the respiratory system, principally by ingestion of milk containing *Mycobacterium bovis*, or through abrasions and injuries to the skin. More often, however, this form of the disease is the result of tubercle bacilli spreading from the primary complex in the lung to other parts of the body via the lymphatics and bloodstream. Before the advent of effective therapy, extrapulmonary tuberculosis often required some form of surgical intervention and was generally referred to as 'surgical tuberculosis'. Fortunately, surgery is rarely indicated today.

Learning outcomes

After studying and reflecting on the material in this chapter, you will be able to:

- discuss the very wide range of clinical forms of extrapulmonary tuberculosis and their serious threats to health and life,
- describe the principal differences in the spread of disease from the pulmonary lesion in primary and post-primary tuberculosis,
- describe the common forms of extrapulmonary tuberculosis and their complications,
- describe the principal forms of disseminated tuberculosis,
- outline the diagnostic problems posed by extrapulmonary tuberculosis.

Tuberculosis may develop in any organ or tissue of the body but, in practice, disease is more likely to develop in some organs and systems than in others. As mentioned in the previous chapter, the term extrapulmonary (or non-pulmonary) tuberculosis is used in this book to include disease outside the lungs and pleurae, although in the USA pleural tuberculosis is classified as a form of extrapulmonary tuberculosis. The organs and systems most usually affected are the superficial lymph nodes, central nervous system, bones and joints, genito-urinary tract, abdomen and skin. In some patients, especially those who have a condition that suppresses the immune responses, the disease may become widely disseminated and involve many organs and tissues.

The number of cases of extrapulmonary tuberculosis relative to pulmonary tuberculosis varies between ethnic communities in a country and is, in part, due to age differences. In England and Wales, for example, extrapulmonary tuberculosis is relatively more common in patients of Indian subcontinent ethnic origin and there are also differences in the type of disease in the various ethnic groups (Table 9.1).

TABLE 9.1 Extrapulmonary tuberculosis in indigenous European and Indian subcontinent ethnic groups in south-east England, 1977–1991

	European (%)		Indian subcontinent (%)	
	1977–83	1984–91	1977–83	1984–91
Lymphadenopathy	30.3	36.6	55.6	59.6
Genito-urinary	37.6	27.2	6.8	8.4
Bone and joint	19.5	19.7	24.7	19.2
Abdomen	5.1	7.8	7.8	8.3
Central nervous system	6.7	4.4	4.3	3.7
Disseminated	0.8	4.2[a]	0.7	0.6
Total number of patients	1470	861	1914	1794
Extrapulmonary cases as percentage of all cases of tuberculosis	21.3	18.9	49.5	45.1

[a]Increase in disseminated disease in this group relates to emergence of HIV.

SUPERFICIAL LYMPH NODES

A swollen lymph node may be the first sign of tuberculosis. The most frequently affected site is the neck, and tuberculous cervical lymphadenitis has for centuries, though for reasons that have defied explanation, been known as **scrofula**. It was also known as the King's Evil, on account of the belief that a touch from the reigning monarch was curative and that the healing gift was passed from one monarch to his or her successor.[1] In *Macbeth* (Act 4, Scene 3), Shakespeare mentions the King's Evil and also the golden medallion or 'touch piece' which the monarch gave to those who he had touched:

> Tis called the evil;
> A most miraculous work in this good king
> Which often, since my here-remain in England,
> I've seen him do. How he solicits heaven
> Himself knows best; but strangely-visited people
> All swol'n and ulcerous, pitiful to the eye,
> The mere despair of surgery, he cures,
> Hanging a golden stamp about their necks
> Put on with holy prayers; and 'tis spoken,
> To the succeeding royalty he leaves
> The healing benediction.

In England, this rather pleasant custom ended rather abruptly when Queen Anne (1665–1714) failed to cure the somewhat choleric and bombastic Samuel Johnson, but in France it persisted until the Revolution in the late eighteenth century.

Scrofula may be due to primary infection of the pharynx or tonsil by milk-borne *M. bovis*, in which case the nodes involved are around the angle of the jaw and, sometimes, on the face in front of the ear. In other cases, scrofula appears to be due to an upward extension of a tuberculous complex in the chest, in which case the involved nodes are those just above the collar bone (supraclavicular nodes).

For reasons that are not clear, supraclavicular lymphadenopathy is a common presentation of tuberculosis in patients of Indian subcontinent ethnic origin living in the UK and other industrially developed nations (see Table 9.1).[2] Most such patients are aged 20–40 years, and women are affected more than men. Lesions of pulmonary tuberculosis are often evident on chest X-rays. In the USA, lymphadenopathy and other forms of extrapulmonary tuberculosis are likewise relatively more common in women and the non-white population.[3]

In the early stages, the involved lymph nodes are rubbery in texture and usually painless and the patients often feel well. As the condition progresses, the nodes undergo central necrosis and are fluctuant on palpation. The disease may spread out of the lymph nodes, with sinus formation and spreading lesions on the skin resembling lupus vulgaris (see below). This condition is called **scrofuloderma**.

Localized or more generalized lymphadenopathy is a common manifestation of tuberculosis in patients infected with the human immunodeficiency virus (HIV; see Chapter 10). Lymphadenopathy in children, especially in those under the age of 5 years, may be due to one of the species of environmental mycobacteria (see Chapter 11).

Tuberculosis is just one cause of lymph node enlargement. Other causes include various bacterial and viral infections, lymphomas, metastatic cancer and sarcoidosis. Histological examination of biopsies or cytological examination of fine-needle aspirates is more helpful diagnostically then acid-fast staining or culture.[4]

Treatment is by standard short-course chemotherapy. In some cases, the affected lymph nodes enlarge, sometimes extensively, during therapy. This is due to immunological hypersensitivity reactions rather than a recurrence of the disease, and usually responds to steroid therapy.

CENTRAL NERVOUS SYSTEM

Tuberculosis of the central nervous system is a serious and life-threatening condition and two main forms are seen: tuberculous meningitis and space-occupying lesions in the brain or spinal cord.[5] The former is the more common and, worldwide, most cases occur in young children, although people of any age may be affected, particularly those who are immunosuppressed. In children it is usually a manifestation of primary tuberculosis and there may be radiological evidence of a primary pulmonary complex.

Tuberculous meningitis is a very serious condition and must be regarded as a medical emergency, as any delay in commencing treatment may lead to death, or to survival with serious neurological consequences such as blindness, deafness, paralysis or all three.

The condition is characterized by inflammation of the meninges – the membranes enclosing the brain and spinal cord – particularly at the base of the brain. This inflammation causes the secretion of a thick exudate which may strangulate the cranial nerves, particularly those leading to the eyes and ears, causing blindness and deafness. The exudate may also block the flow of cerebrospinal fluid, resulting in raised intracranial pressure and hydrocephalus – a common complication of this disease. In addition, the inflammation may involve the arteries at the base of the brain, leading to infarction of areas of the brain with subsequent convulsions and paralysis.[6]

Tuberculous meningitis is classified into three stages.

- *Stage 1*. The patient is fully conscious and rational. Symptoms are non-specific and include general malaise, low-grade fever, apathy, irritability, mood changes, depression and intermittent headache. There are no focal neurological signs and little or no evidence of meningitis. Symptoms may be limited or even absent in those with HIV infection or other causes of immunosuppression.
- *Stage 2*. The patient is mentally confused and/or has focal neurological signs, and may have severe and persistent headache, vomiting and/or an aversion to light (photophobia).
- *Stage 3*. The patient is stuporose or in a coma and/or has complete hemiplegia, paraplegia or quadriplegia.

For diagnosis, it is necessary to obtain a sample of cerebrospinal fluid for laboratory tests, including a thorough microscopical search for acid-fast bacilli, although these are found in less than a third of patients. It is essential to start treatment immediately, so this should be done if there is the slightest suspicion of the diagnosis. In a recent study in Denmark, treatment was commenced in the absence of a definitive bacteriological diagnosis in 85 per cent of patients with tuberculous meningitis.[7]

BONES AND JOINTS

This is a common form of tuberculosis of children in the developing nations and, although any bone or joint may be involved, about half the cases affect the spine. Other common sites are, in order of frequency, the large joints of the lower limb (hip, knee and ankle) and those of the upper limb (shoulder, elbow and wrist). Immunosuppressed people may develop many lesions throughout the skeleton and these may be mistaken for metastatic carcinoma.[8]

Spinal tuberculosis is also known as **Pott's disease**, named after Sir Percival Pott (1713–1788), who was a surgeon at St Bartholomew's Hospital in London.[9] The disease particularly affects the front parts of the vertebrae, which may collapse, causing a characteristic angular deformity, or **gibbus** (Fig. 9.1). It is therefore a cause of 'hunchback' deformities. The collapse may also crush the spinal cord, leading to hemiplegia. Abscesses may develop and can track a long way through the muscles before emerging as sinuses on the skin. Some sinuses may thus emerge on the thigh, well away from the spinal lesion.

Patients usually present with chronic back pain, stiffness and limitation of movement. Characteristically, they show an inability or unwillingness to pick something off the floor. Signs found on clinical examination include muscle spasm and rigidity, fluctuating abscesses, sinuses and spinal deformity. About half the patients show neurological signs due to inflammation of, or pressure on, the spinal cord. Both clinical and X-ray signs may be minimal and fail to reveal the true extent of the disease. Where available, computerized tomography (CT) or magnetic resonance imaging (MRI) gives a more accurate picture of the extent of the disease. Bacteriological and histological examination of material acquired by biopsy or fine-needle aspiration confirms the diagnosis.

Antituberculosis therapy is always required and surgery is indicated if there is spinal deformity, neurological complications, or both. The most effective surgical way of correcting deformity and relieving neurological complications is to excise all the diseased tissue and to

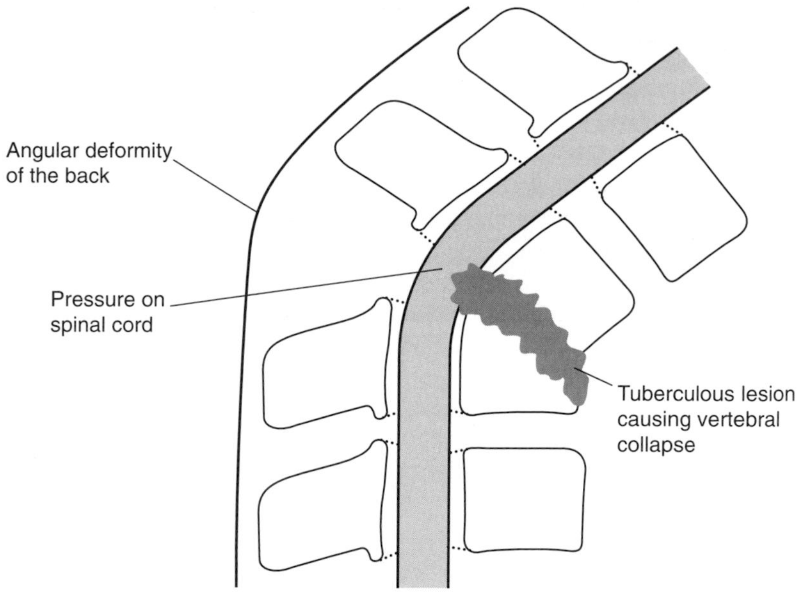

FIGURE 9.1 *Tuberculosis of the spine: lesion in vertebral body leading to wedge-shaped collapse of the vertebra and extension backwards with compression of the spinal cord.*

do bone grafting.[10] However, this – the so-called 'Hong Kong operation' – does require considerable surgical experience and special facilities – neither of which is widely available.

Tuberculosis of other bones and joints is confirmed by bacteriological examination of biopsies of bone or synovium or of aspirated synovial fluid and is treated by standard anti-tuberculosis therapy. Unless the patient experiences undue pain, he or she should be encouraged to keep the joint moving as much as possible during therapy and afterwards. Surgery, including joint replacement, should be considered for patients with persistent pain, deformity or immobility.[10]

RENAL AND GENITAL TRACTS

This form of tuberculosis, which is probably commoner than generally reported, usually begins in the kidney.[11] It occurs later than other forms of extrapulmonary tuberculosis, usually presenting 6–15 years after the initial infection.[12] As it is such a late manifestation of primary tuberculosis, lesions suggestive of tuberculosis are only seen in chest X-rays in about 5 per cent of patients, but they may have a history of the disease. Tubercle bacilli released into the urine from renal lesions cause secondary lesions in the ureters, bladder and, in males, in the epididymis, testes, seminal vesicles and prostate (Fig. 9.2).

Patients may complain of frequency of urination, pain on urination (dysuria), pain in the suprapubic region and blood in the urine, all of which occur in other forms or urinary tract infection. However, many patients just have vague backache, and their disease may not be diagnosed until renal function is impaired. A few patients present with renal colic, which can be extremely painful, but only a minority (less than 10 per cent) of patients feel generally

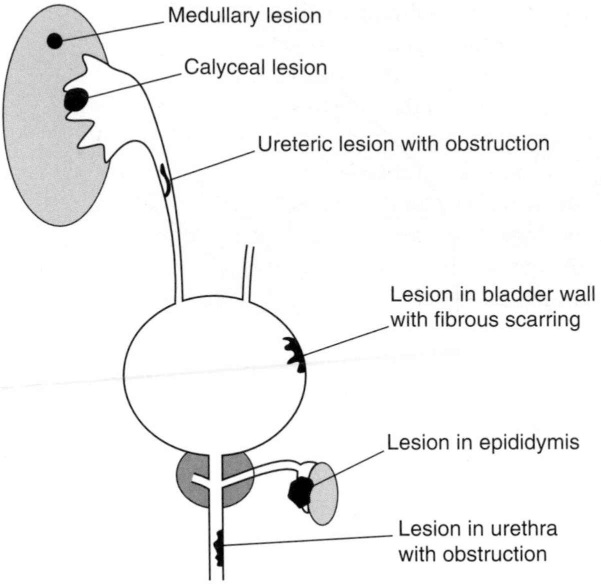

FIGURE 9.2 *Tuberculosis of the male genito-urinary tract and obstructive complications: initial lesion in the kidney with spread to ureter, bladder, epididymis and urethra.*

unwell. The first sign of the disease in males may be a swollen testis or epididymis, or infertility.

If diagnosis is delayed, extensive destruction of the kidney or obstruction of a ureter may lead to renal failure. Fibrosis of the bladder reduces its volume. One form of tuberculosis of the kidney, **tuberculous interstitial nephritis**, runs a very 'quiet' course and may cause severe renal failure before diagnostic signs and symptoms are evident.[13] Tuberculosis should therefore be considered in all cases of renal failure when there is no other obvious cause.

In contrast to tuberculosis of the genital tract in men, the condition in women is not due to seeding from the kidney but to direct spread by the bloodstream from the primary focus of disease in the lung. The disease usually begins in the Fallopian tubes and may spread to the uterus or to the peritoneal cavity (see below). Many patients are infertile. Patients may present with pelvic pain, heavy menstrual periods or amenorrhoea. Others present with ascites, abdominal distension and weight loss, sometimes leading to an initial diagnosis of ovarian cancer.[14] The symptoms are, however, often minimal and the disease may only be detected on examination for the cause of infertility.

Treatment of renal or genital tuberculosis is by standard antituberculosis chemotherapy. Surgery may be required for augmentation of a shrunken bladder or for relief of obstruction of the ureter or urethra,[15] although such obstruction may respond to treatment with steroids.

THE ABDOMEN

There are two main forms of abdominal tuberculosis: intestinal and peritoneal.[5,16] Primary intestinal tuberculosis is usually caused by drinking cows' milk containing *M. bovis* and is therefore rarely seen in the industrially developed nations, where bovine tuberculosis has been almost eradicated. The commonest site of the primary lesion is the ileocaecal region and it causes thickening or hypertrophy of the intestinal wall in the affected region. The local lymph nodes are enlarged (analogous to the hilar lymph node enlargement in primary pulmonary tuberculosis). The thickened intestinal wall and enlarged nodes cause a tender mass, which may be felt on palpation of the right iliac fossa. Patients may develop intestinal obstruction, fistula formation, peritonitis and, rarely, massive and sometimes fatal rectal bleeding.

In post-primary tuberculosis, tubercle bacilli in swallowed sputum may cause gastrointestinal lesions. These usually occur in the stomach and small intestine and are characterized by ulceration rather than hypertrophy. There is therefore a risk of intestinal perforation leading to peritonitis. Some patients present with sub-acute intestinal obstruction due to strictures and scarring and, in a few, the bacilli lodge in anal fissures, leading to abscess and fistula formation.

Tuberculous peritonitis is the result of perforation of intestinal tuberculous ulcers and, as mentioned above, direct spread from the primary focus of disease via the bloodstream or spread from a lesion in a Fallopian tube. The disease is most often seen in young women and older alcoholic men, in whom, even if treated, mortality is high.[17] Diagnosis is not easy, as the symptoms are vague and non-specific.[18,19] Ascites is common. If available, ultrasonography or CT scanning demonstrates thickened intestinal walls and enlarged lymph nodes,[18] and colonoscopy enables biopsies to be obtained from the caecal region – a common site of lesions in primary disease. Aspirated peritoneal fluid is usually negative on examination, but biopsy of the peritoneum by laparoscopy or through a small midline abdominal incision under local anaesthetic is the most effective way of making the diagnosis.[19]

Treatment is by standard chemotherapy. Surgery is only required if there is intestinal obstruction or massive rectal bleeding.

THE SKIN

Skin tuberculosis may be caused by primary accidental inoculation of tubercle bacilli into the skin; implantation of bacilli in coughed-up sputum into minor abrasions around the mouth, a condition termed **tuberculosis orificialis cutis**; direct extension from underlying lesions, such as scrofuloderma over tuberculous lymph nodes (see above); and dissemination to the skin via the bloodstream (Table 9.2).[20] In addition, there are several very uncommon, poorly understood and quaintly named conditions under the umbrella name of **tuberculides**.[21] These may represent some form of hypersensitivity reaction and manifest as small skin lesions, sometimes with necrotic centres, which disappear when the underlying disease is treated.

Traditionally, primary inoculation tuberculosis was an occupational hazard of butchers,

TABLE 9.2 The principal forms of skin involvement in tuberculosis

Primary lesions	Traumatic inoculation into dermis or epidermis
Secondary lesions	Inoculation into skin from endogenous source, especially tuberculous sputum
	Lesions due to haematogenous dissemination, e.g. miliary skin nodules, lupus vulgaris
	Lesions due to lymphatic spread, e.g. satellite lesions proximal to primary skin lesion
	Lesions secondary to involvement of underlying structures, e.g. scrofuloderma
Immunological phenomena	Erythema nodosum
	Tuberculides

anatomists and pathologists and has been called 'prosector's or butcher's wart'.[22] Some recent cases have occurred in medical laboratory workers following 'needlestick' and other minor injuries. It is usually a benign and self-limiting condition, but antituberculosis therapy must always be given. **Brawl chancre** is the name given to a very rare form of skin tuberculosis affecting the knuckles and acquired by punching a patient with open tuberculosis in the teeth. Skin tuberculosis has been reported after circumcision, ear piercing and tattooing when the 'operator' had open tuberculosis.

A classical form of skin tuberculosis, one that is now seldom seen in industrially developed nations, is **lupus vulgaris**. The origin of the name, usually translated as 'common wolf', is obscure and dates back to the eleventh century. Some writers suggest that lupus is a corruption of 'lepros' and that Biblical leprosy may have been skin tuberculosis. It is a slowly progressive and very chronic condition, usually occurring on the nose, cheeks or neck and characterized by red-brown nodules, which may ulcerate. If untreated, it may lead to severe disfigurement such as loss of the nose. It has been suggested that lupus vulgaris is caused by *M. bovis* rather than *M. tuberculosis*, as the very few cases seen in the UK in recent years were caused by the former organism.

Before the introduction of antituberculosis therapy, which is the current treatment, skin tuberculosis was treated by large doses of vitamin D and ultraviolet radiation, with success in many cases.

OTHER FORMS OF EXTRAPULMONARY TUBERCULOSIS

Lesions of tuberculosis may develop in any organ and tissue but, in the absence of immunosuppression and widespread dissemination (see below), muscles are rarely affected. Solitary tuberculous nodules occasionally occur in the breast and thyroid and are easily mistaken for cancer. Involvement of the adrenal glands leads to reduced production of adrenal steroid hormones – a condition termed **Addison's disease**, described by Thomas Addison (1793–1860), a physician at Guy's Hospital, London.

Tuberculous laryngitis is due to implantation of bacilli from tuberculous sputum and is thus secondary to open pulmonary disease. In the days before effective chemotherapy, this was a serious and very painful complication of tuberculosis, often requiring cautery or more radical surgery.

Involvement of the heart muscle is extremely rare, but **tuberculous pericarditis** is not uncommon, particularly in certain geographical regions. Even if it is successfully treated, this condition may have serious long-term sequelae, as fibrous scarring and calcification may compress the heart, leading to cardiac failure. This condition, termed **constrictive pericarditis**, may be prevented to some extent by prescribing steroids at the same time as antituberculosis therapy. For unknown reasons, tuberculous pericarditis is more common in some regions than others. For example, it used to be frequently seen in Transkei in southern Africa, hence the name **Transkei heart**.[23]

DISSEMINATED TUBERCULOSIS

This is now commonly seen in HIV-infected patients, as described in Chapter 10, but is also seen in those with other causes of immunosuppression, including renal failure, post-transplant immunosuppressive therapy and chemotherapy for cancer. It is also seen in the very young and in elderly patients and occasionally in those with no obvious predisposing cause. The clinical manifestations, histological appearance, rate of progression and outcome critically depend on the integrity of the immune defences, and two main forms have been described: **miliary** and **cryptic disseminated** tuberculosis.

Miliary tuberculosis

Patients with this form of tuberculosis have relatively good immune responses and so they are able to produce granulomas around the disseminated tubercle bacilli. Thus affected tissues and organs contain numerous small granulomatous lesions that resemble millet seeds, and the name miliary tuberculosis is derived from the Latin word *milium* – a millet seed.

Historically, this was a disease of young children, but it is now seen in those of all ages. Although often rapidly progressive, miliary tuberculosis may be surprisingly chronic, particularly in adult patients.[24] Symptoms include fever, malaise and weight loss. Involvement of the central nervous system may cause headache. Chest X-rays reveal numerous minute lesions, giving the lung fields a 'snowstorm' appearance, and there are often small pleural effusions. Acid-fast bacilli are seen in sputum in about half the patients, but the best way to make the diagnosis is to obtain a biopsy of the lung through a fibreoptic bronchoscope. The kidneys are usually affected and acid-fast bacilli are detectable in urine in about a quarter of patients. Enlargement of the liver and spleen is detected by palpation of the abdomen in about a quarter of patients. Examination of the eye through an ophthalmoscope may reveal characteristic millet seed-like granulomas on the retina.

Patients respond well to standard antituberculosis therapy, but corticosteroids are also often given, and may be life-saving in those who are very ill and in a state of collapse.

Cryptic disseminated tuberculosis

This occurs in the elderly and in those who are immunosuppressed.[25] In contrast to miliary tuberculosis, there is little or no granuloma formation; instead, the lesions take the form of minute necrotic foci containing numerous acid-fast bacilli. Such lesions are too small to be seen on chest X-rays, so the lung fields look deceptively normal – hence the name. Patients may be very ill, but symptoms are often non-specific and, because of weak immunity, the tuberculin test is usually negative. The course of the disease is often rapidly progressive and many patients die without a diagnosis being made. If suspected, diagnosis is confirmed by finding acid-fast bacilli on microscopical examination of biopsies of lung, liver or bone marrow.

Summary

Extrapulmonary tuberculosis manifests in a myriad of forms and poses a serious challenge to diagnosis. It has, indeed, been remarked that if one knows tuberculosis, one knows all of medicine (although the same has been said of syphilis). In many cases, just one organ or system is involved, although some patients also have pulmonary lesions. In other cases, the disease is widely disseminated and, depending on the immune status, may present in the classical miliary form or as the cryptogenic disseminated form, which is difficult to diagnose. In addition to therapy, there are many aspects of caring for patients with various forms of extrapulmonary tuberculosis, such as surgical care and attention to residual neurological and orthopaedic problems.

Prologue to the next chapter

In this and the previous chapter, the 'classical' features of tuberculosis within and beyond the lung have been described. Over the last two decades, however, the global epidemiology and the very nature of tuberculosis as seen in many countries have been dramatically changed by the evolution and spread of HIV infection and acquired immunodeficiency syndrome (AIDS). Indeed, HIV infection and tuberculosis have been termed 'the cursed duet'. At present, most HIV-related tuberculosis is seen in Africa, but HIV infection is increasing at an alarming rate in other countries where tuberculosis is rife. Knowledge of the particular problems and challenges posed by HIV-related tuberculosis is therefore essential for all those involved in caring for patients with the latter disease.

REFERENCES

1. Wiseman R. A treatise of the King's Evill. In *Eight chirurgical treatises*. London: Tooke and Meredith, 1696. Reprinted in Major RH. *Classic descriptions of disease*, 3rd edn. Springfield, IL: Charles C Thomas, 1959, 54–8.
2. Kennedy DH. Extrapulmonary tuberculosis. In Ratledge C, Stanford JL, Grange JM (eds), *The biology of the mycobacteria*, Vol. 3. New York: Academic Press, 1989, 245–84.
3. Yang Z, Kong Y, Wilson F et al. Identification of risk factors for extrapulmonary tuberculosis. *Clin Infect Dis* 2004; **38**: 199–205.
4. Lau SK, Wei WI, Hsu C et al. Efficacy of fine needle aspiration in the diagnosis of tuberculous cervical lymphadenopathy. *J Laryngol Otol* 1990; **104**: 24–7.
5. Ormerod P. Non-respiratory tuberculosis. In Davies PDO (ed.), *Clinical tuberculosis*, 3rd edn. London: Arnold, 2003, 125–53.
6. Donald PR, Shoeman JF, Cotton MF et al. Missed opportunities for the prevention and early diagnosis of tuberculous meningitis in children. *S Afr J Epidemiol Inf* 1990; **5**: 76–8.
7. Bidstrup C, Andersen PH, Skinhoj P, Andersen AB. Tuberculous meningitis in a country with a low incidence of tuberculosis: still a serious disease and a diagnostic challenge. *Scand J Infect Dis* 2002; **34**: 811–14.
8. Ormerod LP, Grundy M, Rathman MA. Multiple tuberculous bone lesions resembling metastatic disease. *Tubercle* 1989; **70**: 305–7.
9. Khoo LT, Mikawa K, Fessler RG. A surgical revisitation of Pott's distemper of the spine. *Spine J* 2003; **3**: 130–45.
10. Taor WS. Surgery for bone and joint tuberculosis. In Coombs R, Fitzgerald RH (eds), *Infection in the orthopaedic patient*. London: Butterworths, 1989, 307–11.
11. Eastwood JB, Dilly SA, Grange JM. Tuberculosis, leprosy and other mycobacterial diseases. In Cattell WR (ed.), *Infections of the kidney and urinary tract*. Oxford: Oxford University Press, 1996, 291–318.
12. Ustvedt HJ. The relationship between renal tuberculosis and primary infection. *Tubercle* 1947; **28**: 22–5.
13. Morgan SH, Eastwood JB, Baker LRI. Tuberculous interstitial nephritis – the tip of an iceberg. *Tubercle* 1991; **71**: 5–6.
14. Chow TW, Lim BK, Vallipuram S. The masquerades of female pelvic tuberculosis: case reports and review of literature on clinical presentations and diagnosis. *J Obstet Gynaecol Res* 2002; **28**: 203–10.

15. Ramanathan R, Kumar A, Kapoor R et al. Relief of urinary tract obstruction in tuberculosis to improve renal function. Analysis of predictive factors. *Br J Urol* 1998; **81**: 199–205.
16. Marshall JB. Tuberculosis of the gastrointestinal tract and peritoneum. *Am J Gastroenterol* 1993; **88**: 989–99.
17. Sheer TA, Coyle WJ. Gastrointestinal tuberculosis. *Curr Gastroenterol Rep* 2003; **5**: 273–8.
18. Tshibwabwa-Tumba E, Mwaba P, Bogle-Taylor J et al. Four year study of abdominal ultrasound in 900 Central African adults with AIDS refered for diagnostic imaging. *Abdom Imaging* 2000; **25**: 290–6.
19. Rai S, Thomas WM. Diagnosis of abdominal tuberculosis: the importance of laparoscopy. *J R Soc Med* 2003; **96**: 586–8.
20. Harahap M (ed.). *Mycobacterial skin diseases*. New Clinical Applications series – Dermatology. London: Kluwer, 1989.
21. Morrison JGL, Fourie ED. The papulonecrotic tuberculide – from Arthus reaction to lupus vulgaris. *Br J Dermatol* 1974; **91**: 273–7.
22. Grange JM, Noble WC, Yates MD, Collins CH. Inoculation mycobacterioses. *Clin Exp Dermatol* 1988; **13**: 211–20.
23. Strang JI. Tuberculous pericarditis in Transkei. *Clin Cardiol* 1984; **7**: 667–70.
24. Proudfoot AT, Akhtar AJ, Douglas AC, Horne NW. Miliary tuberculosis in adults. *BMJ* 1969; **2**: 273–6.
25. Proudfoot AT. Cryptic disseminated tuberculosis. *Br J Hosp Med* 1971; **5**: 773–80.

FURTHER READING

Kennedy DH. Extrapulmonary tuberculosis. In Ratledge C, Stanford JL, Grange JM (eds), *The biology of the mycobacteria*, Vol. 3. New York: Academic Press, 1989, 245–84.

Ormerod P. Non-respiratory tuberculosis. In Davies PDO (ed.), *Clinical tuberculosis*, 3rd edn. London: Arnold, 2003, 125–53.

CHAPTER 10

Tuberculosis and the HIV/AIDS pandemic

Introduction

Over the past two decades, human immunodeficiency virus (HIV) infection has emerged as the most important and widespread risk factor for the progression from latent infection by the tubercle bacillus to active tuberculosis. Throughout the world, tuberculosis is the most frequent opportunistic infection in people with HIV disease. Unusual (atypical) manifestations of tuberculosis are common in HIV-infected people and this often leads to confusion and delays in diagnosis and treatment. Because of this, and because active tuberculosis stimulates HIV replication, even when tuberculosis is treated effectively, the prognosis of such HIV-infected patients is poor. Each year, HIV infection causes an extra 1 million cases of tuberculosis worldwide, and 30 per cent of deaths in people with the acquired immunodeficiency syndrome (AIDS) are attributable to tuberculosis. At the present time, countries in Africa bear the greatest burden of HIV-related tuberculosis. They will, however, soon be overtaken by the more populous regions in South and South-East Asia, where there is an accelerated growth in national epidemics of HIV infection.

Tuberculosis, especially in immunocompromised patients, confronts nurses and other healthcare practitioners with a range of complex issues, including infection prevention and control and supporting adherence to therapy. HIV-related tuberculosis is a particular challenge in view of the many other social and psychological burdens borne by patients and their families and the overstretching of scarce healthcare resources in those countries most affected.

Learning outcomes

After studying and reflecting on the material in this chapter, you will be able to:

- describe why the HIV/AIDS pandemic has had, and is having, a very serious adverse effect on the global prevalence of tuberculosis,

- discuss the severe threat to global health if measures to contain both tuberculosis and HIV infection are not considerably strengthened,
- outline the clinical features of HIV-related tuberculosis, their relation to the degree of immunosuppression and the diagnostic problems that they cause,
- identify the particular problems encountered in the drug treatment of HIV-related tuberculosis,
- discuss the many barriers to the effective management of HIV-related tuberculosis, particularly in high-prevalence regions, and the steps required to overcome these barriers.

TUBERCULOSIS IN HIV-INFECTED PEOPLE

The epidemiological relationship between tuberculosis and human immunodeficiency virus (HIV) infection is described in Chapter 1, but is briefly reviewed here. Most people who overcome a primary infection by the tubercle bacillus have about a 5 per cent risk of developing post-primary tuberculosis at some time during the rest of their lives, but in a person co-infected with HIV, the risk is around 8 per cent each year. Thus the annual risk of a co-infected person developing tuberculosis is more than 20 times higher than that of someone infected by the tubercle bacillus alone. If an HIV-infected person, especially one with end-stage disease, i.e. acquired immunodeficiency syndrome (AIDS), becomes infected or re-infected by the tubercle bacillus, their risk of developing overt tuberculosis is very high. Furthermore, the time between infection and disease is 'telescoped' from several years or even decades to just a few months. This has led to a number of 'explosive' mini-epidemics of tuberculosis in communities with many HIV-infected people and in institutions providing care for patients with HIV disease.

Historically, most cases of tuberculosis in adults are ascribed to reactivation of endogenous infection, but the use of 'fingerprinting' has shown that many cases of new and recurrent tuberculosis are due to recent infection.[1] This is particularly the case in HIV-infected individuals owing to their lowered ability to prevent infection progressing to active disease. On the other hand, patients with HIV-related tuberculosis are no more infectious than those who are not infected with HIV.[2] Indeed, as pulmonary cavity formation is reduced (see Chapter 5 and below), they may, as a group, be less infectious.

In the year 2003, there were an estimated 40 million HIV-infected people worldwide. Given that one-third were co-infected with tubercle bacilli and that they had an 8 per cent risk of developing tuberculosis in that year (see above), it may be calculated that HIV infection would have been the predisposing cause of more than 1 million cases of tuberculosis in that year. Although AIDS now ranks among the leading infectious causes of death worldwide, the direct cause of death in a third of these patients is tuberculosis.

Globally, around 12 per cent of all cases of tuberculosis are now HIV related. At the present time, the impact of the HIV epidemic on tuberculosis is most severe in sub-Saharan Africa, where, in the last decade of the twentieth century, almost a quarter of the estimated 15 million new cases of tuberculosis were HIV related.[3] As a direct consequence, the prevalence of tuberculosis doubled, trebled or even quadrupled in some African countries over this time period. In Zambia, for example, the prevalence of tuberculosis was fairly constant between 1964 and 1984, with around 7000 new reported cases annually. In 1995, however, 40 000 new cases were reported and three-quarters of these were HIV related. Depending on the country, between 20 and more than 70 per cent of cases of tuberculosis in sub-Saharan Africa are HIV related. Thus, a diagnosis of tuberculosis in this region alerts the medical staff to the distinct possibility of HIV infection. Children as well as adults are affected – between 10 and 40 per cent of children under the age of 14 with tuberculosis in Zambia and Côte d'Ivoire are also infected with HIV. Tuberculosis is foremost among the causes of maternal death in Zambia, where one in four pregnant women are HIV infected.[4]

At present, the greatest impact of HIV on tuberculosis is seen in Africa but the population size (around 750 million in 1998) is relatively small compared to that of the Indian subcontinent, China and South-East Asia. Most of the world's cases of tuberculosis occur in these more highly populated regions, where, unless the present upsurge of HIV infection is controlled, there could be very serious tuberculosis problems in the near future.

HIV DISEASE – A BRIEF SYNOPSIS

The natural history of HIV infection and subsequent disease is comprehensively described elsewhere,[5] but a brief review is required here in order to understand the impact this infection has on tuberculosis. Following HIV infection, predictable immunopathological changes and resultant clinical events can be expected to occur during a continuum from initial infection through to end-stage disease (AIDS) and death. This anticipated course of events occurring in the absence of specific antiretroviral therapy is known as the **natural history of HIV disease** and it incorporates three components:

- HIV infection,
- the interaction of continuing high-level viral replication with the immune system (immunopathogenesis),
- the clinical consequences of a failing immune system.

HIV infection

The HIV belongs to a class of viruses known as **retroviruses**. The genomes of these viruses are composed of two identical copies of single-stranded ribonucleic acid (RNA). Attached to the viral genome are molecules of an enzyme unique to retroviruses known as **reverse transcriptase**. When HIV infects a human cell, this enzyme facilitates the synthesis, or transcription, of a chain of deoxyribonucleic acid (DNA) corresponding to the viral RNA, a process known as **reverse transcription**. Then, with the assistance of another viral enzyme, **integrase**, this unit of DNA (known as a **provirus**) is inserted into a chromosome within the nucleus of the cell it has infected, where it may lie dormant for months or years. However, the infected cell is eventually activated by the immune system and viral replication is initiated. Proviral DNA undergoes **forward transcription** to yield copies of the original viral RNA, and various viral proteins are produced. A third viral enzyme, **protease**, helps to package the new proteins into the component parts of a maturing virus, which bursts through the cell membrane by a process known as 'budding', eventually leading to the death of the infected cell.

HIV immunopathogenesis

This continuing productive viral infection of immune system cells, principally CD4+ T-lymphocytes (helper cells), results in billions of new virions being released from infected cells every day. These viruses swarm throughout the body, intent only on further massive viral replication. This unrelenting destruction of CD4+ cells leads to a progressive and ultimately fatal suppression of the immune system. Each stepwise decline in the level of CD4+ cells is matched by a corresponding increase in the level of virus in the peripheral blood (plasma **viral load**). This is illustrated in Figure 10.1, which shows how the clinical consequences of HIV infection can be staged.

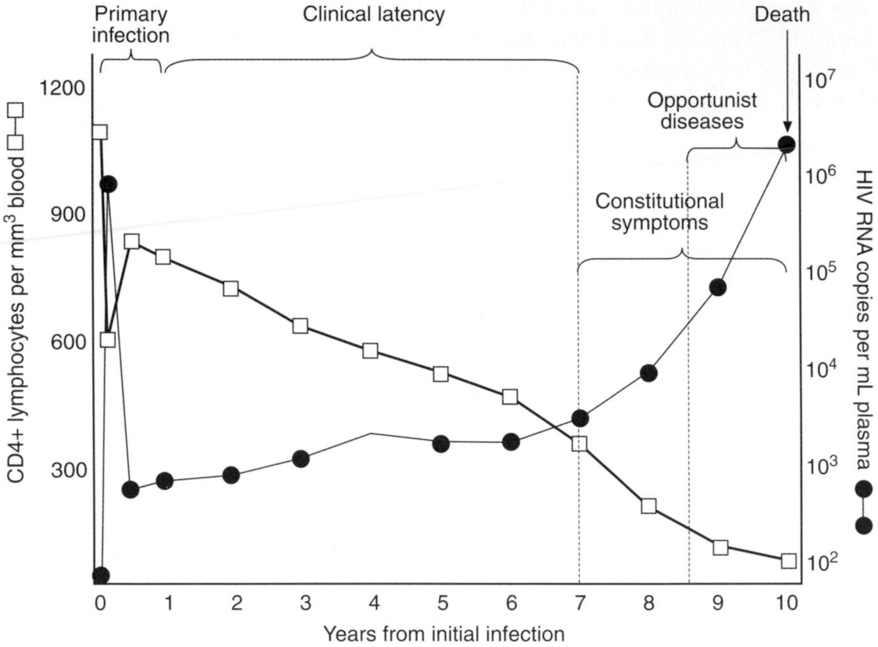

FIGURE 10.1 *The clinical course of HIV infection and disease in relation to the CD4+ lymphocyte count (□) and viral load (●).*

CLINICAL CONSEQUENCES OF HIV INFECTION

The stages of HIV disease are related to the CD4+ cell count, the plasma viral load and the clinical consequences of continuing viral replication causing progressive CD4+ cell destruction (see Fig. 10.1). There are three distinct stages: primary infection, clinical latency and symptomatic disease.

Primary infection

Primary infection refers to the first few months following initial infection. During this period, the viral load is high and the rate of CD4+ cell destruction is rapid, with a consequent fall in the level of these cells in peripheral blood. However, the immune system detects the infection, and vigorous ensuing immune responses slow down the rate of viral replication, in turn causing a decline in viral load. Towards the end of this period, infected individuals **seroconvert**, i.e. serological tests for HIV antibodies become positive. It is important to note that infected individuals will test negative for these antibodies until around 8–12 weeks following initial infection. Although seronegative, they are infected and infectious (especially since they have a high viral load during the first 2 months of infection).

Clinical latency

Following recovery from primary infection, the CD4+ cell count increases somewhat but it does not regain its pre-infection level of approximately 1000 cells per cubic millimetre (mm^3) of peripheral blood. Most infected people then enter a stage of clinical latency lasting several years, unless their underlying nutritional or health status is poor (which is common in the developing world), in which case they may more rapidly progress to end-stage disease. In the developed world, most people are relatively asymptomatic during this stage of clinical latency. Naturally, serological tests for HIV antibodies are positive at this stage and remain so for the remainder of the person's life. During this period, there is, however, unrelenting viral replication, a slowly rising plasma viral load and a corresponding progressive loss of CD4+ cells. When the CD4+ cell count falls below 350–200 cells/mm^3, infected individuals will develop symptomatic disease.

Symptomatic disease

Most infected people will experience ill-health as the CD4+ cell count falls below 350 cells/μL. A variety of diverse constitutional symptoms and signs characterize **early symptomatic disease**, including oropharyngeal candidiasis (thrush), diarrhoea, herpes zoster (shingles), night sweats and intermittent low-grade fevers. As the CD4+ cell count continues to fall and the plasma viral load continues to increase, patients succumb to a variety of serious opportunistic infections and cancers, including tuberculosis, recurrent bacterial pneumonia, pneumonia caused by the fungus *Pneumocystis carinii*, toxoplasmosis of the brain, a severe wasting syndrome and Kaposi's sarcoma. These (and many other conditions) are all AIDS-defining illnesses in HIV-infected people, and it is only during this stage of **late symptomatic disease** that a person is said to have AIDS.

Following initial infection, HIV replication never ceases and the resulting cellular pathology, e.g. continuing CD4+ cell destruction, causes a persistent, progressive and ultimately profound immunodeficiency. Although there is a period of clinical latency, there is never a period of cellular and microbiological latency. Consequently, the entire continuum from infection to late symptomatic disease and death is now generally referred to as **HIV disease**.

THE NATURE OF TUBERCULOSIS IN HIV-INFECTED INDIVIDUALS

The clinical, radiological and pathological characteristics of tuberculosis in those infected with HIV are greatly, but not entirely, dependent on the degree of immunosuppression, which, in turn, is related to the depletion of CD4+ lymphocytes and the viral load.[6] Tuberculosis may develop at any time after infection by HIV infection and often develops soon after infection and before other HIV-related opportunist infections and AIDS-defining conditions occur.

Pulmonary tuberculosis

In patients with relatively high CD4+ lymphocyte counts and a low viral load, the characteristics of tuberculosis are generally similar to those in people not infected with HIV. As immune responses become progressively compromised, as shown by a declining CD4+ cell count and a rising viral load, atypical forms of tuberculosis become relatively more common.[7,8] Being atypical, such cases are not easily diagnosed or readily distinguished from the various other opportunistic infections such as *Pneumocystis carinii* pneumonia, bacterial pneumonia, nocardiosis and fungal infections to which such patients are prone. Pulmonary tuberculosis in the more severely immunosuppressed patients is usually characterized on radiology by extensive and rapidly changing pulmonary infiltrates of non-specific appearance spreading into the lower lobes of the lung, pleural effusions, little or no cavity formation and enlargement of the mediastinal lymph glands.[8] In some cases, the radiological appearance is deceptively normal. Those with no cavity formation are often sputum smear negative and even techniques such as bronchoscopy with bronchoalveolar lavage and induction of sputum only permit a bacteriological diagnosis in about a third of patients. The differences in the clinical and radiological characteristics of post-primary pulmonary tuberculosis in non-immunosuppressed and immunosuppressed patients are summarized in Table 10.1.

TABLE 10.1 Comparison of the clinical and radiological characteristics of post-primary tuberculosis in non-immunosuppressed and immunosuppressed patients

Characteristic	Non-immunosuppressed	Immunosuppressed
Pulmonary cavitation	Very frequent	Limited or absent
Localization by fibrosis	Marked	Limited
Intrathoracic lymphadenopathy	Infrequent	Frequent
Pleural effusions	Infrequent	Very frequent
Miliary disease	Infrequent	Frequent
Atelectasis	Infrequent	Frequent
Lymphatic and haematogenous dissemination	Infrequent	Frequent
Adverse drug reactions	Infrequent	Frequent
Tuberculin test	Positive	Small reaction or negative
Relapse after therapy	Infrequent	Frequent
Death during therapy	Infrequent	Frequent

Studies in Africa have shown that, although atypical presentations are more common in the severely immunosuppressed, exceptions occur.[8,9] Thus, for unknown reasons, some patients with low CD+ cell counts have tuberculosis of 'classical' radiological appearance. Tuberculin reactivity is often diminished or absent in patients with HIV-related tuberculosis, particularly in the more severely immunosuppressed, especially in those with low CD4+ cell counts (less then 200 cells/mm^3).[3] However, tuberculin reactivity is not absolutely related to the CD4+ cell count, and exceptions to this principle are not uncommon.

Extrapulmonary tuberculosis

Patients with HIV-related tuberculosis are more likely to develop extrapulmonary manifestations of the disease such as widespread lymph node involvement, bone and skin lesions, pericarditis, meningitis and widely disseminated disease.[10,11] Lymph node enlargement due to tuberculosis is usually asymmetrical and in some cases lymph nodes may enlarge rapidly, suggesting an acute bacterial infection. These features distinguish tuberculous lymphadenopathy from the non-specific persistent generalized lymphadenopathy (PGL) that commonly develops in HIV-infected people.

Some patients with extrapulmonary tuberculosis have focal signs and symptoms, whereas others just have non-specific constitutional symptoms, such as fever, night sweats and weight loss, which also occur in other opportunistic infections. Weight loss may be severe. In Africa, the severe wasting associated with AIDS is termed 'slim disease' and, although in some cases it may be due to intestinal disease as many patients have chronic diarrhoea, around a half are found to have disseminated tuberculosis at autopsy.[12] As granuloma formation is suppressed, the characteristic millet seed-like lesions of miliary tuberculosis are uncommon in HIV-related disseminated tuberculosis. Instead, there are numerous minute lesions throughout many tissues and organs – a condition termed **cryptogenic disseminated tuberculosis** (see Chapter 9). This is not easily diagnosed, as chest radiographs often appear deceptively normal. Many cases are only diagnosed at autopsy, exposing the pathologist and technical staff to a serious risk of infection.

The tuberculin test is often negative, especially in those with cryptogenic disseminated tuberculosis.[13] If disseminated tuberculosis is suspected, blood should be cultured for mycobacteria (where facilities exist), as it is positive in a third to half of such patients.[14]

Tuberculosis in HIV-infected children

As described in Chapter 8, the diagnosis of tuberculosis in children is far from easy and it is even more difficult in those who are infected with HIV, even in countries with advanced diagnostic facilities.[15,16] Many of the features of the disease are common to other frequently encountered HIV-related opportunistic infections such as *Pneumocystis carinii* pneumonia. As a general rule, however, the clinical differences described above between tuberculosis in HIV-infected and non-infected adults are not so great in children.

Acid-fast bacilli are not usually seen in specimens (even when adequate ones can be obtained), radiological appearances are often non-specific and tuberculin tests are frequently negative. Even when the most sophisticated diagnostic facilities are available, the diagnosis can only be confirmed bacteriologically in about half the cases. Specimens suitable for bacteriological examination may be obtained from unusual sites. For example, cases of tuberculosis of the ear have been reported among HIV-infected children, and in some of these cases the diagnosis was made on examination of ear swabs.[17]

Children of all ages are affected and many are treated on clinical suspicion alone. Clearly, many children will receive inappropriate treatment, while others with vague and atypical symptoms will not receive treatment. There is an urgent need for improved diagnostic criteria.

Because of the difficulty of diagnosing tuberculosis in HIV-infected children, the exact incidence of this disease, relative to other infectious diseases, is uncertain. The reported percentage of such children with tuberculosis depends on the skill and experience of the clinician and the effort put into making the diagnosis.

TREATMENT OF TUBERCULOSIS IN HIV-INFECTED INDIVIDUALS

Treatment of tuberculosis in the HIV-infected person is identical in principle to that of the non-infected person. The bacteriological cure rates achieved by regimens and supervision according to World Health Organization (WHO) principles are very similar in the two groups of patients.[18] It is preferable to treat patients on a daily, rather than an intermittent, basis, as there is some evidence that antituberculosis drugs (notably rifampicin) are less well absorbed in HIV-infected patients.

Owing to their increased susceptibility to the development of disease after re-infection, those who are HIV infected are more likely to develop tuberculosis again, particularly in countries and communities where the risk of re-infection is high. In some localized epidemics of HIV-related tuberculosis, notably in the USA, a higher than expected incidence of drug and multidrug resistance has been encountered.[19] HIV infection itself does not generate drug resistance – this is due to other factors, notably the use of poor drug regimens and inadequate supervision of therapy. If resistance has developed, however, HIV facilitates its spread, as infected people are much more likely to develop tuberculosis after infection and the course of the disease is greatly accelerated. The risk is greatest in confined communities such as hospital wards and prisons, in which mini-epidemics have occurred. Fortunately, drug resistance is relatively uncommon in Africa, where most cases of HIV-related tuberculosis are currently encountered. Worrying, though, is the high incidence of drug resistance in parts of India, Eastern Europe, China and South-East Asia, where the spread of HIV infection is accelerating.

Patients who are infected with HIV are more likely to develop adverse reactions to the antituberculosis drugs. Dermal reactions to thiacetazone are particularly common, and fatal exfoliative dermatitis may develop.[20] For this reason, as well as because of its limited efficacy, thiacetazone should never be given to HIV-infected people. In addition, many patients will be on other drugs for the prevention and treatment of various HIV-related infections and, in some countries, patients will receive antiretroviral agents. This increases the risk of adverse drug reactions and interactions, which make it more likely that the patient will fail to complete therapy unless supported by caring and encouraging supervisors. Adverse drug reactions and interactions and their management are reviewed in Chapter 12.

THE GENERAL MANAGEMENT OF PATIENTS WITH HIV-RELATED TUBERCULOSIS

The management of these patients is much less straightforward than that of those who are not infected with HIV. The former, despite effective antituberculosis treatment, have a much higher risk of becoming ill and dying during or after therapy. As tuberculosis, as well as HIV infection, suppresses immune responses, illness and death due to other infections is common. In sub-Saharan African countries, around a third of HIV-infected smear-positive tuberculosis patients die within a year of starting antituberculosis therapy, and a quarter of the survivors die during the following year.[21] Those who are smear negative have an even worse outlook, due to a combination of diagnostic delays and more severe immunosuppression. Despite these grim figures, the treatment of HIV-related tuberculosis prolongs survival by, on average, 2 years,[7] and sometimes by up to 7 years, and is therefore highly worthwhile. In countries where highly active antiretroviral therapy (HAART) is provided, the risk of other opportunistic infections is reduced and survival time is increased.[22]

As mentioned above, HIV-infected patients with tuberculosis are more likely to develop adverse drug reactions and interactions than those who are not infected with HIV. Also, owing to the stigmatizing nature of the diagnosis, and the fatalistic attitude this may induce in some regions, HIV-infected patients are less likely to complete their course of treatment than those who are not infected with HIV.

The increased risk of patients acquiring other opportunist infections requiring therapy by antibiotics and antifungal agents adds to the complexity and cost of treatment and the time that needs to be devoted to each patient.

There are many barriers to the effective management of tuberculosis, and these are often accentuated where HIV-related tuberculosis is common.[23] Many social, cultural, educational, gender-related and economic issues have a negative impact on access to the diagnosis and subsequent care that are essential to prevent needless suffering and death. In many African countries, the increase in the number of patients in the wake of the HIV pandemic has not been matched by a strengthening of the resources for the care of these patients. As a consequence, severe organizational problems for the supervision of therapy in the community are encountered. Also, many patients are too ill to be treated in their homes and, as a result, hospitals are becoming overcrowded. Not only does this make it increasingly difficult to maintain high standards of nursing care, it also increases the risk of transmission of various infections from patient to patient. In many sub-Saharan African countries, the large increase in the number of patients with tuberculosis due to the HIV/AIDS pandemic threatens to overwhelm National Tuberculosis Control Programmes.

The inability to provide adequate standards of care, together with the resulting suffering and high mortality, understandably has an unsettling effect on the morale and motivation of healthcare providers. (In this context, the institution of effective antiretroviral therapy has a very positive effect on staff morale, as they see their patients living rather than dying.) The health of the staff of clinics and hospitals is also a key factor in the provision of effective services. In this context, the healthcare providers usually have the same incidence of HIV infection as the general population, which, in some African cities, may exceed 30 per cent. The resulting time off work due to illness and eventual death is having a negative effect on health services, including tuberculosis control services. The establishment of adequate healthcare facilities, as well as the provision of effective antiretroviral agents to rectify the underlying immune defect, at no cost to the patients, is a critical strategic goal in most countries throughout the world.

Summary

By greatly enhancing the risk of infection by the tubercle bacillus progressing to active disease, and by accelerating the progression, infection by HIV has had a very serious impact on the global prevalence of tuberculosis. In the year 2003, HIV was responsible for 1 million additional cases of tuberculosis, and 12 per cent of all cases were HIV related. Also, tuberculosis was the cause of 30 per cent of the estimated 3 million deaths due to AIDS. The combination of tuberculosis and HIV infection has therefore justly been termed 'a deadly partnership' and 'the cursed duet'. Africa is particularly affected at present but, unless control measures for both HIV infection and tuberculosis are greatly enhanced, an even more devastating situation could develop in Asian countries. Owing to the increase in the prevalence of tuberculosis caused by HIV infection, healthcare provision requires strengthening, but, in practice, this rarely happens. HIV-related tuberculosis is therefore a serious challenge to the conscience of humanity.

Prologue to the next chapter

Not only has the HIV/AIDS pandemic led to a substantial increase in the prevalence of tuberculosis, it has also, by compromising protective immunity, led to an increase in the prevalence of serious disease due to certain species of mycobacteria that normally live harmlessly in the environment. Disease caused by these mycobacteria, the so-called environmental mycobacteria, is also associated with other forms of immunosuppression, underlying chronic lung disease and penetrating skin injuries, but some cases occur in people with no apparent underlying condition. In the next chapter, this increasingly important group of mycobacteria and the varied range of lesions and infections – from localized abscesses to potentially fatal widespread dissemination – that they cause are described.

REFERENCES

1. Sonnenberg P, Murray J, Glynn JR et al. HIV-1 and recurrence, relapse, and reinfection of tuberculosis after cure: a cohort study in South African mine workers. *Lancet* 2001; **358**: 1687–93.
2. Cruciani M, Malena M, Bosco O et al. The impact of human immunodeficiency virus type 1 on infectiousness of tuberculosis: a meta-analysis. *Clin Infect Dis* 2001; **33**: 1922–30.
3. Ahmed Y, Mwaba P, Chintu C et al. A study of maternal mortality at the University Teaching Hospital, Lusaka, Zambia: the emergence of tuberculosis as a major non-obstetric cause of maternal death. *Int J Tuberc Lung Dis* 1999; **3**: 675–80.
4. World Health Organization. *Global tuberculosis control*. WHO/CDS/2001.287. Geneva: World Health Organization, 2001.
5. Pratt RJ. *HIV & AIDS: a foundation for nursing and healthcare practice*, 5th edn. London: Arnold, 2003.
6. Bocchino M, Sanduzzi A, Bariffi F. *Mycobacterium tuberculosis* and HIV co-infection in the lung: synergic immune dysregulation leading to disease progression. *Monaldi Arch Chest Dis* 2000; **55**: 381–8.
7. Harries AD, Maher D. *TB/HIV: a clinical manual*. WHO/TB/96.200. Geneva: World Health Organization, 1996.
8. Tshibwabwa-Tumba E, Mwinga A, Pobee JOM, Zumla A. Radiological features of pulmonary tuberculosis in 963 HIV-infected adults in three Central African hospitals. *Clin Radiol* 1997; **52**: 837–41.
9. Saks AM, Posner R. Tuberculosis in HIV positive patients in South Africa: a comparative radiological study with HIV negative patients. *Clin Radiol* 1992; **46**: 387–90.
10. Nambuya A, Sewankambo N, Mugerwa J et al. Tuberculous lymphadenitis associated with human immunodeficiency virus infection in Uganda. *J Clin Pathol* 1988; **41**: 93–6.
11. Gilks CF, Brindle RJ, Otieno LS et al. Extrapulmonary and disseminated tuberculosis in HIV-1-seropositive patients presenting to the acute medical services in Nairobi. *AIDS* 1990; **4**: 981–5.
12. Lucas SB, de Cock KM, Hounnou A et al. Slim disease in Africa: the contribution of tuberculosis. *BMJ* 1994; **308**: 1531–3.
13. Diagbouga S, Fumoux F, Ledru E et al. Lack of direct correlation between CD4+ lymphocyte counts and induration sizes of the tuberculin skin test in human

immunodeficiency virus type 1 seropositive patients. *Int J Tuberc Lung Dis* 1998; **2**: 317–23.
14. Schaefer R, Goldberg R, Sierra M, Glatt AE. Frequency of *Mycobacterium tuberculosis* bacteremia in patients with tuberculosis in an area endemic for AIDS. *Am Rev Respir Dis* 1989; **140**: 1611–13.
15. Chintu C, Luo C, Bhat G et al. Impact of the human immunodeficiency virus type-1 on common paediatric illnesses in Zambia. *J Trop Pediatr* 1995; **41**: 348–53.
16. Donald PR, Fourie B, Grange JM (eds). *Tuberculosis in childhood.* Pretoria: JL van Schaik, 1995.
17. Schaaf HS, Geldenduys A, Gie RP, Cotton MF. Culture-positive tuberculosis in human immunodeficiency virus type 1-infected children. *Pediatr Infect Dis J* 1998; **17**: 599–604.
18. Jones BE, Otaya M, Antoniskis D et al. A prospective evaluation of antituberculosis therapy in patients with human immunodeficiency virus infection. *Am J Respir Crit Care Med* 1994; **150**: 1499–502.
19. Frieden TR, Sterling T, Pablos-Mendez A et al. The emergence of drug resistant tuberculosis in New York City. *N Engl J Med* 1993; **328**: 521–6.
20. Nunn P, Kibuga D, Gathua S et al. Cutaneous hypersensitivity reactions due to thiacetazone in HIV-1 seropositive patients treated for tuberculosis. *Lancet* 1991; **337**: 627–30.
21. Cantwell MF, Binkin NJ. Impact of HIV on tuberculosis in sub-Saharan Africa: a regional perspective. *Int J Tuberc Lung Dis* 1997; **1**: 205–14.
22. Hung CC, Chen MY, Hsiao CF et al. Improved outcomes of HIV-1-infected adults with tuberculosis in the era of highly active antiretroviral therapy. *AIDS* 2003; **17**: 2615–22.
23. World Health Organization. *Tuberculosis in the era of HIV. A deadly partnership.* Geneva: World Health Organization, 1996.

FURTHER READING

Blinkhoff P, Bukanga E, Syamalevwe B, Williams G. *Under the Mupundu tree. Volunteers in home care for people with HIV/AIDS and TB in Zambia's copperbelt.* Strategies for Hope Series, No. 14. London: Actionaid, 1999.

Harries AD. The association between HIV and tuberculosis in the developing world with a special focus on sub-Saharan Africa. In Davies PDO (ed.), *Clinical tuberculosis*, 3rd edn. London: Arnold, 2003, 253–77.

Harries AD, Maher D. *TB/HIV: a clinical manual.* WHO/TB/96.200. Geneva: World Health Organization, 1996.

Pozniak A. The association between HIV and tuberculosis in industrialized countries. In Davies PDO (ed.), *Clinical tuberculosis*, 3rd edn. London: Arnold, 2003, 278–93.

Pratt RJ. *HIV & AIDS: a foundation for nursing and healthcare practice*, 5th edn. London: Arnold, 2003.

Ustianowski A, Mwaba P, Zumla A. Tuberculosis and HIV – perspectives from sub-Saharan Africa. In Porter JDH, Grange JM (eds), *Tuberculosis – an interdisciplinary perspective.* London: Imperial College Press, 1999, 283–311.

Zumla A, Grange JM. Tuberculosis and co-infection with the human immunodeficiency virus. In Madkour M (ed.), *Tuberculosis.* Berlin: Springer, 2003, 455–81.

Zumla A, Malon P, Henderson J, Grange JM. The impact of the human immunodeficiency virus (HIV) infection epidemic on tuberculosis. *Postgrad Med J* 2000; **76**: 259–68.

CHAPTER 11

Human disease due to the environmental mycobacteria

Introduction

As discussed in Chapter 2, the principal mycobacterial diseases are tuberculosis and leprosy, but, much less frequently, disease is caused by species of mycobacteria that normally exist freely in the environment and are therefore called environmental mycobacteria (EM). They are also called opportunist mycobacteria and, particularly in the USA, non-tuberculous mycobacteria.

Learning outcomes

After studying and reflecting on the material in this chapter, you will be able to:

- compare and contrast the epidemiology of tuberculosis and leprosy and the diseases caused by EM,
- describe the wide range of diseases due to EM and the characteristics of the patients in which they occur,
- identify the key role of the microbiology laboratory in the diagnosis of these diseases and the importance of collecting suitable specimens and of distinguishing between disease and contamination,
- discuss the particular association of one group of EM (the *Mycobacterium avium* complex) with the acquired immunodeficiency syndrome (AIDS).

Unless infection occurs as a result of penetrating injuries, disease due to environmental mycobacteria (EM) is usually, though not invariably, associated with some form of immunosuppression or, in the case of the lung, with some underlying disease process. Careful investigation of patients who appear immunologically normal may reveal minor immune defects.[1] In recent years, the number of cases of human disease due to EM has increased because of the higher number of people with various severe forms of immunosuppression, including human immunodeficiency virus (HIV) infection and AIDS, renal failure and that caused by post-transplant immunosuppressive therapy. In addition, the distribution of these mycobacteria in the environment is not constant, their number and species being affected by various changing ecological factors, and this is reflected in the patterns of disease and its causative organisms in given regions.[2]

The diagnosis depends critically on the isolation of EM and their identification, which are usually undertaken in specialist reference laboratories. These processes may be accomplished by means of a set of simple tests such as rate and temperature range of growth, pigment production in the light and dark, detection of enzyme activities and susceptibility to antibacterial agents. More sophisticated techniques include analysis of the lipid composition of the bacterial cell walls and detection of specific deoxyribonucleic acid (DNA) or ribonucleic acid (RNA) sequences in the chromosomes of the bacteria. The principal species involved in human disease are described in Chapter 2 (see Table 2.3).

Diseases due to the EM can be placed in five groups:

- pulmonary disease
- lymphadenopathy
- skin lesions
- localized extrapulmonary lesions
- disseminated disease.

The principal manifestations of disease in these five groups and the causative species are summarized in Table 11.1.

TABLE 11.1 The principal manifestations of disease due to environmental mycobacteria

Site	Disease	Causative species
Pulmonary	Non-specific disease resembling tuberculosis (including 'Lady Windermere syndrome' and 'hot tub lung')	Many species
Lymph nodes	Cervical in children aged 5 years or under; localized or widespread in immunocompromised patients	Many species
Skin	Buruli ulcer	*M. ulcerans*
	Swimming pool granuloma	*M. marinum*
	Chronic lesions resembling lupus vulgaris	*M. kansasii*, *M. haemophilum*, occasionally others
	Post-traumatic or post-injection abscesses	*M. abscessus*, *M. chelonae*, *M. fortuitum*, rarely *M. terrae*
Localized extrapulmonary lesions	Non-specific disease resembling tuberculosis	Many species
Disseminated disease	HIV related	*M. avium* complex, occasionally *M. genevense*
	Non-HIV related	Many species

PULMONARY DISEASE

Many species of EM cause pulmonary disease which, in its clinical and radiological features, is very similar to pulmonary tuberculosis.[3] Most cases of pulmonary disease due to EM occur in middle-aged and elderly men with a history of lung disease, especially industrial dust disease, chronic bronchitis, bronchiectasis, rheumatoid lung and cancer. Pulmonary disease due to EM has emerged as a serious problem among gold miners in South Africa, a problem exacerbated by the growing incidence of HIV infection in these workers.[4] HIV-infected patients are susceptible to cavitating and non-cavitating lung disease due to EM, notably members of the *M. avium* complex (MAC). Lung disease due to EM is also a recognized complicating condition in children and young adults with cystic fibrosis.[5]

A minority of cases of lung disease due to EM occur in people (mostly women) who are otherwise apparently healthy. It has been suggested that such disease in women is associated with suppressed clearance of sputum due to the tendency for polite and genteel ladies to cough very softly and quietly. For this reason, the disease in women has been called the **Lady Windermere syndrome**, after the fastidious aristocrat in Oscar Wilde's play *Lady Windermere's fan*.[6] A strange and unexplained association between the disease and bathing in hot tubs has also been observed and this condition has been termed **hot tub lung**.[7]

As EM are common in the environment, they are often present in the upper respiratory tract as contaminants and they may colonize lung tissue damaged by other disease processes. Isolation of these EM from sputum may therefore cause diagnostic confusion, as it is not easy to distinguish between these and organisms causing disease. Guidelines for diagnosis have been published by the American and British Thoracic Societies.[8,9] In general, repeated isolation of EM from sputum samples with many colonies on the culture medium is strongly suggestive of disease in a patient with appropriate clinical and radiological signs. Exceptions occur, and it is sometimes necessary to use a bronchoscope to obtain washings, brushings or biopsies from lesions seen on chest X-rays or computerized tomography (CT) scans.[10] Assessment of the significance of EM is especially problematical in HIV-infected individuals.[11]

In some cases, false diagnosis of pulmonary disease due to EM has been traced to the collection of sputum into unsterile containers (see Chapter 7). In other cases, false diagnosis has been traced to inadequate cleaning and sterilization of bronchoscopes.

LYMPHADENOPATHY

Lymphadenitis due to EM is a well-recognized disease of children. Cases rarely occur in the first year of life, most being seen in the second year, after which the incidence declines and the condition is rarely seen in children over the age of 5 years. In other respects the affected children appear healthy, but one study suggests that they may have minor defects in their cell-mediated immune responses.[12] The disease usually affects lymph nodes in the upper part of the neck and the pre-auricular nodes (those in front of the ear). These are the nodes that drain the pharynx and tonsils, suggesting infection from the environment by the oral route. Various species of EM have been isolated. Lymphadenitis due to EM in adolescents and adults is usually associated with clear causes of immunodeficiency such as HIV infection.

SKIN LESIONS

There are two named mycobacterial skin diseases, **Buruli ulcer** and **swimming pool granuloma** (also called fish tank granuloma and, in a few publications, fish fancier's finger), which are caused, respectively, by *M. ulcerans* and *M. marinum*. There are also various non-specific skin infections usually associated with trauma and caused by a range of species.

Buruli ulcer is a very unpleasant disease, characterized by massive necrosis of the skin and underlying fat leading to enormous ulcers which are deeply undermined. Uniquely for a mycobacterial disease, a bacterial toxin is responsible, at least in part, for the extensive necrosis. Although the disease may resolve spontaneously after several months or years, with healing of the ulcers, extensive scarring often causes severe disfigurement and crippling deformities. The causative organism, *M. ulcerans*, lives in the environment and is thought to be introduced into the skin through minor injuries, principally caused by spiky or thorny vegetation. The disease occurs in certain regions, usually low-lying marshy ones, in Africa, Asia, South America and Australia. In the last few years, the prevalence of Buruli ulcer has increased greatly in some parts of West Africa, where it has become a major public health problem. The World Health Organization (WHO) has published an extensive and well-illustrated review of this disease.[13]

As suggested by the name swimming pool (or fish tank) granuloma, *M. marinum* infects minor skin lesions acquired while swimming in pools and cleaning aquaria.[14] The lesions, which usually occur on the knees and elbows of swimmers and the fingers of aquarium handlers, resemble the lesions of chronic skin tuberculosis (lupus vulgaris, see Chapter 9). Secondary lesions sometimes develop along the superficial lymphatics draining the affected part. This is called **sporotrichoid spread**, as it is a characteristic feature of the fungal infection sporotrichosis. Similar skin lesions are very occasionally caused by *M. kansasii*, *M. malmoense* and *M. haemophilum*, the last mentioned usually in immunocompromised patients.

Other forms of post-inoculation disease due to EM occasionally occur.[15] Abscesses, either as single cases or in small outbreaks, have followed the injection of vaccines or other materials contaminated by the rapidly growing species *M. abscessus*, *M. chelonae* and *M. fortuitum*. The same species have caused serious postoperative wound infection, especially following the insertion of contaminated artificial heart valves, peritonitis in patients with renal failure receiving peritoneal dialysis, and corneal infection (keratitis) in wearers of contact lenses. *M. terrae*, as suggested by the name, is found in soil and is a rare cause of wound infection after skin-penetrating injuries acquired while farming or gardening.

LOCALIZED EXTRAPULMONARY LESIONS

These are similar to those seen in tuberculosis, but are very uncommon. Involvement of the bone, kidney, central nervous system and, extremely rarely, other organs has been described.

DISSEMINATED DISEASE

Disseminated disease due to MAC has been a common AIDS-related illness in the industrially developed nations, but, for unknown reasons, it is much less frequently seen in Africa.[16] The introduction of **highly active antiretroviral therapy** (HAART) has reduced this opportunist disease considerably in those nations that can afford such therapy.[17] Prophylactic therapy against other HIV-associated infections such as toxoplasmosis also reduces the risk of developing disseminated MAC disease.[18] The disease affects many organs and massive infiltration of the intestine may occur, leading to malabsorption of nutrients and debilitating diarrhoea. The diagnosis is made by isolating MAC from blood, bone marrow, faeces or organ biopsies. Other EM such as *M. genevense* also cause disseminated AIDS-related disease, but, for unknown reasons, MAC are by far the most common cause.

Disseminated disease due to EM is also seen in patients with other causes of immunosuppression, notably those with renal failure and transplant recipients receiving immunosuppressive therapy. In contrast to such disease in those with HIV-related immunosuppression, a range of species of EM is involved, including the rapidly growing species *M. abscessus*, *M. chelonae* and *M. fortuitum*. Families in which children suffer immune defects rendering them very susceptible to disseminated disease due to EM as well as Bacille Calmette–Guérin (BCG) following vaccination (but not apparently to tuberculosis) have been described and pose serious management problems.[19]

Summary

There is a large range of presentations of human disease caused by various species of EM. Some have features resembling tuberculosis or pyogenic infections, but two species, *M. marinum* and *M. ulcerans*, cause recognizable and named conditions. Disease due to EM is often associated with various forms of immunosuppression, notably that caused by HIV infection, and mild forms of immune defects have been described in some patients who, apart from their EM disease, appear healthy on initial examination. Diagnosis is not easy, as, in most cases, bacteriological investigations are essential and, particularly in the case of the lung, genuine disease must be distinguished from colonization or contamination by EM. Although uncommon relative to tuberculosis, especially in developing countries, these diseases are an increasing cause of diagnostic and therapeutic problems in many fields of clinical medicine.

Prologue to the next chapter

Having described tuberculosis in the previous chapters, and disease due to EM in this one, it is now necessary to consider the most fundamental aspect of disease control – namely, therapy. It will become apparent that an understanding of the principles of therapy requires an appreciation of the characteristics of the diseases as well as the nature of the causative bacteria. It will also become apparent that the skill and sensitivity with which therapy is given make an enormous difference to whether the patients complete their therapy and are thereby cured. An understanding of the principles and practice of therapy should therefore be of prime interest and concern to nurses and other healthcare workers.

REFERENCES

1. Greinert U, Schlaak M, Rüsch-Gerdes S et al. Low in vitro production of interferon-γ and tumour necrosis factor-α in HIV-seronegative patients with pulmonary disease caused by non-tuberculous mycobacteria. *J Clin Immunol* 2000; **20**: 445–52.
2. Falkinham JO. The changing pattern of nontuberculous mycobacterial disease. *Can J Infect Dis* 2003; **14**: 281–6.
3. Kourbeti IS, Maslow MJ. Nontuberculous mycobacterial infections of the lung. *Curr Infect Dis Rep* 2000, **2**: 193–200.
4. Sonnenberg P, Murray J, Glynn TR et al. Risk factors for pulmonary disease due to culture-positive *M. tuberculosis* or nontuberculous mycobacteria in South African gold miners. *Eur Respir J* 2000; **15**: 291–6.
5. Oliver A, Maiz L, Canton R et al. Nontuberculous mycobacteria in patients with cystic fibrosis. *Clin Infect Dis* 2001; **32**: 1298–303.

6. Reich JM, Johnson RE. *Mycobacterium avium* complex pulmonary disease presenting as an isolated lingular or middle lobe pattern. The Lady Windermere syndrome. *Chest* 1992, **101**: 1605–9.
7. Khoor A, Leslie KO, Tazelaar HD et al. Diffuse pulmonary disease caused by nontuberculous mycobacteria in immunocompetent people (hot tub lung). *Am J Clin Pathol* 2001; **115**: 755–62.
8. American Thoracic Society Official Statement. Diagnosis and treatment of disease caused by non-tuberculous mycobacteria. *Am J Respir Crit Care Med* 1997; **156**(Suppl.): S1–25.
9. Subcommittee of the Joint Tuberculosis Committee of the British Thoracic Society. Management of opportunist mycobacterial infections: Joint Tuberculosis Committee guidelines 1999. *Thorax* 2000; **55**: 210–18.
10. Ikedo Y. The significance of bronchoscopy for the diagnosis of *Mycobacterium avium* complex (MAC) pulmonary disease. *Kurume Med J* 2001; **48**: 15–19.
11. Raju B, Schluger NW. Significance of respiratory isolates of *Mycobacterium avium* complex in HIV-positive and HIV-negative patients. *Int J Infect Dis* 2000, **4**: 134–9.
12. Nylen O, Berg-Kelly K, Andersson B. Cervical lymph node infections with non-tuberculous mycobacteria in preschool children: interferon gamma deficiency as a possible cause of clinical infection. *Acta Paediatr* 2000; **89**: 1322–5.
13. Asiedu K, Scherpbier R. Raviglione M. *Buruli ulcer. Mycobacterium ulcerans* infection. WHO/CDS/CPE/GBU/2000.1. Geneva: World Health Organization Global Buruli Ulcer Initiative, 2000.
14. Collins CH, Grange JM, Noble WC, Yates MD. *Mycobacterium marinum* infections in man. *J Hygiene* 1985; **94**: 135–49.
15. Grange JM, Noble WC, Yates MD, Collins CH. Inoculation mycobacterioses. *Clin Exp Dermatol* 1988; **13**: 211–20.
16. Morrissey AB, Aisu TO, Falkinham JO et al. Absence of *Mycobacterium avium* complex disease in patients with AIDS in Uganda. *J Acquir Immune Defic Syndr* 1992; **5**: 477–8.
17. Havlir DV, Schrier RD, Torriani FJ et al. Effect of potent antiretroviral therapy on immune responses to *Mycobacterium avium* in human immunodeficiency virus-infected subjects. *J Infect Dis* 2000; **182**: 1658–63.
18. Arasteh KN, Cordes C, Ewers M et al. HIV-related nontuberculous mycobacterial infection: incidence, survival analysis and associated risk factors. *Eur J Med Res* 2000; **5**: 424–30.
19. Remus N, Reichenbach J, Picard C et al. Impaired interferon gamma-mediated immunity and susceptibility to mycobacterial infection in childhood. *Pediatr Res* 2001, **50**: 8–13.

FURTHER READING

Banks J, Campbell IA. Environmental mycobacteria. In Davies PDO (ed.), *Clinical tuberculosis*, 3rd edn. London: Arnold, 2003, 439–48.

Grange JM. *Mycobacteria and human disease*, 2nd edn. London: Arnold, 1996.

Wansbrough-Jones MH, Banerjee D. Non-tuberculous or atypical mycobacteria. In James DG, Zumla A (eds), *The granulomatous disorders*. Cambridge: Cambridge University Press, 1999, 189–204.

CHAPTER 12

The treatment of tuberculosis and other mycobacterial diseases

Introduction

Tuberculosis is a treatable disease. Modern therapeutic regimens are a brilliant example of 'evidence-based medicine', as they have been fine-tuned by the most extensive clinical investigations ever undertaken into any infectious disease. Investment in the treatment of tuberculosis is one of the most effective and cost-effective ways of securing years of healthy human life. In theory, the modern drug regimens advocated by the World Health Organization (WHO) are very straightforward to understand and administer. In practice, there are many barriers and obstacles in the way of treating and curing patients with tuberculosis, and this accounts for the fact that, worldwide, this disease remains one of the most prevalent preventable causes of death.

Learning outcomes

After studying and reflecting on the material in this chapter, you will be able to:

- outline the evolution of modern short-course therapy for tuberculosis,
- describe the drug regimens advocated by the WHO and discuss the importance of using these simple regimens, and no others,
- identify the principal characteristics of the drugs used in these regimens and describe how they act on the tubercle bacilli in various different physiological states,
- discuss how drug resistance arises and the need for the use of several drugs given together to prevent its emergence,
- outline the therapy of tuberculosis in special situations, such as in pregnant women and in patients with renal or hepatic failure,
- describe the management of drug-resistant and multidrug-resistant tuberculosis, and the serious challenges this poses to disease control,
- list the common adverse drug reactions and interactions and their clinical management,

- discuss how antituberculosis drugs may be used in the prevention of disease in infected people and the merits and problems of such preventive therapy,
- describe the principles of therapy of other mycobacterial diseases and how this resembles and differs from the treatment of tuberculosis.

Throughout the thousands of years during which humankind has suffered from tuberculosis, numerous remedies have been developed. Many, such as purgation and bleeding, were harmful while others, such as a mixture of pigeon's dung and weasel's blood prescribed by John of Gaddesden (1280–1361), were quite disgusting. Sir William Buchan (1729–1805) was almost certainly right in claiming, in his book *The domestic medicine*, first published exactly a century before Robert Koch's discovery of the tubercle bacillus, that none of the numerous remedies then available was more effective than a trip to the Bahamas for the few who could afford it and a glass of milk for the majority who could not.

An exception was the use of cod liver oil, the introduction of which into clinical use around the year 1770 is attributed to Thomas Percival (1740–1804), a physician also known for his work on medical ethics and jurisprudence and the promotion of health care for the poor. This therapy certainly appeared to help in some cases, probably due to its high vitamin D content – a vitamin that is, as explained in Chapter 5, essential for the activation of key immune defence mechanisms. The early records of the Brompton Hospital, London (now the Royal Brompton Hospital, a greatly respected hospital for the treatment of heart and lung disease), showed that cod liver oil was the most widely prescribed remedy. Subsequently, a combination of vitamin D and ultraviolet light was found to be effective in the treatment of skin tuberculosis which, untreated, sometimes caused mutilating deformities of the face.

Surgical treatment also had its vogue in the pre-antibiotic era. The first such operation was that of **artificial pneumothorax**, first used in 1882, the year in which Robert Koch discovered the tubercle bacillus.[1] The rationale of this procedure was that artificial introduction of air into the pleural cavity collapsed the lung, thereby causing closure of the tuberculous cavities and healing by fibrosis. When collapse of the lung was prevented by pleural adhesions, these were divided by electrodiathermy through a cannula – an early example of 'key-hole surgery'. If pulmonary collapse could not be achieved by these relatively simple procedures, surgeons undertook massive operations, known as **thoracoplasties**, involving removal of most of the chest wall on the affected side. Resolution of tuberculosis was reported in some cases, but at the great cost of severe pain, marked deformity and a high incidence of postoperative complications and mortality.

A more rational and gentler approach to the treatment of tuberculosis, but alas one that did not meet with success at the time, was the stimulation of the immune system to combat the disease – an approach known as **immunotherapy**. In 1891, Robert Koch attempted to treat tuberculosis with Old Tuberculin, a concentrated culture filtrate of the medium in which tubercle bacilli had been cultivated. Although a few patients (notably some with skin and laryngeal tuberculosis) responded dramatically, very variable and generally unimpressive therapeutic effects were noted in those with pulmonary lesions, and some patients died of allergic reactions termed 'tuberculin shock'. Other researchers, notably Sir Almroth Wright (rather unkindly nicknamed Sir Almost Right) of St Mary's Hospital, London, also made strenuous but unsuccessful efforts to develop immunotherapy for tuberculosis and Wright's efforts are immortalized in George Bernard Shaw's play *The doctor's dilemma*, in which he is portrayed as Sir Colenso Ridgeon. With the rise in the prevalence of multidrug-resistant tuberculosis, interest is once again turning to immunotherapy and preliminary clinical trials with novel agents have given encouraging results.[2]

The major breakthrough in the search for an effective treatment for tuberculosis came in 1944 when a team led by the Russian microbiologist Selman Waksman, then living in the USA, discovered streptomycin.[3] Clinical trials established that this antibiotic was indeed effective in the treatment of tuberculosis, but they soon also showed that some patients, after an initial good response, underwent relapse of their disease and failed to respond to re-treatment. Studies by the British Medical Research Council led by Sir John Crofton established that these relapses were due to strains of the tubercle bacillus that had mutated to resistance to streptomycin.[3] Fortunately, other potent agents active against tuberculosis, notably isoniazid and *para*-aminosalicylic acid (PAS), were soon discovered. Crofton's research team found that if all three drugs were given, resolution of the disease without relapse due to drug-resistant mutants occurred.

Multiple therapy is essential because resistance to antituberculosis agents occurs at a very low yet constant rate (perhaps 1 in 10 million cell divisions of the tubercle bacillus), even when the drug is not given. If a drug (we could call it drug A) is given, almost all tubercle bacilli will be killed, but a few mutants resistant to drug A will replicate and replace the original population. If drug B is then given, the similar selection occurs but the patient now has recurrent tuberculosis resistant to both drugs A and B (Fig. 12.1). Prescription of drug C will then induce resistance to drugs A, B and C, and so on. The chance of mutations to all three drugs occurring simultaneously in a single bacterium would, however, be 10 million times 10 million times 10 million. Put another way, only one such triple mutation would be found in a mass of tubercle bacilli weighing around 1000 tons! Accordingly, if drugs A, B and C are all given together, assuming that the patient takes his or her medication regularly, the chance that drug resistance will develop is exceedingly remote. Unfortunately, as we shall see in the following chapter, there are many ways in which defects in management allow drug and multidrug resistance to arise.

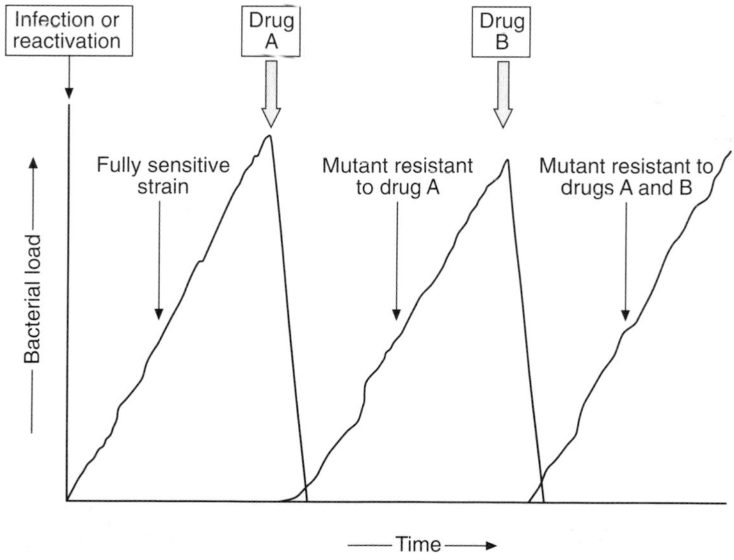

FIGURE 12.1 *The result of treating tuberculosis with single drugs. When drug A is given, almost all tubercle bacilli are killed, but a few mutants resistant to drug A will replicate and replace the original population. If drug B is then given, mutants resistant to drug B as well as to drug A will likewise replicate and replace the previous population.*

The mainstay of therapy between around 1950 and 1970 was streptomycin, isoniazid and PAS. Streptomycin was given by intramuscular injection for the first 3 months of treatment and the other two were given orally for a total of 18–24 months. This therapy was burdensome and distressing for the patient, particularly as the large amounts of PAS required had to be taken in divided daily doses and often caused severe gastrointestinal upsets. Patients therefore often failed to adhere to their treatment regimens and relapse of disease was common.

MODERN SHORT-COURSE ANTITUBERCULOSIS THERAPY

The next major breakthrough in the therapy of tuberculosis came in the late 1960s with the discovery of rifampicin, or rifampin as it is known in the USA. This drug made it possible to develop orally administered regimens lasting the much shorter time of 6 months. Although 6 months' therapy is very long compared with courses of antibiotics for many acute infections, it is considerably shorter than the former 18–24 months and is therefore called **short-course therapy**. As a result of many detailed clinical trials, again mostly by the British Medical Research Council, the highly effective rifampicin-based regimens in use today were developed.[4,5]

The antituberculosis drugs

Drugs active against tuberculosis are usually called antituberculosis agents, although in some publications, such as the *British National Formulary* (available online at <www.BNF.org>), they are termed antituberculous agents.

These agents are either antibiotics (naturally occurring antimicrobial agents produced by various bacteria or fungi, or semi-synthetic derivatives of these agents) or chemicals synthesized in the laboratory. Some antituberculosis drugs have a wide spectrum of antibacterial activity, whereas others are only active against mycobacteria, or even just against the *Mycobacterium tuberculosis* complex. They are also divisible into the first-line drugs that are used in the standard modern short-course regimens described below and the second-line drugs used for treating drug-resistant tuberculosis or cases in which adverse drug reactions prevent the use of one or more of the first-line drugs.

Modern short-course antituberculosis drug regimens

The first-line antituberculosis drugs, i.e. those used in the standard modern short-course regimens, include rifampicin, isoniazid, pyrazinamide, ethambutol and streptomycin.

The WHO has divided cases of tuberculosis into four treatment categories,[6] with regimens suitable for each category, as shown in Table 12.1. The regimens for the first three categories of patient consist of intensive phases lasting for 2 months, followed by continuation phases lasting 4 or 6 months. In order to understand the rationale for the two-phase therapy regimen, and the drugs used in each phase, it is necessary to consider the dynamics of the destruction of tubercle bacilli in the lesions of human tuberculosis.

The dynamics of antituberculosis therapy

The aim of antituberculosis therapy is not just to cure the patients but also to render them non-infectious as quickly as possible and to prevent relapse of the disease. Modern short-

TABLE 12.1 The WHO-recommended short-course antituberculosis drug regimens in four categories of patients

Treatment category	Definition	Initial intensive phase[a] (daily or, in some regimens, three times each week)	Continuation phase[a]
I	New smear-positive pulmonary disease; new smear-negative pulmonary tuberculosis with extensive lung involvement; new severe forms of extrapulmonary disease	2 EHRZ (SHRZ) 2 EHRZ (SHRZ) 2 EHRZ (SHRZ)	4 HR 4 H_3R_3 6 HE
II	Smear-positive pulmonary disease: relapse, treatment failure or treatment after interruption	2 SHRZE/1 HRZE 2 SHRZE/1 HRZE	5 HRE 5 $H_3R_3E_3$
III	New smear-negative pulmonary disease (other than Category I); new less severe forms of extrapulmonary disease	2 HRZ 2 HRZ 2 HRZ	4 HR 4 H_3R_3 6 HE
IV	Chronic cases, i.e. still bacteriologically positive after supervised re-treatment	Second-line drugs required according to WHO guidelines in specialized centers	

[a]The way of writing the regimens is standard: the number before the initials of the drugs indicates the duration of the treatment phases in months, and subscripted numbers following the initials indicate the number of times weekly that the drugs are given. (Absence of a subscripted number indicates that the drugs are given daily.) Thus, for example, 2 EHRZ/4 H_3R_3 means that ethambutol (E), isoniazid (H), rifampicin (R) and pyrazinamide (Z) are given daily for 2 months, followed by isoniazid and rifampicin three times weekly for a further 4 months. (S) = streptomycin.

course regimens are designed to achieve all three aims. The way in which tubercle bacilli are killed by antituberculosis drugs in the human body is quite different from the way they are killed in a culture medium. To understand how the drugs work to cure a patient with post-primary pulmonary tuberculosis – the commonest form of the disease seen in most clinical situations – it is useful to think of the tubercle bacilli as being in three different 'compartments', as described in Chapter 5 (see Fig. 5.8).[7]

- *Compartment 1*. Rapidly replicating bacilli on the wall of the well-oxygenated pulmonary cavity. In typical open, infectious, pulmonary tuberculosis, the great majority of the bacilli are in this compartment.
- *Compartment 2*. Slowly replicating bacilli in the acidic and poorly oxygenated closed lesions.
- *Compartment 3*. Dormant or near-dormant bacilli in dense and anoxic lesions and within the acidic and hostile macrophages.

The antituberculosis drugs are divisible into those that prevent replication of tubercle bacilli at the concentrations achievable in tissues but do not kill them (bacteriostatic agents), those that actually kill the bacilli (bactericidal agents) and those that sterilize the lesions. There is an important difference between bactericidal and sterilizing drugs as, although both will kill tubercle bacilli in the test tube, some of the former are only active against bacilli in certain 'compartments' in the human body. Thus, for example, streptomycin is only active in neutral or slightly alkaline environments, such as the wall of the cavity, and pyrazinamide is only active in acid environments, such as inflamed necrotic tissue, so that, while both are bactericidal, neither on its own is capable of killing all the bacilli in the lesions and thereby sterilizing them.

In the first few days of therapy, isoniazid in particular but also rifampicin and ethambutol (and, if used, streptomycin) destroy almost all the rapidly replicating bacilli in the slightly alkaline wall of the cavity. This has the important effect of rapidly rendering the patient non-infectious because it is these bacilli that enter the sputum and are coughed out. During the next few weeks, the less actively replicating bacilli in the acidic, hypoxic inflamed lesions are killed by rifampicin and pyrazinamide. After 2 months, only a small number of dormant or near-dormant bacilli remain, but it is essential that all these are killed or the disease will return. The best drug by far for this purpose is rifampicin, which is therefore the principal drug in the continuation phase in the most effective regimens. At first view it might seem strange that isoniazid is given as a companion drug in the continuation phase, as this drug only kills actively replicating tubercle bacilli. The reason that it is used is that it will kill any rifampicin-resistant mutants that might arise and commence replication. The dynamics of bacillary killing during therapy are shown in Figure 12.2.

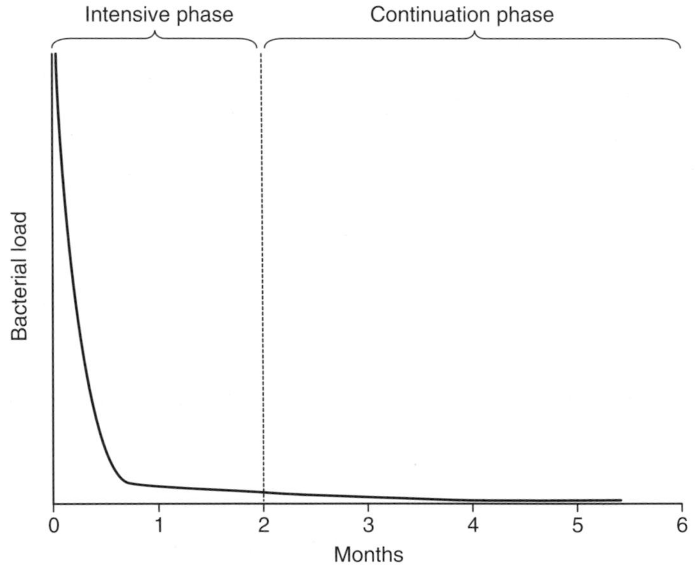

FIGURE 12.2 *The dynamics of bacillary killing during modern short-course therapy.*

Pyridoxine (vitamin B6) is sometimes given to patients with tuberculosis, usually at a dose of 10 mg/day, as it greatly reduces the risk of the neurological side effects of isoniazid. National guidelines should be consulted on its use: some national programmes recommend that it should be routinely prescribed to patients with liver disease, renal failure requiring dialysis, pregnant women, alcoholics, those infected with human immunodeficiency virus (HIV), the malnourished and the elderly.

TREATMENT OF DRUG-RESISTANT TUBERCULOSIS

The treatment of drug-resistant tuberculosis requires the use of alternative agents.[8,9] These include older agents such as ethionamide (etionamide) and the closely related prothion-amide (protionamide), cycloserine, capreomycin and *para*-aminosalicylic acid, and more recently discovered classes of drugs including fluoroquinolones, such as ofloxacin and sparfloxacin, and the newer macrolides, including clarithromycin and azithromycin. There is limited evidence that the antileprosy drug clofazimine (Lamprene) and combinations of penicillins and β-lactamase inhibitors, such as amoxicillin with sulbactam, are also of use. These drugs tend to more toxic, more expensive and less active than the first-line drugs. Accordingly, therapy must often be continued for much longer than standard regimens – for 9 months to 1 year after the sputum becomes bacteriologically negative. Supervision of therapy requires great skill in order to ensure that patients take the drugs, despite various side effects, over prolonged periods of time. Failure to complete treatment will lead to recurrence of the disease and the generation of strains of tubercle bacilli resistant to even more drugs.

In many situations, the mortality from multidrug-resistant tuberculosis (MDR TB) is high, but with careful management a high proportion of patients may be cured.[10] In some areas with a high incidence of MDR TB, the so-called 'DOTS-Plus' strategy has been introduced, as described in the following chapter. Ideally, the drug resistance of all isolated tubercle bacilli should be established by reference laboratories. Where such facilities are not available, empirical drug regimens based on the predominant patterns of drug resistance in a given region are designed.

In the latter case, patients with relapsing disease who are suspected of having drug-resistant tuberculosis should be treated with combinations of drugs that they have not received before. In practice, it is often very difficult to find out which drugs a patient has received before. The 'golden rule' of therapy of relapsing disease is that a single new drug must *never* be given 'blindly' to such a patient, as this is a certain way of generating additional drug resistance.

Thus, the treatment of drug-resistant, and especially multidrug-resistant, tuberculosis is challenging, complex and costly. Guidelines for the management of MDR TB have been published by the WHO.[8]

TREATMENT OF TUBERCULOSIS IN SPECIAL SITUATIONS

The short-course regimens described above are suitable for all forms of pulmonary and extrapulmonary tuberculosis. To be on the safe side, however, some physicians continue the treatment of patients with tuberculous meningitis and spinal tuberculosis for an additional 2 months. Patients with other conditions, notably impaired liver and kidney function, require modified regimens and monitoring of their therapy. Special considerations also apply to pregnant women.

Renal insufficiency

As they are fully metabolized in the body tissues or eliminated in the bile, the first-line drugs rifampicin, isoniazid and pyrazinamide and the second-line drugs ethionamide and prothionamide can be given in their usual doses.[11] Patients receiving isoniazid are at increased risk of neurological complications, including encephalopathy, but the risk is reduced by the prescription of pyridoxine (vitamin B6, see above). Ethambutol is mainly excreted by the kidney but may be used in reduced doses. Streptomycin and related aminoglycosides are entirely eliminated by, and have toxic effects on, the kidney and should be avoided.

Impaired liver function

Patients may safely receive isoniazid, ethambutol and streptomycin. Pyrazinamide should be avoided if possible, although the evidence that it is toxic in patients with impaired liver function is rather weak. Care is required with rifampicin, and liver function tests should be regularly carried out in those with known or suspected impairment of liver function, including alcoholics, the elderly, malnourished children and children below 2 years of age. Opinions differ as to whether regular liver function tests should be performed on all patients being treated for tuberculosis, where facilities exist. Some workers consider them unnecessary, whereas others argue that their use prevents a few deaths from liver failure.[12]

Antituberculosis therapy must be stopped if jaundice develops and only started again when the jaundice has resolved. In many cases, restarting treatment does not lead to a return of the jaundice. Patients who are seriously ill with tuberculosis may be treated safely with streptomycin and ethambutol even if they have jaundice.

Pregnancy

The first-line drugs appear to be safe during pregnancy and standard short-course regimens may therefore be used. There is a small risk of damage to fetal nerves by isoniazid, but this is preventable by giving pyridoxine (vitamin B6). Streptomycin and the rarely used viomycin should not be given during pregnancy, as they may damage the inner ear of the fetus, leading to deafness. Ethionamide and prothionamide should also be avoided, as there is some evidence that they may cause fetal deformities. The treatment of multidrug-resistant tuberculosis in pregnancy poses serious problems, but limited evidence indicates that even those with disease resistant to many drugs can, with care and attention, be treated successfully with no harm to the infants.[13]

DRUG FORMULATIONS

Most modern regimens are based on a four-drug intensive phase and a two-drug continuation phase. The drugs may be given as single tablets, but **combination preparations** containing two, three and four drugs are available and help with compliance as the patients only have to take a few pills daily, rather than up to 16 in the intensive phase if single drugs are taken. They also ensure that the patients receive all of the drugs, and thus lower the risk of the development of drug resistance. The management of the supplies of drugs is also simplified, although treatment centres will also need supplies of single drugs for those patients whose regimens require modification on the basis of adverse drug reactions.

Only combination formulations that have been evaluated by World Health Organization (WHO)-approved laboratories should be used, as the production of such formulations is not straightforward.[14] Suitable formulations can be obtained, at a very reasonable price, from the Global Drug Facility managed by the WHO Stop TB Partnership.[15]

ADVERSE DRUG REACTIONS

Almost all drugs are capable of causing some form of adverse reactions in some patients, and the antituberculosis drugs are no exception.[16–18] In general, only a small minority of patients react adversely to the drugs in modern short-course regimens. Adverse reactions are more of a problem with the second-line drugs used to treat drug-resistant tuberculosis. Patients over the age of 60 years and those infected with HIV are more likely to develop serious adverse drug reactions.[19] The adverse effects of the various drugs are described under the individual drug descriptions in Box 12.1.

BOX 12.1 The antituberculosis agents and their adverse effects

First-line drugs

Isoniazid has powerful activity against replicating tubercle bacilli but is not active against dormant or near-dormant bacilli. Cross-resistance with other antituberculosis agents does not occur. It is converted to an inactive form by the process of acetylation, which is under genetic control, with some people being rapid acetylators and others slow acetylators. The status does not affect the efficiency of standard short-course antituberculosis therapy, but adverse side effects and interactions with other drugs are more evident in slow acetylators.

Adverse side effects are uncommon and mostly involve the nervous system. They include restlessness, insomnia and muscle twitching and, rarely, psychiatric disorders. Patients with liver and renal disease, pregnant women, alcoholics, human immunodeficiency virus (HIV) patients, the malnourished and the elderly are at particular risk, but the risk is greatly reduced by prescription of pyridoxine (vitamin B6) 10 mg daily.

Isoniazid occasionally causes hypersensitivity skin reactions, especially in those infected with HIV.

Rifampicin (*rifampin* in the USA) is the most powerful antituberculosis agent currently in use, and effective concentrations are obtained in all tissues. It is one of a group of chemically similar agents termed rifamycins. Cross-resistance to other antituberculosis agents, other than related rifamycins, does not occur. Patients should be warned that rifampicin is red coloured and that it gives this colour to urine, tears and sweat.

Adverse reactions include mild itching and redness (erythema of the skin), which usually resolve spontaneously. Some patients suffer from gastrointestinal upsets, which are reduced by taking rifampicin with food. Liver function may be impaired in alcoholics and those with other liver diseases. If laboratory facilities are available, liver function tests including assay of serum bilirubin should be done monthly on these patients. A few patients on rifampicin develop the so-called 'flu syndrome', with fever, chills, headache, bone pain and, in some cases, a mild thrombocytopenic purpura. For unknown reasons, this is more common in those on intermittent than on daily treatment. More serious but very uncommon adverse events include respiratory collapse, low platelet counts leading to purpura and haemorrhages, haemolytic anaemia and renal failure. Again, these are more frequent in those on intermittent dosage regimens. If any of these serious adverse events occur, rifampicin must be stopped immediately and never given again. Corticosteroid therapy is required for life-threatening respiratory collapse.

Ethambutol is particularly active during the early, intensive, phase of treatment and there is some evidence that it enhances the activity of other antituberculosis agents by increasing the permeability of the cell wall of the tubercle bacillus.

Its most important side effect is inflammation of the optic nerve (optic neuritis), which may cause irreversible blindness. Although this is a very rare complication if the recommended maximum dose (25 mg/kg daily) is given for no longer than 2 months, it is a very serious one, and national codes of practice for the detection and prevention of ocular toxicity should be strictly followed. Patients should be told to stop therapy and to seek medical advice if they notice any change in their vision or perception of colour. This drug should not be given to young children and others unable to understand or follow this advice. Other uncommon adverse effects include peripheral neuritis, joint pain, low platelet counts and jaundice.

Pyrazinamide is an important first-line drug and is active against tubercle bacilli in acidic inflammatory lesions.

Adverse effects are uncommon and include gastrointestinal upsets and loss of appetite, aching joints and sensitivity of the skin to light. A few patients develop gout, which requires treatment with allopurinol. Contrary to early reports, toxic effects on the liver rarely occur except in patients with pre-existing liver disease.

Streptomycin is a member of the aminoglycoside group of antibiotics. Although occasionally used in short-course antituberculosis regimens, it has the great disadvantage that it must be given by intramuscular injection, with the risk of transmission of HIV and other viruses. Protective gloves should be worn by nurses when streptomycin injections are administered, to avoid sensitization dermatitis.

Its main adverse effects are on the inner ear, leading to vertigo and deafness, which may be permanent if the drug is not stopped when symptoms commence. The hearing of the child may be impaired if streptomycin is given to a pregnant woman. Kidney damage may also occur.

Second-line drugs

These are used in patients with drug-resistant tuberculosis and in those with adverse reactions to first-line drugs. They are mostly less effective, more toxic and more expensive than the first-line drugs.

Fluoroquinolones are a group of agents, including ciprofloxacin, ofloxacin and sparfloxacin, that have been evaluated for the treatment of drug-resistant tuberculosis.

Azithromycin and *clarithromycin* are newer members of the macrolide family, of which the best known is erythomycin. The newer macrolides are increasingly used to treat tuberculosis and disease due to some environmental mycobacteria, as described in Chapter 10.

Ethionamide and *prothionamide* are closely related to each other and to isoniazid, although no cross-resistance with the latter is seen. Their activity is much less than that of isoniazid, being just bacteristatic agents. Many patients develop distressing gastric irritation, which is improved to some extent by taking the drugs at bedtime.

Other aminoglycosides, including kanamycin and amikacin, are active against tubercle bacilli. Like streptomycin, they must be given by intramuscular injection and have adverse toxic effects on the inner ear and kidney.

Capreomycin and *viomycin* are of limited availability and rarely used. Although unrelated structurally to the aminoglycosides, they show partial cross-resistance to them. Also, in common with the aminoglycosides, they must be given by intramuscular injection and have similar adverse toxic effects on the inner ear and kidney.

Para-aminosalicylic acid is one of the earliest antituberculosis agents; it has only limited bacteristatic activity. Gastrointestinal upsets are common; it is of limited availability and very rarely used nowadays.

Thiacetazone is a weak drug with the single advantage of cheapness. It is a frequent cause of skin rashes, particularly in patients of Chinese ethnic origin. The incidence of severe and life-threatening skin reactions is unacceptably high in people infected with HIV. For this reason, together with its weak activity, thiacetazone should be dropped from the list of drugs used to treat tuberculosis.

Cycloserine is a rather weak bacteriostatic drug that frequently causes unpleasant neurological and psychiatric side effects, including headache, dizziness, depression and confusion. Its use should be avoided whenever possible.

Other agents: among the rifamycin group of antibiotics, rifabutin and rifapentine are being evaluated as alternatives to rifampicin in some circumstances. The former is used as an alternative to rifampicin in HIV-infected patients receiving antiretroviral therapy. There is limited evidence that the antileprosy drug clofazimine (Lamprene) and amidopenicillins in combination with β-lactamase inhibitors, such as amoxicillin with sulbactam, are effective in the treatment of tuberculosis.

The principal adverse drug reactions are hypersensitivity reactions affecting the skin, toxic effects on the liver and neurological complications. Patients receiving rifampicin may develop an influenza-like disease – the so-called 'flu syndrome' – which, paradoxically, occurs more frequently in those receiving the drug twice or three times weekly than in those receiving it daily.

Hypersensitivity reactions of the skin are usually seen between the second and fourth week of treatment and may be mild (just itching), moderate (a rash and fever) or severe. Patients with severe hypersensitivity reactions may, in addition to the rash and fever, have circulatory collapse, enlargement of lymph nodes, liver and spleen, and swelling of the conjunctivae, the lips and the mucous membranes of the mouth. The name **Stevens–Johnson syndrome** is given to a generalized and severe rash with peeling of the skin and ulceration of the conjunctivae and the mucous membranes of the mouth and genital organs. This serious and life-threatening syndrome is common in HIV-infected patients and particularly so in those receiving thiacetazone.[20]

Mild itching is usually self-limiting and is relieved by antihistamines. When more severe reactions occur, therapy should be stopped. Corticosteroid therapy is required if serious systemic effects, particularly circulatory collapse, are present. Once the hypersensitivity reaction has subsided, antituberculosis therapy should be recommenced with other drugs, but never thiacetazone. As first-line drugs are much more effective than alternative agents, attempts should be made to re-introduce them, though with great care and under strict observation. This is done by giving small challenge doses of these drugs, commencing with the drug least likely to have caused the reaction, and increasing to regular doses over a few days, as shown in Table 12.2.

It is possible to desensitize patients who react adversely to isoniazid or rifampicin, by giving one-tenth of the standard dose of the drug and increasing the dose by one-tenth each day until the regular dose is reached. It is very important that desensitization is *only*

TABLE 12.2 Sequence of re-introduction and challenge doses for recommencing antituberculosis therapy

Agent	Likelihood of the drug causing a reaction and sequence of re-introduction	Challenge dose		
		Day 1	Day 2	Day 3
Isoniazid	Least/first	50 mg	300 mg	300 mg
Rifampicin	↓	75 mg	300 mg	Full dose
Pyrazinamide	↓	250 mg	1 g	Full dose
Ethambutol	↓	100 mg	500 mg	Full dose
Streptomycin	Greatest/last	125 mg	500 mg	Full dose

attempted in specialist centres and under very close clinical observation. Desensitization must *never* be attempted in HIV-infected patients.

ADVERSE DRUG INTERACTIONS

In addition to causing adverse effects, several of the antituberculosis drugs inhibit or enhance the effects of other drugs and this has serious clinical implications.[21,22] Drug interactions are a particular problem in patients infected with HIV, as they may be taking several drugs for the treatment of bacterial and fungal infections and, in some regions, they may be receiving antiretroviral agents.

The principal interactions between the antituberculosis drugs and other drugs are listed in Table 12.3. Most of the drug interactions involve rifampicin and the related drugs rifabutin and rifapentine because these induce the production by the liver of certain enzymes, called **cytochromes**, which play an important part in the metabolism of many drugs. Examples

TABLE 12.3 Interactions between antituberculosis drugs and other therapeutic agents

Drugs with effects opposed by rifampicin	Antiretroviral agents	Opioids
	Azathioprine	Oral contraceptives
	Corticosteroids	Phenytoin
	Cyclosporin	Propranolol
	Diazepam	Quinidine
	Digoxin	Theophylline
	Haloperidol	Tolbutamide
	Imidazoles	Warfarin
Drug enhancing the effects of rifampicin	Trimethoprim-sulfamethoxazole (Cotrimoxazole)	
Drug with effects opposed by isoniazid	Enflurane	
Drugs with effects enhanced by isoniazid	Phenytoin	Carbamezapine
Drug enhancing the effects of isoniazid	Insulin	
Drugs opposing the effects of isoniazid	Prednisolone	Antacids (inhibit absorption)
Drugs with effects enhanced by streptomycin	Neuromuscular blocking agents	
Drug enhancing the effects of quinolones	Cimetidine	
Drugs with effects enhanced by quinolones	Aminophylline	Theophylline
Drugs opposing the effects of quinolones	Antacids, iron preparations, sucralfate, didanosine (all inhibit absorption)	

include the more rapid metabolism of oral contraceptives, so women receiving rifampicin should be given advice on alternative means of contraception. Rifampicin and related drugs also reduce the levels and effectiveness of the azole anti-fungal drugs such as ketoconazole and fluconazole and of dapsone, which is given to some HIV-infected patients to prevent *Pneumocystis carinii* pneumonia. Revised doses of these agents may therefore be required.

The induction of cytochromes by rifampicin lowers the levels of some antiretroviral agents used in the treatment of HIV disease, notably the protease inhibitors such as saquinavir, indinavir, nelfinavir and ritonavir. This not only reduces the effectiveness of these agents, but also increases the risk of the HIV developing resistance to them. Conversely, and by a similar mechanism, the protease inhibitors enhance the metabolism of rifampicin and related agents, and adjustments to the dosage of these may be required.

The current edition of *British National Formulary* is a useful source of up-to-date information on the dosages, side effects and interactions of the antituberculosis drugs.

The treatment of tuberculosis in patients receiving antiretroviral therapy is therefore fraught with problems, particularly as antiretroviral regimens are frequently modified as new agents are introduced. Specialist advice, or reference to the latest guidelines issued by the Centers for Disease Control and Prevention, Atlanta, Georgia, is therefore required.[23] Some regimens in use at the time of writing are summarized in Table 12.4. As a general rule, priority should be given to the treatment of tuberculosis and to delay antiretroviral therapy until 3 weeks after completion of the antituberculosis therapy, by which time rifampicin will have been cleared from the plasma.

TABLE 12.4 Antituberculosis drug regimens with concomitant antiretroviral regimens

Antituberculosis regimen	Months of therapy	Antiretroviral therapy
Rifampicin	6	Triple non-nucleoside reverse
Isoniazid	6	transcriptase inhibitors (NRTI)
Pyrazinamide	2	
Ethambutol	2	
Rifabutin	6	nelfinavir, indinavir, amprenavir,
Isoniazid	6	efavirenz or nevirapine
Pyrazinamide	2	
Ethambutol	2	

PREVENTIVE ANTITUBERCULOSIS THERAPY

In addition to their use in the treatment of tuberculosis, antituberculosis drugs are sometimes given prophylactically to prevent the development of tuberculosis in those at high risk of infection, such as infants born to mothers with the disease. **Preventive therapy** differs from **prophylactic therapy** in that it is given to those already infected, usually demonstrated by tuberculin reactivity, to prevent them from developing overt disease.[24]

The most widely used form of preventive therapy is isoniazid alone (monotherapy), usually for 9 or 12 months. Use of a single drug has been justified by the assumption that there will be so few replicating bacilli in a person with latent tuberculosis that the chance of an isoniazid-resistant mutant arising is extremely small. Isoniazid monotherapy has been widely used in the USA, where it has been shown to be effective and, as in most regions of that country the risk of exogenous re-infection is very low, protection is long lasting. The problems encountered in the use of isoniazid monotherapy include ensuring adherence and the occurrence of liver toxicity, particularly in those aged over 35 years. Some workers therefore recommend that preventive therapy should only be given to those under the age of 35.[24] Clearly, isoniazid monotherapy will be ineffective in people infected by isoniazid-resistant (including MDR) tubercle bacilli. Understandably, therefore, nurses caring for patients with MDR TB have justified anxiety in countries where staff protection against tuberculosis is based on isoniazid monotherapy rather than Bacille Calmette–Guérin (BCG) vaccination.

Preventive therapy has played only a small part in the control of tuberculosis in countries with a high incidence of the disease because of the difficulty of supervising therapy, which is essential for supporting adherence.[25] However, as the chance of a person dually infected with the tubercle bacillus and HIV developing tuberculosis is very high, the use of preventive therapy has received serious consideration. Although several studies have shown that preventive therapy with isoniazid is effective in such dually infected individuals, the protection is short lived. Accordingly, repeated courses of preventive therapy, or even such therapy continued for the remainder of the patient's life, may be required. For reasons that are not clear, the degree of prevention is related to the immune status of the patient, being greatest in those who are tuberculin positive and who have relatively high lymphocyte counts. Thus the WHO recommends that preventive therapy should only be given to HIV-infected people who are tuberculin positive.[26]

The usual preventive regimen for those who are dually infected is isoniazid monotherapy for 9 months. Continuation to 12 months confers no significant advantage. Other regimens, including rifampicin for 4 months or rifampicin plus pyrazinamide for 2 months, have the advantage of short duration,[27] but the latter causes an unacceptably high incidence of severe liver toxicity and is no longer recommended.[28]

In general, though, only a small minority of dually infected patients receive preventive therapy, as the need for supervision adds yet another burden to the already overburdened health services. It is very important to ensure that HIV-infected people receiving preventive therapy do not have active tuberculosis, as the regimens developed for preventive therapy are not powerful enough to cure active tuberculosis and their use could encourage the development of drug resistance.

As the policies and regimens for preventive therapy vary from country to country, national guidelines should be consulted.

THE USE OF STEROIDS IN THE TREATMENT OF TUBERCULOSIS

Steroids have no direct action on the tubercle bacillus but they are sometimes used to prevent or treat the complications of tuberculosis or its therapy.[29] There is some evidence that the addition of steroids to standard antituberculosis regimens hastens clinical recovery and healing of pulmonary lesions,[30] but such treatment is rarely given. The use of steroids for treating serious reactions to antituberculosis drugs has been briefly mentioned above. Steroids are also used to reduce gross enlargement of lymph nodes, which may occur during therapy as a result of hypersensitivity reactions and which may cause respiratory obstruction. They are also used to prevent complications due to scarring, especially narrowing of the ureter and shrinkage of the bladder in renal tuberculosis and constriction of the heart by fibrous tissue during the resolution of tuberculous pericarditis. On very rare occasions, involvement of the adrenal glands by tuberculosis leads to adrenal failure (Addison's disease), requiring steroid replacement therapy.

TREATMENT OF OTHER MYCOBACTERIAL DISEASES

Leprosy

In common with tuberculosis, and for the same reasons, leprosy is treated with multidrug regimens. Unlike tuberculosis, leprosy shows a very distinct 'spectrum' of immunological and clinical features with, at one pole of the spectrum, marked immune reactivity and very few leprosy bacilli (tuberculoid leprosy) and, at the other, little or no immune responsiveness and enormous numbers of bacilli in the skin and other tissues (lepromatous leprosy), and various stages in between. For practical clinical management, patients are assessed by making small and very superficial incisions in the skin, gently scraping out some tissue fluid and making smears of this on microscope slides (so-called slit-skin smears). Patients are divided into those in whom acid-fast bacilli cannot be seen microscopically in these smears and those in whom they can be seen. These are termed, respectively, paucibacillary (PB) and multibacillary (MB) patients. The former are treated with rifampicin and dapsone for 6 months and the latter with rifampicin, dapsone and clofazimine (Lamprene) for 1 to 2 years.[31] An alternative regimen based on a combination of rifampicin, ofloxacin and minocycline (ROM) is advocated as a single dose for single-lesion PB leprosy and as monthly doses for 24 months for MB patients who refuse to take clofazimine because of its side effects, especially skin discolouration.[32]

Environmental mycobacteria

Because they are relatively uncommon, there have been few clinical trials to assess therapy for the various diseases due to environmental mycobacteria (EM). One such trial of acquired immunodeficiency syndrome (AIDS)-related disseminated disease due to the *M. avium* complex (MAC) showed that one of the newer **macrolides**, azithromycin or clarithromycin, in combination with ethambutol was effective.[33] Limited experience has shown that the above regimen is also useful for the treatment of pulmonary and other infections in non-immunosuppressed patients due to the more commonly encountered EM – MAC, *M. kansasii*, *M. xenopi* and *M. malmoense*.[34] An alternative in these patients is a regimen of rifampicin, isoniazid and ethambutol. Laboratory tests for susceptibility to antibacterial agents are of limited value, as their results show poor correlation with clinical responses to treatment.[35] **Highly active antiretroviral therapy** (HAART) plays an important role in the treatment of AIDS-related mycobacterial disease.[36] Indeed, there is some evidence that reduction of the viral load and reversal of the decline in immune competence by use of HAART may contribute more to the remission of disease due to EM than antibacterial therapy.[37]

Disease due to the rapidly growing species *M. abscessus*, *M. chelonae* and *M. fortuitum* is treated by various antibacterial agents, including co-trimoxazole, doxycycline, macrolides, amikacin and cephalosporins. The choice of drugs is based on limited and largely anecdotal experience and the results of drug susceptibility tests. The duration of therapy is determined by clinical response.[34]

Summary

The great majority of patients with tuberculosis can be effectively treated, provided that a few simple principles are observed. Drug resistance is a tragedy that has arisen because the established simple principles were not observed and now poses a serious and increasing barrier to the eventual conquest of this disease. The modern short-course regimens are based on an understanding of the nature of the disease and the way in which the bacilli behave in various physiological 'compartments'. Modern regimens are suitable for adult patients with all forms of tuberculosis and, with certain modifications, for children, pregnant women and those with complicating factors such as HIV infection and hepatic and renal disease. Nobody need be denied effective therapy for tuberculosis. Adverse drug reactions and interactions may occur, but strategies for their management are available and they do not prevent the cure of the patient. The use of drugs to prevent the development of tuberculosis in those at risk of infection or who are already infected is a topic of some controversy, but there are circumstances in which preventive therapy is used. The growing problem of HIV-related tuberculosis raises the need to give careful consideration to the more widespread use of such preventive therapy. The therapy for leprosy resembles, in principle, that for tuberculosis except that the regimen used depends on the bacterial load. With the exception of MAC infection in AIDS patients, therapy for disease due to EM has not been subjected to rigorous clinical trials, but there is considerable anecdotal evidence to serve as a guide to therapy.

Prologue to the next chapter

As in many circumstances in life, what seems really simple in principle can prove very difficult in practice. Paradoxically, modern short-course therapy is the most effective and cost-effective remedy for any chronic infectious disease, yet tuberculosis has been declared a global emergency. In reality, there are many barriers between the availability of effective drug regimens and the cure of the patient with tuberculosis. Foremost among these are inadequate tuberculosis control services in many parts of the world, difficulties in accessing even simple primary health care, poor medical practice resulting in the prescription of the wrong drugs, and a failure, for a whole host of reasons, for the patient to complete the course of therapy. In recent years, all these issues have been of great concern to international agencies and have culminated in the launch of the first phase of the WHO's Global Plan to Stop Tuberculosis, which is the principal theme of the next chapter.

REFERENCES

1. Goldstraw P. The surgery of tuberculosis. In Davies PDO (ed.), *Clinical tuberculosis*, 3rd edn. London: Arnold, 2003, 224–41.
2. Stanford JL, Stanford CA, Grange JM, Nguyen Ngoc Lan, Etemadi A. Does immunotherapy with heat-killed *Mycobacterium vaccae* offer hope for multi-drug-resistant pulmonary tuberculosis? *Respir Med* 2001; **95**: 444–7.
3. Ryan F. *Tuberculosis: the greatest story never told* (in the USA: *The forgotten plague*). Bromsgrove: Swift, 1992.

4. Wing Wai Yew. Chemotherapy of tuberculosis: present, future and past. In Davies PDO (ed.), *Clinical tuberculosis*, 3rd edn. London: Arnold, 2003, 191–210.
5. Rieder HL. *Interventions for tuberculosis control and elimination*. Paris: International Union Against Tuberculosis and Lung Disease, 2002.
6. World Health Organization. *Treatment of tuberculosis: guidelines for national programmes*, 2nd edn. Geneva: World Health Organization, 1997.
7. Mitchison DA. The role of individual drugs in the chemotherapy of tuberculosis. *Int J Tuberc Lung Disease* 2000; **4**: 796–806.
8. World Health Organization. *Multidrug resistant tuberculosis (MDRTB). Basis for the development of an evidence-based case-management strategy for MDRTB within the WHO's DOTS strategy*. Geneva: World Health Organization (Communicable Diseases), 1999.
9. Crofton J, Chaulet P, Maher D. *World Health Organization guidelines for the management of drug-resistant tuberculosis*. Geneva: World Health Organization, 1997.
10. Zumla A, Grange JM. Multidrug resistant tuberculosis – can the tide be turned? *Lancet Infect Dis* 2001; **1**: 199–202.
11. Eastwood JB, Dilly SA, Grange JM. Tuberculosis, leprosy and other mycobacterial diseases. In Cattell WR (ed.), *Infections of the kidney and urinary tract*. Oxford: Oxford University Press, 1996, 291–318.
12. Mitchell I, Wendon J, Fitt S, Williams R. Antituberculosis therapy and acute liver failure. *Lancet* 1995; **345**: 555–6.
13. Shin S, Guerra D, Rich M et al. Treatment of multidrug-resistant tuberculosis during pregnancy: a report of 7 cases. *Clin Infect Dis* 2003; **36**: 996–1003.
14. Fox W. Drug combinations and the bioavailability of rifampicin. *Tubercle* 1990; **71**: 241–5.
15. World Health Organization Global Drug Facility. *Frequently asked questions about the 4-drug fixed-dose combination tablet recommended by the World Health Organization for treating tuberculosis*. WHO/CDS/STB/2002.18. Geneva: World Health Organization, 2002.
16. Peloquin CA. Clinical pharmacology of the antituberculosis agents. In Davies PDO (ed.), *Clinical tuberculosis*, 3rd edn. London: Arnold, 2003, 172–90.
17. Grange JM, Zumla A. Antituberculosis agents. In Cohen J, Powderly WG (eds), *Infectious diseases*, 2nd edn. London: Elsevier Health Sciences, 2003, Section 7, 1851–67.
18. Grange JM. Antimycobacterial agents. In Finch RG, Greenwood D, Norrby SR, Whitley RJ (eds), *Antibiotic and chemotherapy*, 8th edn. Edinburgh: Churchill Livingstone, 2003, 426–40.
19. Yee D, Valiquette C, Pelletier M et al. Incidence of serious side effects from first-line antituberculosis drugs among patients treated for active tuberculosis. *Am J Respir Crit Care Med* 2003; **167**: 1472–7.
20. Chintu C, Luo C, Bhat G et al. Cutaneous hypersensitivity reactions due to thiacetazone in Zambian children infected with tuberculosis and the human immunodeficiency virus. *Arch Dis Child* 1993; **68**: 331–4.
21. Grange JM, Winstanley PA, Davies PDO. Clinically significant drug interactions with antituberculosis agents. *Drug Saf* 1994; **11**: 242–51.
22. Yew WW. Clinically significant interactions with drugs used in the treatment of tuberculosis. *Drug Saf* 2002; **25**: 111–33.
23. Centers for Disease Control and Prevention (CDC). Prevention and treatment of tuberculosis among patients infected with human immunodeficiency virus: principles of therapy and revised recommendations. *MMWR* 1998; **47**(RR20): 1–51. Also available online at <http://www.cdc.gov/epo/mmwr/preview/mmwrhtml/00055357.htm>.

24. Israel HL. Chemoprophylaxis for tuberculosis. *Respir Med* 1993; **87**: 81–3.
25. Hawken MP, Muhindi DW. Tuberculosis preventive therapy in HIV-infected persons: feasibility issues in developing countries. *Int J Tuberc Lung Dis* 1999; **3**: 646–50.
26. World Health Organization Global Tuberculosis Programme and UNAIDS. *Policy statement on preventive therapy against tuberculosis in people living with HIV*. Geneva: World Health Organization, 1998.
27. Wilkinson D, Squire SB, Garner P. Effect of preventive treatment for tuberculosis in adults infected with HIV: systematic review of randomised placebo controlled trials. *BMJ* 1998; **317**: 625–9.
28. Report. Update: Adverse event data and revised American Thoracic Society/CDC Recommendations against the use of rifampin and pyrazinamide for treatment of latent tuberculosis infection – United States, 2003. *MMWR* 2003; **52**(31): 735–9.
29. Alzeer AH, FitzGerald JM. Corticosteroids and tuberculosis: risks and use as adjunct therapy. *Tuber Lung Dis* 1993; **74**: 6–11.
30. Smego RA, Ahmed NA. Systematic review of the adjunctive use of systemic corticosteroids for pulmonary tuberculosis. *Int J Tuberc Lung Dis* 2003; **7**: 208–13.
31. World Health Organization. *Chemotherapy of leprosy*. Technical Report Series No. 847. Geneva: World Health Organization, 1994.
32. World Health Organization. *Seventh WHO Expert Committee on Leprosy*, June 1997. Geneva: World Health Organization, 1997.
33. Dunne M, Fessel J, Kumar P et al. A randomized, double-blind trial comparing azithromycin and clarithromycin in the treatment of disseminated *Mycobacterium avium* infection in patients with human immunodeficiency virus. *Clin Infect Dis* 2000; **31**: 1245–52.
34. Subcommittee of the Joint Tuberculosis Committee of the British Thoracic Society. Management of opportunist mycobacterial infections: Joint Tuberculosis Committee guidelines 1999. *Thorax* 2000; **55**: 210–18.
35. Heginbothom ML. The relationship between the in vitro drug susceptibility of opportunist mycobacteria and their in vivo response to treatment. *Int J Tuberc Lung Dis* 2001; **5**: 539–45.
36. Baril L, Jouan M, Agher R et al. Impact of highly active antiretroviral therapy on onset of *Mycobacterium avium* complex infection and cytomegalovirus disease in patients with AIDS. *AIDS* 2000; **14**: 2593–6.
37. Havlir DV, Schrier RD, Torriani FJ et al. Effect of potent antiretroviral therapy on immune responses to *Mycobacterium avium* in human immunodeficiency virus-infected subjects. *J Infect Dis* 2000; **182**: 1658–63.

FURTHER READING

Centers for Disease Control and Prevention (CDC). National Center for HIV, STD, and TB Prevention. *Updated guidelines for the use of rifamycins for the treatment of tuberculosis among HIV-infected patients taking protease inhibitors or nonnucleoside reverse transcriptase inhibitors*. Updated January 20, 2004. Atlanta, GA: CDC. Also available online at <http://www.cdc.gov/nchstp/tb/tb_hiv_drugs/toc.htm>.

Davies PDO (ed.). Drug-resistant tuberculosis. From molecules to macro-economics. *Ann N Y Acad Sci* 2001; **953**: 87–253.

International Union Against Tuberculosis and Lung Disease. *Management of tuberculosis. A guide for low income countries*. Paris: International Union Against Tuberculosis and Lung Disease, 2002.

Rieder HL. *Interventions for tuberculosis control and elimination*. Paris: International Union Against Tuberculosis and Lung Disease, 2002.

Wing Wai Yew. Chemotherapy of tuberculosis: present, future and past. In Davies PDO (ed.), *Clinical tuberculosis*, 3rd edn. London: Arnold, 2003, 191–210.

World Health Organization. *Treatment of tuberculosis: guidelines for national programmes*, 2nd edn. Geneva: World Health Organization, 1997.

World Health Organization. *Multidrug resistant tuberculosis (MDRTB). Basis for the development of an evidence-based case-management strategy for MDRTB within the WHO's DOTS strategy*. Geneva: World Health Organization (Communicable Diseases), 1999.

World Health Organization Stop TB Partnership. *The Global Plan to Stop Tuberculosis*. Geneva: World Health Organization, 2001.

New evidence-based guidance for treating tuberculosis will be published by National Institute for Clinical Excellence (NICE) in England in February 2006 and will be available on their website: http://www.nice.org.uk

CHAPTER 13

The Global Plan to Stop Tuberculosis

And the pity, nay the horror of it all, is that the backsliding [in tuberculosis control] is most noticeable precisely where militant activity should be most conspicuous.

Leonard Williams, 1908.

Introduction

After years of neglect, the declaration of tuberculosis as a global emergency by the World Health Organization (WHO) in 1993, followed by a decade of intensive advocacy by the WHO and various governmental and non-governmental organizations, has led to a serious global commitment to eradicate tuberculosis. This commitment has been linked to a 'massive effort' to conquer the three infectious diseases that pose the greatest threat to human health and life: tuberculosis, human immunodeficiency virus/acquired immunodeficiency syndrome (HIV/AIDS) and malaria. A major development in respect to the first of these has been the formulation of the *Global Plan to Stop Tuberculosis*, with the first phase running from the year 2001 to 2005. Not only is the WHO taking practical steps to ensure that countries are able to establish effective tuberculosis control programmes, it also disseminates up-to-date news, knowledge and information through various media, including the Internet.

Learning outcomes

After studying and reflecting on the material in this chapter, you will be able to:

- define and distinguish between DOT and DOTS,
- describe the WHO DOTS strategy for the global control of tuberculosis,
- outline the targets set for the diagnosis and treatment of tuberculosis within DOTS programmes and the progress towards reaching these targets,
- discuss the international efforts being directed towards the control of tuberculosis and other major diseases affecting the poorer nations.

During the latter half of the twentieth century, there was a general opinion that tuberculosis was nearing extinction in the industrially developed nations, and that in time socio-economic improvements in the developing nations would likewise lead to its extinction worldwide. Many institutions devoted to the conquest of tuberculosis were closed, including the British Medical Research Council's Tuberculosis and Chest Diseases Unit, which had played a very major role in the development of modern short-course drug regimens. In the words of Peter Davies, a leading British authority on this disease, 'If one wished to find a symbol of the way the developed world has turned its back on the problems of disease in the developing world, which had seen little change in the incidence of disease among its people, then this closure would perhaps be the most poignant'.[1]

In the 1980s, at the time of the closure of the British Medical Research Council's Tuberculosis and Chest Diseases Unit, ominous trends, including the impact of human immunodeficiency virus (HIV) infection, were inducing many experts to challenge the prevalent complacent assumptions. Accordingly, by the early 1990s, the WHO was re-establishing a very serious interest in tuberculosis.[2] This renewal of interest led, in 1993, to the unprecedented declaration by the WHO that tuberculosis was a global emergency. This was no empty slogan, as it heralded a period of intense advocacy and activity.

As a direct consequence, in 1998, the *Global Plan to Stop Tuberculosis* (GPSTB) was launched in Bangkok and rapidly grew into an extensive network of numerous governmental, non-governmental and academic organizations with a secretariat based at the WHO headquarters in Geneva.[3] (Full details are available on the GPSTB website <www.stoptb.org>.) The basis of the GPSTB programme is the WHO DOTS strategy. DOTS is an acronym of *Directly Observed Therapy, Short Course* and is the 'brand name' of a five-point control strategy formally introduced in 1994.[4] It was pioneered by Dr Karel Styblo, a greatly respected epidemiologist and physician who for many years worked for the International Union Against Tuberculosis and Lung Disease. The political implications of the use of a 'brand name' for promoting the DOTS strategy for global tuberculosis control have been critically analysed by Ogden and her colleagues.[5]

The strategic objectives of the GPSTB are to:

- *expand* the DOTS programme so that eventually all those with tuberculosis will be effectively diagnosed and treated;
- *adapt* the programme to face the challenges of HIV-related tuberculosis and multidrug resistance;
- *improve* the control of the disease by developing new diagnostic tests, drugs and vaccines;
- *strengthen* the partnership so that the control strategies are effectively applied.[3]

THE WHO DOTS STRATEGY

DOTS is sometimes confused with DOT, which is short for *Directly Observed Therapy*, but there is an important difference between them. Although DOT is a key component of DOTS, the latter is much more comprehensive. In *An expanded DOTS framework for effective tuberculosis control*, published in 2002,[6] the five essential elements of the DOTS strategy are as follows.

- *Sustained political commitment* to increase human and financial resources and to make tuberculosis control a nationwide activity integral to national health systems.
- *Access to quality-assured tuberculosis sputum microscopy* for case detection among people

presenting with, or found through surveys to have, symptoms of tuberculosis (most importantly, prolonged cough). Special attention is necessary for case detection among HIV-infected people and other high-risk groups, such as people in institutions.

- *Standardized short-course chemotherapy for all cases of tuberculosis under proper case-management conditions including direct observation of therapy*: proper case-management conditions imply technically sound and socially supportive treatment services.
- *Uninterrupted supply of quality-assured drugs* with reliable procurement and distribution systems.
- *Recording and reporting system enabling outcome assessment* of each and every patient and assessment of the overall programme performance.

A number of key operations for the establishment of the expanded DOTS strategy are defined, including the development of the structure of the tuberculosis control programme, future development plans, preparation of programme manuals and the training and supervision of staff. DOTS is a rational, common-sense and straightforward strategy, although (as described in Chapter 14) encouraging patients to adhere to, or to comply with, their treatment requires more than simple observation of pill-taking, which, if conducted in an authoritative or insensitive manner, may indeed set up barriers to the completion of treatment.

Experience in several countries, including China,[7] leaves no doubt that the DOTS strategy, when properly applied, is effective and has the potential to reduce the death rate and the incidence of the disease. Cure rates of more than 85 per cent have been reported and in Peru, where there is an active DOTS programme with very wide coverage of the population, the incidence of tuberculosis is declining by around 7 per cent annually.

As a strategy for saving lives and maintaining the health of economically productive young adults in the developing nations, DOTS is among the most cost effective of all health interventions. Tuberculosis has a devastating economic impact on a household in a developing country. On average, a family loses 30 per cent of its income if a money-earner develops tuberculosis, and 15 years of income if that person dies of the disease. Tuberculosis is not merely a disease of poverty, it is a generator of poverty and, accordingly, tuberculosis control is a way of combating poverty.[8] As the drugs for curing a patient of the disease can now be purchased for around US$10, financial investment in tuberculosis control is soon repaid in terms of economic gain to the society. In general, patients treated within DOTS programmes do much better than those treated outside these programmes, with cure rates of, respectively, more than 80 per cent and less than 30 per cent. Thus, in addition to saving lives, DOTS reduces the recurrence rate of the disease, treatment failure leading to the emergence of drug resistance, and the spread of infection in the community.

The benefits of the DOTS strategy are thus well established, and the huge challenge facing the global community is to ensure that all patients with tuberculosis have access to diagnosis and treatment within this strategy. In March 2000, in the so-called Amsterdam *Declaration to Stop TB*, the targets of diagnosing 70 per cent of sputum smear-positive patients and curing 85 per cent of those diagnosed by the year 2005 were set. An additional target is to reduce the global burden of tuberculosis, in terms of prevalence and death rates, to half of its year 2000 level by 2005. More detailed targets and milestones have been established by the *Stop TB Working Group on DOTS Expansion*, which also offers advice and support to countries pledged to achieving these targets.[3,6]

The expansion of the application of DOTS between 1990 and 2000 was (as shown in Fig. 13.1) rapid and impressive.[9] The 22 countries with the highest burden of tuberculosis have

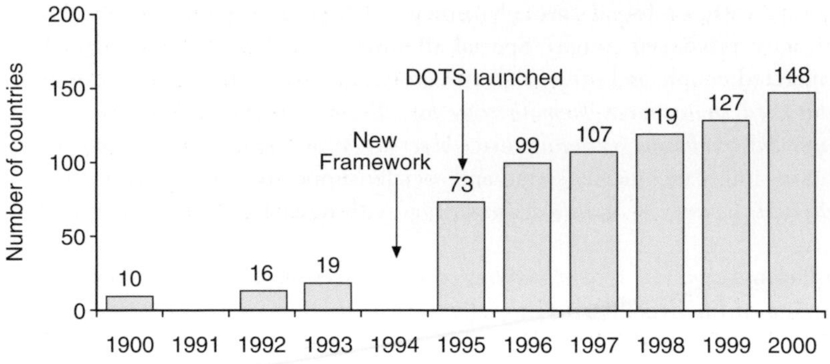

FIGURE 13.1 *The rapid and impressive DOTS expansion between 1990 and 2000. Data from the World Health Organization.*[9]

adopted the DOTS strategy and, by the end of the year 2001, 95–100 per cent of the population had access to DOTS programmes in ten of these countries.[10] Unfortunately, worldwide, most of the countries achieving high coverage are rather small ones, and among the larger countries only Vietnam and Peru had achieved the Stop TB targets for tuberculosis control. By the end of 2003, more than 10 million tuberculosis patients had been successfully treated within DOTS programmes in 155 countries in the 10 years since the formal introduction of the DOTS strategy in 1994. Notwithstanding, in the year 2003, only one in three patients with tuberculosis were detected and treated within DOTS programmes. The target of 50 per cent detection by the year 2003 was therefore not met, and dramatic improvements in the adoption of this strategy will be needed if the global targets are to be reached by the year 2005, particularly in view of the challenges posed to tuberculosis control by the HIV/acquired immunodeficiency syndrome (AIDS) pandemic.[11,12]

The expanded DOTS strategy is aimed at all those with tuberculosis.[13] Reliance on sputum microscopy alone is, however, inadequate for the diagnosis of tuberculosis in children, as few produce sputum containing sufficient acid-fast bacilli to be detected microscopically. It could be argued that detection of infectious adults indirectly benefits children, as source cases are detected and rendered non-infectious. Nevertheless, better tools for the diagnosis of all patients with tuberculosis, irrespective of their age or type of disease, are urgently required, and this issue is being addressed by a Working Group on New TB Diagnostics within the GPSTB.[3]

THE GLOBAL ALLIANCE FOR TB DRUG DEVELOPMENT

Although, in the absence of drug resistance, the standard modern drug regimens for tuberculosis are highly effective, new drugs are required in order to develop even shorter regimens and to combat the increasing threat of multidrug resistance. Unfortunately, the development and evaluation of new drugs are very costly, and pharmaceutical companies are unwilling to embark on research programmes that are unlikely to bring financial gains. As a result, only a very small research effort has been put into new treatments for diseases that cause so much suffering and death in the developing nations, compared to the 'lifestyle' illnesses of the wealthier nations. Fortunately, altruism has prevailed and, in October 2000, *The Global*

Alliance for TB Drug Development was launched in Bangkok at the International Conference on Health Research for Development.[14] The members of this new alliance, including governments, non-government organizations (NGOs), pharmaceutical companies and funding agencies, made a pledge to apply recent scientific breakthroughs to the development of new cost-effective antituberculosis drugs that will shorten the duration of treatment or otherwise simplify its completion, improve the treatment of latent infection by the tubercle bacillus, and be effective against multidrug-resistant tuberculosis (MDR TB).

THE GLOBAL TB DRUG FACILITY (GDF)

This initiative, launched in March 2001 as a project of the *Global Partnership to Stop TB (GPSTP)*, is intended to increase access to high-quality antituberculosis drugs. Its aim is to provide drugs to treat up to 11.6 million tuberculosis patients over the next 5 years, and to assist nations to reach the WHO global tuberculosis control targets by 2005.[15]

DOTS-PLUS

As discussed in Chapter 1, drug and multidrug resistance is a serious and increasing threat to the global control of tuberculosis. Patients with MDR TB are treatable and curable if resources are available.[16] A project in Peru showed that, with financial and technical support including laboratory assessment of drug resistance, patients with MDR TB could be managed effectively in a relatively poor nation.[17] As a result, the so-called DOTS-Plus strategy for the management of MDR TB is under serious consideration by the WHO, and the GPSTB has established the Working Group on DOTS-Plus for MDR TB and, as the subject is in pressing need of further operations research, this working group has established a 'Green Light Committee' (GLC) to assess and evaluate pilot projects in the management of MDR TB. In addition, the working group has published guidelines for establishing DOTS-Plus pilot projects for the management of MDR TB,[18] which will be updated periodically to reflect developments in this subject.

Two DOTS-Plus models are currently under investigation: one is based on individualized treatment regimens according to drug susceptibility determined in the laboratory, and the other is based on the use of empirical treatment regimens. The former is preferable, though more costly. DOTS-Plus strategies are in a state of evolution, and up-to-date WHO publications should be consulted for developments and guidelines. It is important that DOTS-Plus programmes are only introduced in regions where optimal DOTS strategies are already in place. The establishment of a DOTS-Plus programme at the expense of a DOTS programme can have a detrimental effect on tuberculosis control.[19]

THE MASSIVE EFFORT CAMPAIGN

Clearly, the campaign to stop tuberculosis and other major diseases will prove very costly, and the involvement of leading funding organizations has therefore been a prime objective of the WHO, culminating in the establishment of the *Advocacy Forum for Massive Effort Against Diseases of Poverty*. The first meeting of this forum, now known as the *Massive Effort Campaign*, sponsored by the WHO and the Joint United Nations Programme on HIV/AIDS

(UNAIDS), was held in October 2000 in the Swiss city of Winterthur. A statement published on the Advocacy Forum's website (www.winterthurhealthforum.ch) was impressive:

> This year – at the start of a new millennium – a movement is building that has the power to break the vicious cycle of poverty and disease. For the first time in history, the international community has the financial means, the medications, and the know-how to take a stand against a small number of diseases that cause tremendous suffering and economic loss. This massive effort against the diseases of poverty, which unites partners in unique ways, is moving the world from words to action – action that can facilitate sustainable development, stimulate economic growth, ensure greater global public health security and, most importantly, save human lives.

The three principal diseases targeted by the *Massive Effort Campaign* are tuberculosis, HIV/AIDS and malaria, which account for at least one in ten of all deaths worldwide. The global economic burden of these diseases was emphasized at the foundation meeting of the *Massive Effort Campaign* and, accordingly, the WHO established the Commission on Macroeconomics and Health to study the link between health and economic development. It was estimated that by 2015–2020, an annual investment of US$66 billion into the application of existing technologies would not only save 8 million lives each year, but would also generate six-fold economic benefits – a saving of more than US$360 billion a year.

It was also estimated that the cost of applying existing technologies to this saving of human lives and economic benefits in low-income and middle-income countries would, in the year 2007, amount to US$34 for each person annually. This compares very favourably with the average of US$2000 spent annually on health care for every person in the industrialized countries! Further details are available on the user-friendly *Massive Effort Campaign* website: <www.MassiveEffort.org>.

WORLD TB DAY

On 24th March 1882, Robert Koch announced his discovery of the cause of tuberculosis. This date has therefore been declared 'World TB Day' and it provides a special focus of the advocacy activities of all those concerned in the struggle against this disease. In many countries, nurses have been actively involved in advocacy and public awareness campaigns on World TB Day and the WHO has published useful guidelines that emphasize the four key elements of advocacy: documenting the situation, packaging the message, working with the media, and mobilizing other people.[20,21] Further useful information and a library of images suitable for presentations are available online at <www.who.int>.

Local organizations and charities, such as *TB Alert* in the UK, organize various events with the aim of enlightening policy makers, healthcare workers and the general public. Such events often include testimonies from cured patients – the most impressive and powerful advocates of all. Indeed, the theme for World TB Day 2003 was 'DOTS cured me – it will cure you too!'

THE INTERNATIONAL UNION AGAINST TUBERCULOSIS AND LUNG DISEASE

The International Union Against Tuberculosis and Lung Disease (UNION or, formerly, IUATLD) is a non-governmental voluntary organization, founded in 1920, with a headquarters in Paris, and is open to corporate and individual membership. Its prime concerns are the prevention and control of tuberculosis, but it is also involved in various aspects of lung disease and advocacy against smoking. The Union provides technical and material support to tuberculosis control initiatives in developing countries and conducts and supports operational and applied research through its scientific sections. It undertakes educational activities, including regional and international conferences, and it publishes a monthly journal, the *International Journal of Tuberculosis and Lung Disease*, and a newsletter that is available electronically, as well as various technical guides, slide presentations and other educational materials that are available on its two excellent websites – <www.iuatld.org> and <www.tbrieder.org>.

Summary

The WHO DOTS strategy is of proven effectiveness in detecting and treating patients with tuberculosis, particularly those who are infectious, with cure rates of more than 85 per cent. Although many countries have adopted the DOTS strategy, coverage is often not complete, and only around a third of all patients are diagnosed and treated within this strategy. Progress in implementing the strategy worldwide has been slow and, unless there is a major increase in commitment, the targets set for diagnosing 70 per cent of patients, and curing 85 per cent of those diagnosed, in the year 2005 will not be achieved. The *Massive Effort Campaign* may be able to obtain the funding necessary to implement DOTS on a wider scale. Meanwhile, advocacy plays a very important role in raising awareness of the serious public health problems posed by tuberculosis, and nurses are of key importance in this activity, with a special focus on World TB Day.

Prologue to the next chapter

One of the points in the five-point DOTS strategy is direct observation of therapy. Some form of supervision of therapy is deemed essential, as a failure to comply with, or adhere to, therapy is a major cause of treatment failure, recurrence of disease, prolonged infectivity and the emergence of drug resistance. The exact procedures used for supervision require very careful consideration and modification according to local anthropological factors. Insensitive and authoritarian supervision may be worse than useless. As nurses are particularly well placed to undertake careful and humane supervision of therapy as part of a holistic approach to patient care, this subject is considered in detail in the next chapter.

REFERENCES

1. Davies PDO. Preface. In Davies PDO (ed.), *Clinical tuberculosis*. London: Chapman and Hall, 1994, xvii–xix.
2. Kochi A. The global tuberculosis situation and the new control strategy of the World Health Organization. *Tubercle* 1991; **72**: 1–6.
3. Stop TB Partnership. *Progress Report on The Global Plan to Stop Tuberculosis*. Geneva: World Health Organization, 2004.
4. World Health Organization. WHO report on the tuberculosis epidemic. *TB – a global emergency, low priority*. Geneva: World Health Organization, 1994.

5. Ogden J, Walt G, Lush L. The politics of 'branding' in policy transfer: the case of DOTS for tuberculosis control. *Soc Sci Med* 2003; **57**: 179–88.
6. World Health Organization. *An expanded DOTS framework for effective tuberculosis control.* Geneva: World Health Organization, 2002.
7. China Tuberculosis Control Collaboration. Results of directly observed short-course chemotherapy in 112,842 Chinese patients with smear-positive tuberculosis. *Lancet* 1996; **347**: 358–62.
8. World Health Organization. *Scaling up the response to infectious diseases, a way out of poverty*. Geneva: World Health Organization, 2002.
9. World Health Organization. *Global tuberculosis control.* WHO Report 2002. WHO/CDS/TB/2002.295. Geneva: World Health Organization, 2002.
10. World Health Organization. *Tuberculosis (TB Advocacy Report 2003)*. WHO/CDS/TB/2003.321. Geneva: World Health Organization, 2003.
11. Veron LJ, Blanc LJ, Suchi M, Raviglione MC. DOTS expansion: will we reach the 2005 targets? *Int J Tuberc Lung Dis* 2004; **8**: 139–46.
12. Elzinga G, Raviglione MC, Maher D. Scale up: meeting targets in global tuberculosis control. *Lancet* 2004; **363**: 814–19.
13. World Health Organization. *Treatment of tuberculosis: guidelines for national programmes*, 3rd edn. Geneva: World Health Organization, 2003.
14. Global Alliance for TB Drug Development. *The economics of TB drug development*. New York: Global Alliance for TB Drug Development, 2001.
15. Kumaresan J, Smith I, Arnold V, Evans P. Global TB drug facility: innovative global procurement. *Int J Tuberc Lung Dis* 2004; **8**: 130–8.
16. Mukherjee JS, Rich ML, Socci AR et al. Programmes and principles in treatment of multidrug-resistant tuberculosis. *Lancet* 2004; **363**: 474–81.
17. Farmer P, Kim JY. Community based approaches to the control of multidrug resistant tuberculosis: introducing 'DOTS-Plus'. *BMJ* 1998; **317**: 671–4.
18. World Health Organization. *Guidelines for establishing DOTS-Plus pilot projects for the management of multidrug resistant tuberculosis (MDR-TB)*. Geneva: World Health Organization, 2000.
19. Sterling TR, Lehmann HP, Frieden TR. Impact of DOTS compared with DOTS-Plus on multidrug resistant tuberculosis and tuberculosis deaths: decision analysis. *BMJ* 2003; **326**: 574.
20. World Health Organization. *TB advocacy – a practical guide 1999*. Geneva: World Health Organization, 1998.
21. World Health Organization. *Guidelines for social mobilization: planning World TB Day*. Geneva: World Health Organization, 2000.

CHAPTER 14

Adherence to antituberculosis therapy

Introduction

Tuberculosis is largely curable if people with the disease have access to, and are able to adhere to, effective treatment regimens. As with many other diseases, adherence to therapy is beset with numerous difficulties and problems. The emergence of drug-resistant and multidrug-resistant tuberculosis has increased the complexity, toxicity and duration of therapy for such patients, who therefore face additional difficulties in adhering to therapy.

In this chapter we define the term adherence, discuss its importance in the management of tuberculosis, including drug-resistant and multidrug-resistant forms, explore the various factors that facilitate or prevent adherence to therapy by patients, and discuss the use of self-managed therapy and directly observed therapy. Finally, we discuss the approaches that can be used by nurses to assist patients to integrate the taking of their medicines into their everyday activities and to complete their courses of therapy.

Learning outcomes

After studying and reflecting on the material in this chapter, you will be able to:

- discuss with patients and their families the importance of adhering to antituberculosis therapy,
- identify factors in patients' everyday lives that may create barriers to successful adherence,
- assist patients in planning strategies to support and maintain adherence to therapy,
- discuss the appropriate advantages and disadvantages of self-managed therapy and directly observed therapy.

ADHERENCE AS A PARTNERSHIP

Historically, patients have been viewed as 'sleeping partners' in treatment decisions, and their inability to complete prescribed regimens of therapy has been described in the literature as non-compliance.[1] Compliance has been defined as 'the extent to which a person's behaviour (in terms of taking medications, following diets or executing lifestyle changes) coincides with medical or health advice'.[2] This model requires the patient to obey instructions, often without question, and failure to do so is considered to be obstructive or difficult behaviour. Non-compliance is therefore considered to arise from problems associated with the patient rather than from a responsibility that the healthcare providers must share.[3–6]

In recent times there has been a shift from paternalistic and authoritarian models to a partnership model in the approach taken by healthcare professionals to ensure that patients complete their treatment. Consequently it is now generally advocated that the term 'compliance' should be replaced with that of 'adherence', to indicate a greater collaborative involvement of patients in achieving the optimum therapeutic outcome.[7,8] In the UK, The Royal Pharmaceutical Society suggests the use of the term 'concordance' to define the therapeutic partnership.[9] It is felt that this term promotes a better understanding of the health beliefs of both the patient and the healthcare providers and an encouragement of 'the active exchange of information, negotiation and spirit of cooperation'.[10] In this context, the power of belief must never be underestimated. What may appear highly rational within a patient's personal or communal belief system may appear irrational or absurd to a health worker trained in so-called scientific medicine, and vice versa.

ADHERENCE TO THERAPY

Adherence to therapy in any chronic illness has a direct effect on the progression of disease and clinical outcome for the patient. In illnesses such as human immunodeficiency virus (HIV) disease, diabetes, renal failure, hypertension and rheumatoid arthritis, adherence to treatment is estimated to be between 20 and 80 per cent. Factors that are consistently associated with poor adherence include anxiety associated with taking medication, the impact of side effects, health beliefs, complexity of regimens and poor clinician–patient relationships.[11–16] In addition, some authors suggest that decisions by patients not to take medication or follow medical advice are efforts to maintain some level of control over their lives or to cope with illness in their own ways.[17,18] Studies in the USA indicate that adherence to self-administered antituberculosis medication varies from 82 per cent in the general population to 11 per cent among those who are homeless, mentally ill, or who misuse drugs.[19]

The duration of treatment, the need for several different drugs and the importance of therapy for curing patients and preventing transmission of tuberculosis to their families and the wider public make the support and encouragement of adherence to therapy a key issue in the patient's treatment plan. Directly Observed Therapy (DOT) is one of the five key components of the WHO DOTS (Directly Observed Therapy, Short Course) strategy, as discussed in the previous chapter. This is, however, the component that has given rise to the greatest amount of debate and dissonance, as many workers assert that inflexible DOT-based strategies may, under certain circumstances, be ineffective or even counterproductive.

Adherence to therapy is difficult to measure objectively and accurately. The methods used to determine adherence include self-reporting by the patient, estimates by the clinician, pill counts and checking prescription refills. More elaborate methods include the use of electronic devices that track the date and time when patients open and close their medicine containers. These methods make the assumption that reports or estimates are accurate, or that the patient has taken the medications that have been removed from the container. Adherence may also be measured by means of laboratory tests that evaluate blood or urine levels of drugs and these appear to give a more objective assessment of adherence. However, patients may display what is called 'white coat adherence' by taking their medications just before their clinic appointments but less regularly at other times. Alternatively, blood and urine drug levels may be low due to other factors such as impaired bioavailability or sub-optimal prescribing.

Poor adherence to antituberculosis therapy has serious clinical consequences for patients and for the health of the community, as it increases the risk of transmission of the tubercle bacillus.[20] In addition, if patients omit many doses, they may develop drug-resistant and even multidrug-resistant tuberculosis, with serious consequences for themselves and the community.

APPROACHES TO ANTITUBERCULOSIS THERAPY

There are two approaches currently employed in initiating and maintaining antituberculosis therapy. In self-managed therapy (SMT), as its name suggests, control of medication taking is placed with the patient, although it commonly involves support from a specialist nurse or other healthcare provider.

Directly observed therapy (DOT) is derived from the concept of 'entirely supervised administration of medicines', which was first widely applied to tuberculosis during the 1950s (although the question of who actually pioneered it is open to debate). Although the term 'directly observed therapy' implies 'supervised swallowing', the key to success is the establishment of an environment and level of support within which patients feel comfortable and willing to adhere to their treatment schedules. Thus in many countries that have adopted the WHO DOTS strategy, attendant interventions, such as removing socio-economic barriers, providing social support, housing, food tokens and transport vouchers, have proved to be of equal importance to the basic direct observation of therapy.[20–22]

BARRIERS TO ADHERENCE

In early research into adherence to treatment regimens in chronic diseases, attempts were made to identify predictors of adherence and non-adherence. However, these studies provided no evidence that socio-demographic, clinical or lifestyle factors constituted reliable predictors of non-adherence. The only consistent factor found across all studies is depressed mood.[23] For most people, the ability or intention to adhere to treatment regimens is affected by the circumstances of their daily lives. Adherence, or lack of it, is therefore dynamic, changing and varying within the life of an individual patient according to circumstances at given points in time.

Although not predictive of adherence levels, there are a number of factors that need to be considered by patients and clinicians in order to promote adherence, prevent further transmission of infection and cure the disease.

The antituberculosis regimen

Treatment recommendations are described in detail in Chapter 12 for both drug-sensitive and drug-resistant tuberculosis. In general, therapy for drug-susceptible disease lasts for 6 months, with four antituberculosis drugs being used in the intensive phase (first 2 months) and two drugs being used in the continuation phase. Regimens for drug-resistant tuberculosis are longer, generally 12–18 months, and require the use of second-line drugs that are more expensive, more toxic and more likely to cause troublesome adverse effects.

The number of pills that have to be swallowed every day has been identified as a barrier to successful adherence. In the case of drug-susceptible tuberculosis, this difficulty may be reduced by prescribing combination tablets, but patients with multidrug-resistant disease, for which there are fewer standardized regimens, still have to take many pills and therefore require considerable support and encouragement.

PATIENT CHARACTERISTICS

Important factors in adherence to antituberculosis therapy are the cultural backgrounds and health beliefs of the patients and their previous experiences or perceptions of medication. Research in rural South Africa suggests that, in some communities, there are beliefs that tuberculosis is a result of breaking cultural rules and that it can therefore only be treated successfully by traditional healers. People with little experience of modern Western healthcare systems may view healthcare professionals working within such systems, and the medicines they prescribe, with suspicion and distrust. This may prove to be a considerable barrier to the development of the type of partnership that is so important in supporting adherence to therapy. While not being proven predictors of non-adherence, the social and cultural norms of ethnic and immigrant communities need to be understood by healthcare providers so that they can modify their approaches to patients from these communities in ways that will lead to the development of a successful therapeutic partnership.[24,25]

There are suggestions in the literature that the intention of a patient to take medication is directly influenced by the perceived benefits and usefulness of the therapy. As outlined in Chapter 15, patients with HIV disease who are aware of their poor prognosis may see little point in being treated for tuberculosis. In addition, the capacity for self-care is a crucial determinant of the ability of people to follow treatment regimens.[19,24]

The only consistent predictors of poor adherence in the research literature, across many chronic conditions, are depressed mood and mental health problems. Although there is little information concerning the extent of co-morbidity of depression with tuberculosis, it is reasonable to assume that rates of depression in those with this disease are consistent with those in the general community, in which between 3 and 10 per cent of the population suffers from major depression. The symptoms of depression include lack of motivation, poor organization and difficulty in concentrating and remembering, all of which are important to the success of both SMT and DOT.

Social and emotional support is an important factor in ensuring adherence to therapy. The demographic profile of the tuberculosis epidemic in both industrially developed and resource-poor environments, and the increasing number of people with HIV co-infection, mean that many people may have limited social or family networks. The homeless have always been at particular risk of tuberculosis, and this lack of belonging together with an unstable environment create specific challenges for managing treatment adherence. The diagnosis of tuberculosis also carries considerable stigma, which is discussed in greater depth in the next chapter. The fear of being stigmatized and being noticed when taking medication by those outside immediate social networks causes many patients to abscond from therapy. Additional problems arise if members of their family are found to have latent tuberculosis and are, as is the practice in some regions, prescribed supervised preventive therapy.

While there is little consistent evidence that substance or alcohol misuse is a predictor of non-adherence, the chaotic lifestyle of many patients with these problems may increase the difficulties they face in taking medication correctly and on time and in keeping regular clinic appointments.

LEVELS OF KNOWLEDGE AND UNDERSTANDING

If treatment is to be based on the partnership approach discussed earlier in this chapter, it is essential that patients are equipped with the knowledge and understanding to participate in discussions and make individual decisions about the best approach to treatment for them. It is widely accepted that patients who are well informed are more likely to be adherent because they understand the reasoning behind treatment, are aware of the effects of medication, and appreciate the consequences of interrupting or stopping the regimen. Notwithstanding, even the most knowledgeable and well-informed person may forget to take, or may make an informed decision to miss, a particular dose of medication.

HEALTHCARE PROVIDER FACTORS

Many of the early studies into compliance focused on the behaviour and skills of patients, making the assumption that it was they who were 'at fault' when therapy failed. The shift towards partnership and concordance approaches has highlighted that the healthcare provider has clear responsibilities in facilitating adherence. The collaborative nature of treatment decisions is central to supporting adherence and ensuring what has been termed 'patient holding'.[26] The term 'holding' has several meanings (summarized in Table 14.1) and all are of relevance to the treatment of tuberculosis and need to be taken into account when organizing care for patients. Holding requires a degree of engagement between the healthcare provider and the patient that allows for open discussion and the flexibility to review and modify approaches throughout the treatment journey. In order to achieve this level of engagement, the healthcare provider needs to employ a range of interpersonal and clinical skills, including listening, being sensitive to the needs and limitations of the patient, developing an understanding of the patient's situation, avoiding misunderstandings by good communication skills, including the use of interpreters, being able to use a range of media to communicate information that is detailed yet understandable, and to recognize the patient as an equal partner in treatment decisions. Unfortunately, there have been many instances in which the arrogant and overbearing attitudes of physicians and other health workers in state-run health services have induced patients to seek care in the private sector, even though they could ill afford it, and where the prescription of highly inappropriate therapy is commonplace. The 'human touch' in the management of tuberculosis, and indeed of any disease, is so important yet so often overlooked.[27] It is also important that there is continuity of care so that expectations are consistent and experiences shared. There will, of course, always be a small number of patients who refuse treatment but, as a general rule, the quality of a health service is reflected in its ability to hold patients. Instances where patient holding fails should be fully investigated to facilitate the development of alternative and more effective approaches.

TABLE 14.1 Definitions of 'holding' in relation to tuberculosis care

Definition	Relevance to tuberculosis care
To 'keep or detain' a person	The Public Health Act in England can be used to detain people for health care, but this has been shown to be very difficult to administer with any success.
To 'remain secure, intact or in position without breaking or giving way'	Patients need to remain motivated to complete the full course of treatment. Good relationships with patients and a commitment to meeting their individual needs are essential. Supportive partnerships with other agencies must be developed to achieve this.
To 'contain or be capable of containing'	Staffing levels to match the caseload are required so that each patient can be cared for effectively. Proper support of staff is essential so that those requiring their services may have the best possible access to effective care.
To 'have in one's possession' implies the need to 'take responsibility for'	It cannot be assumed that patients are always able to take responsibility for their treatment, and the service has to take responsibility for ensuring that all patients are effectively treated.
To 'carry, support with one's arms' i.e. care for	Although treatment is standardized, care needs to be planned on an individual basis. Patients react differently to their diagnosis and have to make different adjustments to their daily lives. It is essential that each patient's cultural, social and economic circumstances are understood and that they are offered ongoing, accessible and appropriate support and information.

Adapted from Table 25.1 in reference 26.

THE NURSING ROLE IN SUPPORTING ADHERENCE TO ANTITUBERCULOSIS THERAPY

Nursing interventions to support and maintain adherence to antituberculosis therapy need to be available and should be used from the very beginning of the treatment of all patients. In the same way that adherence behaviour is multi-factorial and dynamic, approaches to supporting adherence need to be multi-focused and flexible in order to meet the diverse and often developing needs of individuals.

The nurse is ideally placed to support patients through many of the difficulties that occur during the course of treatment of tuberculosis. These include the decision-making process associated with selecting an SMT or DOT approach to therapy, identifying with patients how best to integrate medication taking into daily routines, providing advice and adjuvant therapy if side effects are experienced, and maintaining general physical and psychological support throughout the period of treatment. Nurses can also provide advice on accessing additional sources of information and support, including support groups, Internet resources, other members of the multi-disciplinary team and social services. While the priority for the healthcare provider may be to ensure that treatment is taken, patients may have a number of over-riding priorities that are of greater concern to them than their disease and hence their treatment. It is important to assess the patient's social and psychological situation and take steps to address these with the patient rather than focusing entirely on the treatment itself. This helps to develop trust and a rapport that enhances the sense of partnership between the healthcare provider and the patient.

ASSESSMENT OF PATIENTS

The concept of concordance and partnership in medication adherence requires an approach that allows a level of individual freedom to choose treatment approaches. In antituberculosis therapy, this choice is limited to some degree in view of the wider public health implications, but it is important that where choices can be made by patients, they are adequately equipped to make them. In order to tailor therapy to meet individual requirements, the nurse needs to have a detailed knowledge of the patient's clinical history, psychological state, lifestyle, health beliefs and available support mechanisms. This information needs to be collected systematically and recorded accurately so that potential barriers to adherence can be identified. Questions that are helpful in assessing patients' perceptions about their disease throughout the course of treatment and that may be used at particular points during treatment and repeated at follow-up visits are shown in Box 14.1.[24]

BOX 14.1 Taking a patient history

- What do you think causes tuberculosis?
- What problems will your illness cause you?
- Why do you think you got sick when you did?
- What does tuberculosis do to your body?
- How severe do you think your illness is?
- What treatment do you think you should receive for tuberculosis?
- What are the most important results you hope to receive from this treatment?
- What are the main problems your illness has caused you?
- What do you fear about your illness?
- How do your family members or close friends feel about your illness?

PROMOTING KNOWLEDGE AND UNDERSTANDING

As outlined above, the knowledge and understanding of the patient are the foundation of all subsequent strategies to support adherence to antituberculosis therapy, and information enables them to participate in the decision-making process and to take responsibility for their choices. Information can be provided in a range of formats and media in order to facilitate understanding and involvement. In immigrant and ethnic populations, it may be necessary to provide information in an appropriate language. While interpreters can be helpful in getting information across in the clinic or home setting, it is always advisable to have information in a written format in an appropriate language so that elements that may be lost in translation or misinterpreted can be clarified. This may entail harnessing the assistance of community groups to ensure that material takes account of cultural and linguistic factors and uses images that are appropriate and acceptable to the patients. Providing information in a variety of formats will help to reinforce messages and can be useful in providing material for discussion and assessing the understanding of the requirements of therapy.

HELPING PATIENTS TO REMEMBER MEDICATION

If patients choose to manage their therapy themselves, it is essential that their healthcare providers closely support them over the first few weeks of therapy in order to assist them to anticipate some of the problems they may face. Many patients state that they simply forget to take medications at certain times. This tendency can be reduced by a process of identifying 'cues' that help to remind them to take their medications at the correct time, thereby overcoming unintentional non-adherence. Cues involve linking the taking of medication to everyday objects or routine behaviours, which vary considerably from region to region and from culture to culture. In an industrially developed country, such cues might be making the first cup of tea in the morning, going to the bathroom, watching particular television programmes or letting the dog out last thing at night. The aim of cueing is to remind the patient to take the medication before carrying out the associated routine. This is clearly far more difficult in patients who may be homeless or who have chaotic lifestyles associated with drug and alcohol abuse.

ORGANIZING MEDICATION

Making medications easily accessible at the correct time of day is one of the practical problems faced by patients. Strategies to help the organization of medications include the provision of daily or weekly dosset boxes that allow the various pills to be taken at the appropriate time without having to negotiate two or three different medication containers. Developing routines associated with organizing medications, such as filling dosset boxes each night or at the beginning of each week, may help some patients adhere better to treatment.

Watch alarms or bleeps can act as reminders to take medications, and some medication containers have built-in alarms. This strategy can be particularly useful for the difficult to remember dose or doses that patients identify as being inconvenient in the normal pattern of their daily lives. Using medication reminder charts makes patients aware of their medication-taking behaviour and they reveal which doses are most likely to be missed. The latter is important, as it may help to determine patterns of missed doses that will help patients and clinicians to develop strategies for overcoming problems. Nurses can also advise on planning ahead for disruptions to daily routines such as social events (religious festivals, weddings and funerals), travel and return to employment.

ADHERENCE PROGRAMMES: DIRECTLY OBSERVED THERAPY

For many patients, a DOT approach may be the most effective method of establishing and maintaining therapy, particularly if the patient is homeless, abuses drugs or alcohol, has mental illness or impairment, is a child or adolescent or has previously found it difficult to adhere to SMT programmes. The concept of DOT as simply consisting of supervised swallowing is not reflected in the literature. The majority of DOT approaches involve a comprehensive set of services delivered by a multi-disciplinary team that include providing clinic appointments that do not disrupt the patient's employment or domestic duties, identifying and supplying voluntary workers and other enablers who encourage patients to attend the clinic and take their medications, take steps to reduce barriers to adherence and provide assistance with housing and finance.[24,28] In fact, these attendant enhancements make it difficult to assess the specific effectiveness of the directly observed component of the overall DOTS strategy.[21,22] In order for DOT to be successful, it is essential that the healthcare provider and the patient are in agreement about the number of visits required as well as the schedule and location of appointments. If a clinic location cannot be agreed on, the healthcare provider must go to the patient in order to deliver DOT. In some regions, DOT workers may be volunteers from the community, such as locally selected women who also have other health-related duties, local religious leaders and storekeepers. A very good example is the programme developed by BRAC, a non-governmental organization in rural Bangaldesh.[29]

DIRECTLY OBSERVED THERAPY VERSUS SELF-MANAGED THERAPY

It should be noted that DOT is the method advocated by the WHO and forms a key part of the DOTS strategy, with which it is often confused. A valid and important argument in support of DOT is that rifampicin is such a valuable drug that stringent measures must be adopted to prevent resistance to it arising. On the other hand, it is important to bear in mind that the world is a very diverse place and that tuberculosis services vary enormously in their quality and their very nature. Several authors have warned about the dangers of dogmatism in tuberculosis control. As outlined in the previous chapter, the WHO DOTS strategy, although being adopted to an ever-increasing degree, was in the year 2004 only available to a third of all tuberculosis patients. While DOT has formed the basis of a number of highly successful control programmes, other studies indicate that this approach may not be the optimal one in all situations. A study in South Africa, for example, revealed that DOT was no better than SMT – indeed, it was slightly, though not significantly, worse.[22] While most authorities are fully supportive of the overall WHO DOTS strategy and acknowledge the very real benefits that have accrued in regions where it has been adopted, many are of the opinion that there is an ongoing need for great flexibility and the evidence-based tailoring of therapeutic strategies to local regions and to individual patients. It must be realized that there are enormous differences in the ability of different populations and, even more so, of different people within populations to access and adhere to curative therapy.[30]

SOCIAL SUPPORT

In addition to formal clinics or structured programmes, it is important to make use of the existing social support networks available to patients. Encouraging patients to involve partners, family members, religious leaders and personal friends in providing practical and informational support can improve adherence to therapy. Practical support may involve providing reminders or checking that medications have been organized correctly. If patients lack established social networks, the use of patients who have been through the experience of treatment for tuberculosis may help to support them through the initial stages of therapy, while structured group programmes may provide the opportunity to construct more supportive networks for themselves. In the tuberculosis control programme run by BRAC in rural Bangladesh, patients or their relatives are required to make a small payment as a bond, which is refunded with interest if treatment is successfully completed. This has been found to act as an incentive to adhere to therapy.[29]

ONGOING MONITORING AND SUPPORT

It is important to check with patients on a regular basis that they are taking their medication on time and in the correct dose. Questions that enable patients to self-report on their own progress should be built in to every interaction with their healthcare provider. This offers patients the opportunity to discuss any difficulties they may be having and, if necessary, to explore the options for switching from SMT to DOT or vice versa. Research shows that patients often find it difficult to remember accurately their behaviour beyond the previous 7 days and it is therefore important that healthcare providers ask questions about taking medications over the past week. Questions such as 'What did you do on Saturday? Did that interfere with how you took your tablets?' can help to prompt patients' memories. In addition to self-report approaches, the measurement of drug levels or detecting the presence of a drug by means of urine tests can be a useful indicator of adherence. As the prime aims of therapy and adherence to it are to cure the patient with attendant alleviation of symptoms and, in the case of open pulmonary tuberculosis, to achieve sputum smear conversion from positive to negative, it is important to provide patients with feedback about their progress and keep them up to date with laboratory results. This will enhance motivation and provide positive reinforcement that they are succeeding in their efforts to adhere.

Summary

Adherence to antituberculosis medication is essential if treatment is to cure patients, reduce the development of drug resistance and protect the community from infection. Although a number of factors contribute to poor adherence, the only factor that is consistently predictive of non-adherence is depression. Within the constraints of wider public health issues, it is crucial that patients are fully informed and involved in deciding the best strategy for curing their infection. The use of SMT or DOT provides a choice for patients if they have insight into the barriers that they may face in adhering to medication regimens, although, for certain patient groups, some form of DOT is required. Nurses need to make an accurate assessment of the barriers and supports to adherence with individual patients and develop treatment plans that will sustain motivation and increase case holding. The use of DOT and interventions such as integrating treatment into daily activities, making medications accessible in the correct dose and at the right time and providing ongoing peer or healthcare provider support will assist in the establishment and sustainability of SMT adherence behaviours. Nurses also need to create a climate of trust and collaboration with patients, so that reasons for non-adherence can be monitored and clinical management can be modified where possible when adhering to regimens is problematic or has an impact on the patient's quality of life. These approaches will help to build a partnership approach to adherence to antituberculosis medication that is crucial to the global management of the tuberculosis pandemic.

Prologue to the next chapter

This chapter has given an insight into the numerous factors that stand in the way of the patient with tuberculosis and his or her cure. Unfortunately, societal attitudes are among the greatest yet most insidious of the numerous factors that operate to deny a patient a return to health. In particular, patients with tuberculosis are often victims of stigma, which, in addition to causing much psychological suffering, can deny patients their basic human rights and their ability to access and complete effective treatment. Indeed, stigma may even prevent the establishment of health services orientated to the needs of such patients. Overcoming the very prevalent attitudes based on fear and ignorance that lead to stigma and its tragic consequences is a very great challenge to all those involved in tuberculosis control in all parts of the world and in all communities, both wealthy and poor. Stigma is therefore the topic of the next chapter.

REFERENCES

1. Addington W. Patient compliance: the most serious remaining problem in the control of tuberculosis in the United States. *Chest* 1979; **76**: 741–3.
2. Dunbar Jacob J, Erlen JA, Schlenk EA et al. Adherence in chronic disease. *Annu Rev Nurs Res* 2000; **18**: 48–90.
3. Haynes RB. Introduction. In Haynes RB, Taylor DW, Sackett DC (eds), *Compliance in health care*. Baltimore: Johns Hopkins University Press, 1979, i–iv.
4. Varni JW, Wallander JL. Adherence to health-related regimes in paediatric chronic disorders. *Clin Psychol Rev* 1984; **4**: 585–96.
5. Donovan JCL, Blake DR. Patient non-compliance: deviance or reasoned decision-making. *Soc Sci Med* 1992; **34**: 507–13.
6. Stimson G. Obeying doctors orders: a view from the other side. *Soc Sci Med* 1975; **8**: 97–104.
7. Sumartojo E. When tuberculosis treatment fails. A social behavioral account of patient adherence. *Am Rev Respir Dis* 1993; **147**: 1311–20.
8. Ogden JA. Compliance versus adherence: just a matter of language? The politics and poetics of public health. In Porter JDH, Grange JM (eds), *Tuberculosis – an interdisciplinary perspective*. London: Imperial College Press, 1999, 213–33.
9. Royal Pharmaceutical Society. *From compliance to concordance: achieving shared goals in medicine taking*. London: Royal Pharmaceutical Society, 1996.
10. Mullen PD. Compliance becomes concordance. *BMJ* 1997; **314**: 691–2.
11. Eraker SA, Kirscht JP, Becker MH. Understanding and improving adherence. *Ann Intern Med* 1984; **100**: 258–68.
12. Meichenbaum D, Turk DC. *Facilitating treatment adherence*. New York: Plenum Press, 1987, 19–39.
13. DiMatteo MR, Friedman HS. Patient cooperation with treatment. In *Social psychology and medicine*. Cambridge, MA: Oelgeschlager, Gunn and Hain Publishers; 1982, 35–58.
14. Paterson DL, Swindells S, Mohr J et al. Adherence to protease inhibitor therapy and outcomes in patients with HIV infection. *Ann Intern Med* 2000; **133**: 21–30.
15. Altice FL, Friedland GH. The era of adherence to HIV therapy. *Ann Intern Med* 1998; **129**: 503–5.
16. Hecht F, Colfax G, Swanson M, Chesney MA. Adherence and effectiveness of protease inhibitors in clinical practice. Paper presented at the 5th Conference on Retroviruses and Opportunistic Infections, February 2–6 1998, Chicago, Illinois.
17. Samet JH, Libman H, Steger KA, Rajeev K. Adherence with zidovudine therapy in patients infected with human immunodeficiency virus, type 1: a cross-sectional study in a municipal hospital clinic. *Am J Med* 1992; **92**: 495–502.
18. Conrad P. The meaning of medications: another look at adherence. *Soc Sci Med* 1985; **20**: 29–37.
19. McDonnell M, Turner J, Weaver MT. Antecedents of adherence to antituberculosis therapy. *Public Health Nurs* 2001; **18**: 392–400.
20. Hill AR, Manikal VM, Riska PF. Effectiveness of directly observed therapy (DOT) for tuberculosis. *Medicine* 2002; **81**: 179–93.
21. Volmink J, Garner P. Systematic review of randomised control trials of strategies to promote adherence to tuberculosis treatment. *BMJ* 1997; **315**: 1403–6.
22. Volmink J, Matchaba P, Garner P. Directly observed therapy and treatment adherence. *Lancet* 2000; **355**: 1345–50.

23. Dunbar Jacob J, Burke LE, Puczynski S. Clinical assessment and management of adherence to medical regimens. In: Nicassio PM, Smith TW (eds), *Managing chronic illness*. Washington, DC: American Psychological Society, 1998, 313–49.
24. Centers for Disease Control. *Improving patient adherence to tuberculosis treatment*. Available at <www.cdc.gov/nchstp/tb/pubs/adherence.htm>.
25. Edington ME, Sekante CS, Goldstein SJ. Patients' beliefs: do they affect tuberculosis control? A study of a rural district of South Africa. *Int J Tuberc Lung Dis* 2002; **6**: 1075–82.
26. Williams G. Patient holding. In Davies PDO (ed.), *Clinical tuberculosis*, 3rd edn. London: Arnold, 2003, 427–35.
27. Chaisson RE, Barnes GL, Hackman J et al. A randomised controlled trial of interventions to improve adherence to isoniazid therapy to prevent tuberculosis in injection drug users. *Am J Med* 2001; **110**: 610–15.
28. Grange JM. DOTS and beyond. Towards a holistic approach to the conquest of tuberculosis. *Int J Tuberc Lung Dis* 1997; **1**: 293–6.
29. Chowdhury AMR, Chowdhury SA, Islam MN et al. Control of tuberculosis through community health workers in Bangladesh. *Lancet* 1997; **350**: 160–72.
30. Farmer P. Social scientists and the new tuberculosis. *Soc Sci Med* 1997; **44**: 347–58.

CHAPTER 15

The stigma of tuberculosis

Introduction

Many problems and difficulties affect the general welfare of patients with tuberculosis and compromise their ability to obtain medical care and to complete a course of treatment. Among the most insidious and damaging of these are the various manifestations of stigma that are widespread throughout the world. The word stigma means 'a distinguishing mark of social disgrace'. Its origin is obscure, but it is thought to date from the time when thieves and other criminals in the Roman Empire were branded on their foreheads as a perpetual sign of their disgrace. The stigma of leprosy is well known and is, in part, associated with the characteristic recognizable physical deformities caused by this disease. Although tuberculosis is rarely the cause of obvious physical deformity, those afflicted often meet with very negative societal attitudes, which add greatly to their suffering. In some regions, the actual and perceived link between tuberculosis and human immunodeficiency virus (HIV) has added a new stigmatizing factor.

Learning outcomes

After studying and reflecting on the material in this chapter, you will be able to:

- describe the nature of stigma associated with tuberculosis and its adverse impact on patients,
- describe the groups of patients who are particularly adversely affected by stigma,
- discuss how stigma may be overcome or minimized in various situations.

THE NATURE AND IMPACT OF STIGMA

Stigma may affect the patient adversely at all stages of the disease – treatment seeking, diagnosis and adherence to therapy – and may persist long after a complete cure.[1] It may also prevent the establishment and maintenance of effective tuberculosis control services as societies may not want to acknowledge the extent, or even the existence, of the disease in their midst.[2]

Tuberculosis is prevalent in populations such as ethnic minority groups, the poor, homeless, 'travellers', prisoners and other institutionalized people already bearing the stigma of social disadvantage and marginalization.[3] These patients often fall victim to what Paul Farmer, a distinguished public health authority, has termed 'structural violence' – the combination of societal features that prevent them from accessing health care and adhering to therapy.[4] Farmer has noted that, 'Throughout the world, those least likely to comply (with therapy) are those least able to comply'. Although such despicable racist views as those of John Haycraft, who, in 1895, praised the tubercle bacillus as a 'friend of our race' because it exterminated the 'underclass', are unlikely to be expressed openly today, they may still be held covertly. As a consequence, tuberculosis is not likely to be given the attention it requires until those who have control over healthcare provision perceive themselves or their political interests to be at risk.[2]

In recent years, the actual or perceived link of tuberculosis with human immunodeficiency virus (HIV) disease has accentuated the stigma in some regions,[5] and this has led to delays in seeking treatment for tuberculosis and to poor adherence to therapy.[6] Patients with HIV disease may conclude that, as their prognosis is bleak, there is no point in adhering to treatment of tuberculosis. Thus such patients are significantly less likely to complete a course of antituberculosis therapy than those not infected by HIV.[7] In addition, healthcare providers may conclude that, as the patients will die of HIV disease, treatment of their tuberculosis is a waste of resources.

The attitudes that generate stigma are usually linked to local belief systems concerning the cause, nature and prognosis of the disease.[1] Some beliefs about the cause of tuberculosis are fairly widespread and include 'germs', alcoholism, nutritional factors, heredity, moral degeneration, curses, karma and divine retribution. Other beliefs are restricted to certain local communities. In a rural district of South Africa, for example, there is a strong belief that tuberculosis is the result of breaking cultural rules that demand abstinence from sex after the death of a family member and after a woman has had a miscarriage.[8] A widespread cause of stigma is the correct belief that the disease is transmissible coupled with the incorrect one that it is incurable. Stigma may affect the patient's family in regions where it is believed that tuberculosis is hereditary, is the result of living in a dirty household or is caused by a curse. Stigma may also be enhanced when a disease is used as a metaphor for some ill in society, although in this respect tuberculosis acquired a somewhat 'romantic' image, especially in Victorian art and literature.[9]

As a consequence of stigma, a diagnosis of tuberculosis may be met with shock, denial, disgust, fear and anger. Shock may prevent patients from fully understanding explanations given to them about their disease and its treatment and it may also induce them to 'shop around' for an alternative diagnosis. Fear and disgust lead to denial, which, in turn, may lead to poor adherence to therapy. Anger may well be directed against the healthcare providers. The authors know of a chest physician in London who was threatened with legal proceedings because she told an 'upper-class' person that he had tuberculosis – a diagnosis that he considered out of the question on account of his social status!

A study in India revealed that the social stigma associated with tuberculosis is the cause of severe psychological disturbances that affect the personal, familial, occupational and social aspects of the lives of many patients.[10] As described in Chapter 5, such psychological stress could, by stimulating excess corticosteroid production, inhibit protective immune responses and enhance tissue-destroying ones.

The effects of stigma are particularly harmful to women (see below) and young people. The Indonesian newspaper the *Jakarta Post* (24th November 2003) carried the story of a boy who, on returning to school after successful therapy, was treated with such disgust and fear that he stopped going to school: 'Once I had this dream of becoming an engineer. Now I no longer have any dreams'.

In addition, 'self-stigma' is widespread and patients often suffer from a deep sense of shame. The edition of the *Jakarta Post* referred to above cited a 41-year-old mother who stated, 'What is killing me is not the tuberculosis but all these feelings of fear and shame because I have this disease'. Another patient reported that she was shocked to learn that she had tuberculosis and so great was her shame that she travelled to another city to obtain treatment. Even in countries such as the USA where many patients understand tuberculosis in medical terms, they may perceive themselves as vectors of the disease and, in one study, almost all patients felt that their friends and even their family shunned them. In response to this, the patients isolated themselves and became secretive about their illness. Thus, nurses may be required to consider and address community attitudes in the industrially developed nations as well as in the developing ones.[11]

ETHNIC MINORITIES

In many of the industrially developed nations, tuberculosis is relatively more common in ethnic minority populations who have migrated from countries where there is a high incidence of the disease. Patients in ethnic minority groups often delay seeking medical attention and fail to adhere to treatment, and in many cases these problems are due to social and cultural factors.[4,12,13] As discussed below, women are particularly vulnerable. An understanding of the social and cultural dimensions of disease is essential for overcoming ignorance, fear and stigma. Also, good communication and mutual trust and respect between the patients and their healthcare providers are essential. Indeed, a failure of health workers to understand the cultural differences in attitudes towards tuberculosis and its treatment may inadvertently lead to an enhancement of stigma, mistrust and a failure to adhere to treatment. Good communication poses problems if the patients and staff do not speak each other's languages, and the use of interpreters, especially members of their extended families, may deny patients their right to privacy. In the UK, this problem has to some extent been overcome by the use of Language Line, a service that provides a three-way communication by telephone between the patient, healthcare provider and an interpreter.[14,15]

The need to reach a greater understanding of the specific problems faced by those in the various ethnic minorities has led to the establishment of the discipline of Transcultural Medicine by a London physician, Dr Bashir Qureshi.[13]

GENDER-RELATED ISSUES

Women's health issues have largely focused on reproductive events, and relatively little attention has been paid to infectious diseases, including tuberculosis.[16] The small amount of research has, however, revealed important gender-related differences in treatment seeking and adherence to therapy for infectious diseases in general. Leprosy and filariasis, both of which may cause disfigurement, have particularly adverse consequences for women, as they seriously reduce their chance of marriage and may lead to their separation from their families. This fear of loss and ostracism is a strong barrier to treatment seeking. More surprisingly, women are also less likely than men to seek treatment for non-disfiguring tropical diseases such as malaria and tuberculosis. This may be due, in part, to differences in ease of access to healthcare services, but fear of loss is also prominent. Unmarried women with tuberculosis, even after its successful treatment, fear that they will never become marriage partners or be employable, and married women fear divorce or enforced separation from their husbands and children.[17] The marriage prospects of healthy women from households in which there is a member with tuberculosis may be reduced in those regions where it is believed that the disease is hereditary.

Worldwide, tuberculosis is the leading cause of death of women in the age range 15–44, the age at which they are having children and bringing up their families.[18] The death of a woman in this age range often has serious social consequences by creating orphans and generating great hardship for families. The very fact that women are raising families may cause them to delay seeking medical attention and to adhere less well than men to treatment. Accordingly, they are more likely than men to die of the disease.

Women in ethnic minorities in industrially developed countries face particular problems in accessing health care.[14,15] In the East End of London, for example, many female tuberculosis patients are of Indian subcontinent ethnic origin and many have recently arrived in the country. In some communities, women find it very difficult to seek medical attention, or even to leave their homes, unless accompanied by a male relative. Furthermore, they often speak little or no English and, accordingly, male relatives often have to serve as interpreters, thereby denying these patients their right of privacy, especially as they may be anxious to conceal the diagnosis of a stigma-bearing disease from their extended families. The use of the Language Line service mentioned above has greatly helped to alleviate this difficulty.

OVERCOMING STIGMA

It is essential that healthcare workers, whether physicians, nurses or voluntary workers, should look beyond the disease and see the patient, for whom the signs and symptoms of tuberculosis may be just part of a complex pattern of 'dis-ease'. The quality of health services, particularly as perceived by the patients, and the friendliness and attentiveness of staff can have an enormous beneficial impact on overall well-being as well as on the successful completion of treatment. In rural South Africa, adherence to therapy was greatly enhanced by voluntary workers who were able to gain the respect and trust of the patients.[19] It has been emphasized that all healthcare providers should act as 'destigmatizers' and that training in social skills is required.[17]

Unfortunately, negative attitudes may be enhanced and compounded by insensitive and inappropriate conduct and attitudes of health workers. An extreme example is of workers in one community health centre who refused to collect sputum from patients with tuberculosis for fear that they too would be infected. Even when healthcare workers take a personal interest in patients and give them advice, this may reflect false belief systems that are very similar to those held by the patients and which may therefore reinforce them. In some cases, the cultural or class distance between patients and their healthcare providers may result in insensitive and harmful comments and attitudes. Case conferences on the stigmatizing and other negative factors encountered by patients facilitate the development of strategies to overcome them and enable healthcare providers to evaluate critically their own attitudes, assumptions and prejudices.

Community involvement can do much to reduce stigma and other factors that create barriers to effective tuberculosis control. Mere education on the nature of tuberculosis and its curability does not necessarily reduce stigma and enhance adherence to therapy. Indeed, explaining the infectious nature of the disease may, as mentioned above, enhance self-stigma, as people may perceive themselves to be vectors of the disease. It is therefore essential that education is based on local surveys of attitudes towards the disease. Many different members of the community can provide psychological and practical support to patients to complete their treatment and, ideally, this aspect of patient care should involve or be instigated by the patients themselves.[20]

In a region of Ethiopia, patients are encouraged to form 'TB clubs'.[21] The members of these clubs elect leaders from their number who arrange supervision of therapy and check for adverse effects of the drugs. The clubs also disseminate information concerning tuberculosis within the local communities. As a result, social ostracism and stigma previously experienced by patients have been largely overcome, while patient attendance for treatment has increased from 68 to 98 per cent. Passive case detection, defaulter tracing, case notification and involvement of the community in general health care have all substantially improved.

There is, however, no single strategy that will overcome the blight of stigma. Techniques that work well in one region may be useless or worse than useless in another. Initiatives and innovations must therefore be based on careful sociological research at the local level. While cultural factors play a central role in determining the impact of tuberculosis control programmes, the provision of caring, locally respected and, above all, highly effective treatment is of even greater importance. If the community sees that patients are readily and permanently cured of tuberculosis, and that the prevalence of the disease is rapidly diminishing, negative attitudes quickly change. Accordingly, the control of tuberculosis must be based on the implementation of both the global DOTS-based control strategy (see Chapter 13) and interventions carefully tailored for the local community.

Summary

Stigma in its various forms has a deleterious effect on patients with tuberculosis, leading to delays in diagnosis and poor adherence to therapy, and on the overall quality of their lives and the effectiveness of healthcare services. The families of the patients may also be adversely affected, and the problem is especially serious for ethnic minority groups and women. Overcoming stigma is central to effective tuberculosis control, requiring, on the part of healthcare providers, an understanding of the social and cultural aspects of the disease, the ability to communicate clearly and the incentive to educate the patients, their families and the community. Probably the best antidote to stigma is the establishment of effective and user-friendly treatment services so that the community sees that patients are successfully and permanently cured.

Prologue to the next chapter

In the previous chapters we considered the basic scientific principles of antituberculosis therapy and the steps being taken by the World Health Organization and other agencies to ensure that therapy will not be denied to any person suffering from this disease. We then considered one of the central components of tuberculosis control – namely, the support of the patients to ensure that they complete their courses of therapy. The many factors, including stigma, that may prevent patients accessing health care and completing therapy were discussed. In the next chapter, we move on to consider the practicalities of establishing health services able to respond effectively to the needs of the community so that patients with symptoms suggestive of tuberculosis present for diagnosis and are supported throughout their treatment. In particular we will consider the key role of the nurse in the effective functioning of these health services.

REFERENCES

1. Rangan S, Uplekar M. Socio-cultural dimensions in tuberculosis control. In Porter JDH, Grange JM (eds), *Tuberculosis – an interdisciplinary perspective*. London: Imperial College Press, 1999, 265–81.
2. Zumla A, Grange JM. Establishing a united front against the injustice of tuberculosis. *Int J Tuberc Lung Dis* 1998; **2**: 179–81.
3. Grange JM, Story A, Zumla A. Tuberculosis in disadvantaged groups. *Curr Opin Pulm Med* 2001; **7**: 160–4.
4. Farmer P. Social scientists and the new tuberculosis. *Soc Sci Med* 1997; **44**: 347–58.
5. Godfrey-Faussett P, Ayles H. Can we control tuberculosis in high HIV prevalence settings? *Tuberculosis (Edinb)* 2003; **83**: 68–76.
6. Ngamvithayapong J, Winkvist A, Divan V. High AIDS awareness may cause tuberculosis patient delay: results from an HIV epidemic area, Thailand. *AIDS* 2000; **14**: 1413–19.
7. Ustianowski A, Mwaba P, Zumla A. Tuberculosis and HIV – perspectives from sub-Saharan Africa. In Porter JDH, Grange JM (eds), *Tuberculosis – an interdisciplinary perspective*. London: Imperial College Press, 1999, 283–311.
8. Edginton ME, Sekatane CS, Goldstein SJ. Patients' beliefs: do they affect tuberculosis control? A study in a rural district of South Africa. *Int J Tuberc Lung Dis* 2002; **6**: 1075–82.
9. Sontag S. *Illness as metaphor* and *AIDS and its metaphors*. London: Penguin, 1991.
10. Bhatia MS, Bhasin SK, Dubey KK. Psychosocial dysfunction in tuberculosis patients. *Indian J Med Sci* 2000; **54**: 171–3.
11. Kelly P. Isolation and stigma: the experience of patients with active tuberculosis. *J Community Health Nurs* 1999; **16**: 233–41.
12. Rubel AJ, Garro LC. Social and cultural factors in the successful control of tuberculosis. *Public Health Rep* 1992; **107**: 626–36.
13. Qureshi B. *Transcultural medicine. Dealing with patients from different cultures*. Dordrecht: Kluwer Academic, 1989.
14. Grange JM, Festenstein F. The human dimension of tuberculosis control. *Tuber Lung Dis* 1993; **74**: 219–22.

15. Festenstein F, Grange JM. Tuberculosis in ethnic minority populations in industrialised countries. In Porter JDH, Grange JM (eds), *Tuberculosis – an interdisciplinary perspective*. London: Imperial College Press, 1999, 313–38.
16. Diwan V, Thorson A, Winkvist A (eds). *Gender and tuberculosis – an international research workshop*. Göteborg: The Nordic School of Public Health, 1998.
17. Liefooghe R, Michiels N, Habib S et al. Perceptions and social consequences of tuberculosis: a focus group study of tuberculosis patients in Sialkot, Pakistan. *Soc Sci Med* 1995; **41**: 1685–92.
18. Hudelson P. Gender differentials in tuberculosis: the role of socio-economic and cultural factors. *Tuber Lung Dis* 1996; **77**: 391–400.
19. Westaway MS, Conradie PW, Remmers L. Supervised out-patient treatment for tuberculosis: evaluation of a South African rural programme. *Tubercle* 1991; **72**: 140–4.
20. Hadley M, Maher D. Community involvement in tuberculosis control: lessons from other health care programmes. *Int J Tuberc Lung Dis* 2000; **4**: 401–8.
21. Getahun H. Partners against tuberculosis: Ethiopia's 'TB clubs'. *Afr Health* 1998; **21**: 20.

FURTHER READING

Ali SS, Rabbani F, Siddiqui UN et al. Tuberculosis: do we know enough? A study of patients and their families in an out-patient hospital setting in Karachi, Pakistan. *Int J Tuberc Lung Dis* 2003; **7**: 1052–8.

Blinkhoff P, Bukanga E, Syamalevwe B, Williams G. *Under the Mupundu tree. Volunteers in home care for people with HIV/AIDS and TB in Zambia's copperbelt*. Strategies for Hope Series, No. 14. London: Actionaid, 1999.

Liefooghe R, Baliddawa JB, Kipruto EM et al. From their own perspective: a Kenyan community's perception of tuberculosis. *Trop Med Int Health* 1997; **2**: 809–21.

Westaway MS, Wolmarans L. Cognitive and affective reactions of black urban South Africans towards tuberculosis. *Tuber Lung Dis* 1994; **75**: 447–53.

CHAPTER 16

The contribution of nurses to tuberculosis control – a public health perspective

Introduction

The principal aim of tuberculosis control is to reduce the pool of infection in the community, thereby preventing the spread of the disease. This can be achieved by identifying people with infectious disease (active cases) early and ensuring that they complete a full and effective course of treatment. This in turn will both cure them and render them non-infectious. There are a variety of methods used to identify people with tuberculosis and these are discussed in this chapter, along with additional preventive measures. The care of patients being treated for tuberculosis is discussed in the following two chapters.

Before implementing any active screening measures or starting an education campaign to encourage people with signs and symptoms suggestive of active tuberculosis to come forward for testing, it is essential that a health service is equipped to respond effectively. The care of patients with tuberculosis may be organized by specialist TB teams or be fully integrated into the department of chest medicine or infectious diseases or, indeed, into general primary care. The term 'health service' is used to refer to any of these circumstances.

If a health service is effective only at case finding but lacks the facilities to monitor and support patients for the duration of their treatment, there is a significant risk that they will receive incomplete or incorrect treatment. This, in turn, may well result in progressive ill-health, continuing infectiousness and the development of drug-resistant tuberculosis.

Learning outcomes

After studying and reflecting on the material in this chapter, you will be able to:

- discuss the measures available to prevent the spread of tuberculosis,
- prioritize different preventive measures,
- describe the roles and responsibilities of nurses working in diverse settings in relation to tuberculosis control.

A variety of guidelines are available to facilitate the development of national, regional and local strategies for the prevention and control of tuberculosis, including those published by the Joint Tuberculosis Committee of the British Thoracic Society (BTS),[1] a number available from the Centers for Disease Control and Prevention (CDC) in the USA (see 'Internet resources' at the end of the chapter), and, especially important, the World Health Organization (WHO), whose guidance forms the basis of tuberculosis control in many countries,[2] especially those in the developing world (see Chapter 13). These and other authoritative guidelines provide advice on the important public health measures essential for tuberculosis control, as listed in Box 16.1.

BOX 16.1 The most important measures that can be taken to control the spread of tuberculosis

- Prompt diagnosis and treatment of active cases (passive case finding)
- Notification of all cases
- Caring support of all patients on treatment
- Isolation of known and suspected infectious cases in in-patient settings
- Screening of high-risk groups (active case finding)
- Outbreak management
- Treatment of latent tuberculosis infection
- Administration of BCG vaccination
- Monitoring of the efficacy of control activities and rectification of weaknesses

PROMPT DIAGNOSIS AND TREATMENT OF ACTIVE CASES (PASSIVE CASE FINDING)

A case of tuberculosis is defined as a patient with symptomatic disease due to infection with a member of the *Mycobacterium tuberculosis* complex. There are two approaches to identifying cases: passive and active case finding.

Passive case finding refers to the diagnosis of tuberculosis among patients who present to health services with symptoms. It is considered to be very cost effective and forms the basis of case detection strategies in most parts of the world. In low-prevalence countries such as the UK, it is recommended that this should be the principal method for the detection of cases of tuberculosis, although some active case finding (discussed below) occurs through the screening of high-risk groups.[3]

The sooner patients with tuberculosis are diagnosed, the sooner they will be able to start treatment, which will rapidly lead to an improvement in their condition and render those with open tuberculosis non-infectious (see Chapter 12). There are a number of factors relating to both the health service and the patient that may slow the process down, and the most common of these are discussed below.

Signs and symptoms

The diagnosis of tuberculosis is often difficult because its symptoms may mimic other conditions such as a chest infection, pneumonia and carcinoma. The resulting delay in diagnosis and treatment leads to patients with open pulmonary tuberculosis remaining infectious for longer (see Chapter 4). This is a common cause of outbreaks in both the community and the hospital.[4] In addition to this, patients with any form of tuberculosis will suffer more extensive damage as the disease progresses and some will die. It is essential, therefore, that all healthcare workers are aware of the signs and symptoms of the disease (Table 16.1) as well as being familiar with the level of tuberculosis in their community and how it is managed by local services. This in turn will lead to a reasonable level of suspicion and the appropriate referral of suspect cases.

TABLE 16.1 Symptoms of tuberculosis

Pulmonary	General
Productive or dry cough for 3 weeks or more	Weight loss
Localized chest pain	Night sweats
Breathlessness	Fever
Haemoptysis	Lethargy
	Fatigue
	Pain at affected area
	Loss of appetite

Patient anxiety

By the time those with suspected tuberculosis arrive at healthcare facilities they will already have realized that they have a problem and will have decided to seek help. If they are not treated well, or are given confusing advice, they may never return or follow the instructions they have been given. While it is acknowledged that all patients should be treated with care and respect, this is especially important when dealing with people who may have tuberculosis. For many people it is a frightening and often stigmatizing disease, as described in Chapter 15.

Tuberculosis has caused serious ill-health in adults and children since the beginning of recorded human history. It has had devastating impacts on different parts of the world at different points in history, which has resulted in the development of powerful cultural beliefs and folklore surrounding the disease. These beliefs can lead people to deny that they may have tuberculosis and may well discourage them from seeking further help. On the other hand, people who have recent experience of the disease, for instance those who have come from a country with a high prevalence of tuberculosis and have seen that treatment is effective, may well understand the importance of being diagnosed and starting treatment. It is essential to assess each patient's response to the possibility of having tuberculosis and to provide the relevant information and reassurance, emphasizing that tuberculosis can be cured.

Even before a diagnosis of tuberculosis is made, it is good practice to refer patients who have particular questions and concerns to the specialist tuberculosis nurse so that they can discuss these in detail. If it turns out that the patient does have tuberculosis, this can form an important basis for a good relationship between the nurse and the patient throughout treatment. If not, then at least they will feel that their concerns have been taken seriously and they have been kept informed while awaiting results.

Index of suspicion

A patient referred to hospital via the chest clinic or a general practitioner (GP) with a suspicion of tuberculosis and who is subsequently found to have this disease will be identified and treated much quicker than the patient who is referred or admitted for conditions unrelated to tuberculosis. Even patients presenting in an accident and emergency department with classic signs and symptoms of the disease may be missed if they do not fall into a known high-risk category or if tuberculosis is not commonly seen in the local area. It is these patients who potentially pose a risk to other patients and healthcare workers if tuberculosis is not identified.

If tuberculosis is suspected, the appropriate steps should be taken to ensure the best likelihood of making a successful diagnosis while maintaining the co-operation of the patient. As discussed in Chapter 7, the most effective way to find out whether someone is suffering from infectious tuberculosis is to use a microscope to look for acid-fast bacilli in his or her sputum (sputum smear microscopy). Patients should be instructed as to how to produce a good specimen and provided with clear information as to when specimens should be obtained and where they need to be taken. (See Chapter 7 for more details about this and other tests used to diagnose tuberculosis.)

Test results: reporting and documentation

The speed with which laboratory results are reported, documented and acted upon can affect a number of crucial elements of patient care. If reporting is slow, it can delay the start of treatment if results are positive and prolong isolation should the results be negative. The longer patients have to wait for results, the more anxiety they suffer, particularly if they are in respiratory isolation. A good relationship with the local laboratory can speed up the process of reporting. This may mean a phone call to check on results rather than waiting for them to come through the hospital mailing system. The process is usually more streamlined where laboratory results are computerized.

At each stage of the diagnostic process, accurate and prompt documentation is essential so that errors, delays, duplication and/or loss of specimens are avoided. This relates to the labelling of specimen containers, the completion of the appropriate request forms, the recording in patients' notes of the times and dates specimens are sent and the prompt documentation of results. In a ward where there is a complete change of staff every shift, it is essential that progress regarding the collection of specimens and receipt of results is updated at each handover. Important aspects of the nurse's role in establishing a correct diagnosis are highlighted in Box 16.2.

Case notification/reporting

'Control of tuberculosis in low prevalence countries is critically dependent on the efficient, effective monitoring and surveillance of disease.'[4] In many countries, notification of all cases of tuberculosis is a legal requirement. It is essential for initiating contact tracing as well as for gathering important information for epidemiological purposes and service provision (see Chapter 1). Around the world, the recording of every case of tuberculosis is required in

BOX 16.2 The role of the nurse in the diagnosis of tuberculosis in different settings

In primary/community care settings

- To assess the patient for signs and symptoms of tuberculosis
- To bring these to the attention of the patient's hospital physician or GP
- To contact the local TB team for advice if necessary

In acute settings

- To assess the patient for signs and symptoms of tuberculosis
- To bring these to the attention of the medical team in charge of the patient's care
- To support the patient
- To ensure the appropriate tests are ordered
- To ensure that results are accurately documented and fed back promptly to both staff and patients
- To liaise with the TB team

In specialist practice

- To assess patients for signs and symptoms of tuberculosis and order the appropriate tests
- To assess the patients' response to their potential tuberculosis diagnosis and offer appropriate information and support
- To liaise with the laboratory to ensure that the TB team is informed promptly of all positive results
- To maintain communication with patients whether in hospital or at home
- To document results promptly and accurately
- To work closely with the physicians managing patients with tuberculosis

order to follow the patient's progress, to collect local tuberculosis data and to monitor the performance of the tuberculosis control programme. Notification or reporting should be done at the moment the patient starts treatment for tuberculosis, without waiting for bacteriological confirmation. Information regarding test results, which may arrive weeks after a patient has started treatment, should be recorded in the patient's notes and also collected on an ongoing basis for wider surveillance purposes. The notification or reporting process is often co-ordinated by nurses working with the TB team and it is therefore essential that they are informed about all patients starting treatment for tuberculosis.

Support and monitoring of patients on treatment

Once treatment has started, patients need adequate support in order to successfully complete the full course of medication prescribed. This is discussed in greater detail in Chapters 14 and 18. The treatment for tuberculosis, although called short-course chemotherapy, lasts at least 6 months and there are many reasons why patients may fail to complete the course. If patients are unable to adhere to treatment, they risk becoming unwell again, being infectious to others and developing drug-resistant disease. Treatment support is therefore a very important preventive measure, and monitoring is essential so that nurses can identify problems at an early stage.

Isolation of known and suspected infectious people in in-patient settings

This topic is covered in detail in Chapters 17 and 20 but is highlighted here as an important preventive measure in that it helps reduce transmission to healthcare workers and other in-patients, who may be very vulnerable to tuberculosis if exposed. It is while patients with infectious pulmonary tuberculosis remain undiagnosed and therefore untreated that they pose the greatest risk of infection to others. This is why it is essential to isolate all patients suspected of pulmonary tuberculosis as well as known cases until either the diagnosis of infectious tuberculosis has been ruled out or they have been started on effective chemotherapy and are showing signs of clinical improvement (in practice, this is often 2 weeks, but this is not universally adhered to).

SCREENING OF HIGH-RISK GROUPS (ACTIVE CASE FINDING)

Active case finding refers to the identification and screening of asymptomatic people who may have been in contact with a person with active tuberculosis. Although people confirmed as having been exposed are at the highest risk of infection and therefore most likely to develop disease subsequently, other people may also be at considerable risk. These include people from within certain groups known to have a higher incidence of tuberculosis than that in the general population and who are therefore more likely to come into contact with tuberculosis, such as, among others, new immigrants and refugees from countries with a high prevalence of tuberculosis,[5,6] prisoners[7] and the homeless.[8]

Contacts

Contact tracing is a vital component of prevention and control strategies for two reasons. First, it permits the detection of people who may have been infected by the patient and could therefore go on to develop tuberculosis, and second, it may identify the person from whom the disease was contracted, who may be unaware of his or her condition and therefore untreated and infectious. Although always a possibility, sources of adult tuberculosis are not often detected, as the patient could have been infected at any previous time in their lives. On the other hand, patients who are children have almost certainly been recently infected by an adult with active disease, such as a member of their household, close relative or family friend.

Contact investigation is usually organized by a tuberculosis or respiratory nurse specialist or health visitor and involves a combination of chest X-ray and tuberculin testing by the Heaf or Mantoux method (see Chapter 7). It can often be a traumatic experience for the patient, so it is essential that the whole process is handled with as much sensitivity and discretion as possible. Every effort must be made to maintain the patient's confidentiality. In some cases, patients will not even want their spouse or close family to know their diagnosis. As previously discussed, reactions to the diagnosis of tuberculosis can vary greatly and it is important to assess each patient on an individual basis in order to provide the appropriate level of support and reassurance.

The number of contacts investigated varies according to the nature of the index case,[9,10] that is, the patient who was originally diagnosed as having tuberculosis. Close contacts are those who have most contact with the patient in terms of both proximity and the amount of time spent together. They usually include people from the same household and very close associates of the index case, such as a partner or frequent visitor to their home. Casual contacts are those with whom the index patient works or meets socially on a regular basis. These will only be screened when the index patient has sputum smear-positive tuberculosis. There may be individual exceptions to this, depending on a particular case and the discretion of the nurse organizing the screening.

In each case, the lifestyle of the index patient needs to be carefully considered, as other places of close contact may be revealed – for example the work environment, an air flight or a shelter for homeless people. It is recommended that close household contacts of a sputum smear-positive patient are identified by the tuberculosis nurse/health visitor within 2 days and are then seen by a physician as soon as possible – within 5 working days of identification.[1] Child contacts under the age of 2 years and immunocompromised contacts should be seen urgently – ideally in the next clinic session. If there is any likelihood of symptomatic contacts being seen in the same clinic environment as immunocompromised patients, a sputum specimen should be obtained and tested for the presence of acid-fast bacilli and/or a chest X-ray should be taken before the patient attends the clinic. This should reduce the risk of transmission to other vulnerable patients.

Hospital contacts

The need to carry out contact screening of other in-patients can be kept to a minimum if there is a high index of suspicion for tuberculosis and if those with both suspected and confirmed infectious pulmonary forms of the disease are isolated appropriately. There may, however, be some patients with non-specific symptoms who are missed and are only found to have infectious tuberculosis after spending some time on the open ward. Current UK guidelines state that, in this event, the risk of other patients being infected as a result is likely to be small.[1] Each case needs to be individually assessed for risk, and decisions about the appropriate course of action should be centred around the index patient's degree of infectivity, the length of time over which other patients were exposed, the proximity of contact and whether any of the patients were particularly susceptible to infection, for example young children or immunocompromised adults. Patients in the same bay as the infected patient (as opposed to all patients on the ward) should be regarded as being at risk only if the index case was coughing and was in the bay for more than 8 hours. Individual risk assessment should be carried out for susceptible patients who were on the same ward but not necessarily in the same bay as the index case, and when the length of stay for the index case exceeded 2 days.

Occupational contacts

Most occupational contacts come under the heading of 'casual contacts', and follow-up is usually only necessary if the index case is sputum smear positive. There may be a need to screen occupational contacts if they are unusually susceptible, if the index case is considered to be highly infectious or in the event of an outbreak. In the last case the Health Protection Agency (HPA) in the UK and similar authorities in other countries would be closely involved in the decision to follow up and screen contacts. Screening of healthcare workers following exposure to a patient with sputum smear-positive disease would not be undertaken routinely unless it was felt that there was a significant risk of transmission. Any staff concerned about having been exposed to tuberculosis would generally be advised to contact their occupational health department for reassurance. In the event of a healthcare worker being diagnosed with tuberculosis, from either occupational exposure or another source, liaison between the physician responsible for treatment, the occupational health department, the HPA or analogous authority and the infection control team is important. If that worker has been at work while infectious, patients and colleagues who have had significant contact will need to be identified and assessed. Because the period during which the index case was infectious is often unknown, it is recommended that contacts be reviewed for the period of time that the index case has had respiratory symptoms, including a cough. In the event of this not being known, contacts from the 3 months preceding the first positive sputum smear or culture result should be traced.

New entrants and other risk groups

Ideally, all immigrants/entrants from high-prevalence countries should be screened for tuberculosis on arrival in their new country of residence. In some countries, such as the Netherlands and the USA, a systematic screening process is in place. In the UK, although it is recommended that all new entrants from high-prevalence countries are screened on or shortly after arrival, in practice this can be difficult to organize, particularly as screening arrangements vary from area to area according to the resources available and the local demography.

TREATMENT OF LATENT TUBERCULOSIS INFECTION

Screening processes that include tuberculin testing will identify people who have been infected with members of the *M. tuberculosis* complex but who have no clinical, bacteriological or radiological signs of active disease, i.e. people with latent tuberculosis infection.[11] A person is considered to be infected with tuberculosis if he or she has a strongly positive Heaf or Mantoux test (see Chapter 7). Those who have previously had Bacille Calmette–Guérin (BCG) vaccination may have up to grade 2 Heaf results or Mantoux reactions of up to 9 mm diameter. Grade 3 and 4 Heaf results and Mantoux reactions of 10 mm or more in diameter suggest infection with *M. tuberculosis* complex. As tuberculin reactivity is affected by ecological factors, especially exposure to environmental mycobacteria, local guidelines should be consulted.

In countries with a low prevalence of tuberculosis, the treatment of latent tuberculosis infection is an important public health intervention, as it can significantly reduce the chances of infected people subsequently developing active disease and becoming sources of infection to others.[3,11,12] As it is not always possible or practical to offer preventive treatment to all those infected with latent tuberculosis infection, assessment is needed to identify those at greatest risk of developing active disease in the future.[13] Issues surrounding the treatment of latent tuberculosis are discussed in more detail in Chapter 12.

People who are prescribed preventive treatment should be under the care of a tuberculosis specialist nurse or health visitor, as they need ongoing support and reassurance. It can be difficult to motivate people who have no clinical signs or symptoms to take drugs (which are sometimes associated with unpleasant side effects) for a long period of time for a disease that they may or may not suffer from in the future. People in this situation need to be monitored regularly and given the opportunity to discuss their situation in detail. They should also be able to access help and advice should they encounter problems, such as developing adverse effects to the drugs.

Vaccination

Vaccination using BCG is discussed in Chapter 6. Nurses working in a variety of settings may be involved in BCG vaccination programmes. Midwives, health visitors and practice nurses are often involved in neonatal vaccination against tuberculosis. In the UK, school nurses run the schools' BCG programme together with community medical officers, while practice nurses and others working in travel clinics will offer BCG to those who have not previously received the vaccine and are travelling to areas of high tuberculosis prevalence. Tuberculosis specialist nurses offer BCG to anyone under the age of 16 who they have screened for tuberculosis for whatever reason and who have been established to have had no previous vaccination and who have a negative reaction to tuberculin. All nurses involved in BCG vaccination should be competent in the procedure (which usually involves the administration of an intradermal injection) and aware of the associated potential adverse reactions (see Chapter 6). Anyone vaccinated with BCG, as well as the parents of young children, should be informed about the appropriate care of the injection site.

Health education

As previously discussed, it is essential to have a health service that has an effective strategy to manage tuberculosis, i.e. one that can promptly and competently diagnose and fully treat people with active disease, before encouraging more people to use it. Increasing demand on a health service struggling to support existing patients with tuberculosis can have serious consequences in terms of poor outcomes, including treatment failure and loss of patients on treatment, resulting in an increase of acquired multidrug resistance.[14]

Health education is an important part of the prevention of tuberculosis transmission in the community and should involve a wide variety of people, including healthcare workers, patients, voluntary groups and local authority agencies. The aim should be to enable people to recognize the signs and symptoms of tuberculosis and to seek help promptly from the appropriate health services.[11] Due to the stigma which is often associated with tuberculosis, it is essential to highlight the fact that it can be treated and cured and that it is not the fatal disease it used to be.

It is also essential that any health education takes account of the health services available and that careful consideration is given to who needs to be involved in the planning and delivery of health education campaigns. Frustration and mistrust will result from inaccurate information being given by people who are not properly informed and who have no connection to the local health services themselves.

It is important to plan health education campaigns strategically and to think carefully about how best to proceed. The International Union Against Tuberculosis and Lung Disease (UNION) recommends that the following questions are asked before embarking on public health education.[14]

- Who should be educated? Which health workers, patients and members of the community should be targeted?
- Why should they be educated? What does each target group need to learn for what purpose?
- Where should they be educated: in medical/nursing schools, health services or a community setting?

- Who needs to be involved in planning and delivering the education: tuberculosis services, doctors, nurses, community leaders etc.? What are the trusted information channels within the target group?
- How should they be educated and by use of what methods: posters, pamphlets, manuals, books, videos, plays etc.? What are the key messages?
- What other methods are available that would be useful: radio, television, campaigns etc.?

Having answered these questions, it will be possible to prioritize the target groups and prepare a structured plan. Careful consideration needs to be given to the presence and types of stigma associated with tuberculosis within particular target groups so that these can be addressed. As described in Chapter 15, stigma can be attached to any number of cultural or commonly held beliefs and myths, and these need to be explored, exposed and challenged. It is important to remember that healthcare workers may hold the same beliefs.

Nurses are often involved in health education in a multitude of different settings and they therefore need to focus on a variety of target groups – for instance school nurses running vaccination programmes and practice nurses involved in travel vaccinations. Tuberculosis specialist nurses/health visitors will often be involved in one-to-one patient education, giving information to families and participating in wider activities involving various staff and community groups.

Summary

There are a number of measures that can be taken to control tuberculosis, all of which are focused on reducing the pool of infection in the community and thereby preventing the spread of the disease. It is important that a locally agreed strategy is in place, which reflects the demography and epidemiology of the area and has clear lines of responsibility associated with the appropriate participants.

Tuberculosis control is a joint effort involving service commissioners, managers, acute and community healthcare workers, local authorities, patients and community groups. It is essential that everyone involved is aware of their role and familiar with the local strategy for preventing tuberculosis. Nurses play an important role at many different levels, especially with regard to the prompt diagnosis of the disease and the supporting of patients through treatment – the two key elements of tuberculosis control.

Prologue to the next chapter

One of the key health institutions involved in the management of tuberculosis is the hospital to which people are referred, either as in-patients or out-patients, when they are showing signs and symptoms of tuberculosis. As well as being referred with suspected tuberculosis for further investigation, patients may present themselves directly at accident and emergency or other departments or they may have been referred for other health reasons. The appropriate management of all these patients is essential to ensure that tuberculosis is diagnosed as quickly as possible and the risks of transmission are thereby reduced. Once diagnosed, the appropriate care of patients during the very early stage of their treatment is essential to ensure that they have trust in the health service and go on to complete their course of medication successfully. The care of patients in hospital will be the subject of the next chapter.

REFERENCES

1. Joint Tuberculosis Committee of the British Thoracic Society. Control and prevention of TB in the UK: Code of Practice 2000. *Thorax* 2000; **55**: 887–901. Also available online at <http://www.brit-thoracic.org.uk/index.asp>.
2. World Health Organization. *WHO framework for effective tuberculosis control.* WHO/TB/94.179. Geneva: World Health Organization, 1994. Also available online at <http://www.who.int/gtb/publications/framework/>.
3. Broekmans JF, Migliori GB, Rieder HL et al. European framework for tuberculosis control and elimination in countries with a low incidence. *Eur Respir J* 2002; **19**: 765–75.
4. Leitch AG. Control of tuberculosis in low-prevalence countries. In Davies PDO (ed.), *Clinical tuberculosis*. London: Chapman and Hall, 1994, 313–24 (cited quotation p. 320).
5. EuroTB. *Surveillance of tuberculosis in Europe. Report on cases notified in 1999*. Paris: Maulde and Renou, 2002.
6. Hardie RM, Watson JM. Screening migrants at risk of tuberculosis. *BMJ* 1993; **307**: 1539–40.
7. Reyes H, Coninx R. Pitfalls of tuberculosis programmes in prisons. *BMJ* 1997; **315**: 1447–50.
8. Citron K, Southern A, Dixon M. *Out of the shadow*. London: Crisis, 1995.
9. Shaw JB, Wynn-Williams N. Infectivity of pulmonary tuberculosis in relation to sputum status. *Am Rev Tuberc* 1954; **69**: 724–32.
10. Rouillon A, Perdrizet S, Parrot R. Transmission of tubercle bacilli: the effects of chemotherapy. *Tubercle* 1976; **57**: 275–9.
11. Clancy L, Rieder HL, Enarson DA, Spinaci S. Tuberculosis elimination in the countries of Europe and other industrialised countries. *Eur Respir J* 1991; **4**: 1288–95.
12. American Thoracic Society, Centers for Disease Control. Targeted tuberculin testing and treatment of latent tuberculosis infection. *Am J Respir Crit Care Med* 2000; **161**: S221–47.
13. Loddenkemper R, Sagebiel D. Control in low-prevalence countries. In Davies PDO (ed.), *Clinical tuberculosis*, 3rd edn. London: Arnold, 2003, 357–80.
14. International Union Against Tuberculosis and Lung Disease (IUATLD). *Tuberculosis programs: review, planning, support: a manual of methods and procedures.* Paris: IUATLD, 1998.

INTERNET RESOURCES

Centers for Disease Control and Prevention (CDC): National Center for HIV, STD and TB Prevention – Division of Tuberculosis Elimination. Produces several guidelines focused on infection prevention and control, case finding, treatment and surveillance: <http://www.cdc.gov/nchstp/tb/>.

International Union Against Tuberculosis and Lung Disease (UNION): <http://www.iuatld.org/full_picture/en/frameset/frameset.phtml>.

World Health Organization: <http://www.stoptb.org>.

CHAPTER 17

The individualized care of patients with tuberculosis

> The unique role of the nurse is to assist the individual, sick or well, in the performance of those activities contributing to health or its recovery (or to peaceful death) that he would perform unaided if he had the necessary strength, will or knowledge. And to do this in such a way as to help him gain independence as rapidly as possible.
>
> *Virginia Henderson*[1]

Introduction

This chapter focuses on caring for patients admitted to hospital for investigation or treatment of tuberculosis and it also provides useful information for nurses planning care for patients who are managed on an out-patient basis. Many patients with tuberculosis will not require admission to hospital and can be appropriately treated as an out-patient with the back-up and support of a specialist multi-disciplinary team of healthcare professionals, usually known as the TB team. Admission to hospital may be necessary if the patient is particularly unwell, has multidrug-resistant tuberculosis or other problems with therapy, is unable to care for him/herself at home or has other serious medical conditions, such as disease caused by infection with the human immunodeficiency virus (HIV). As discussed in the previous chapter, it is essential that nurses are alert to the signs and symptoms of tuberculosis, as a significant number of patients may attend accident and emergency departments or be admitted to hospital with no one considering tuberculosis as a differential diagnosis. The admitting nurse has the primary nursing responsibility to identify patients who may have signs and symptoms suggestive of active pulmonary tuberculosis.[2,3] This applies when admitting any patient to any ward.

As discussed in Chapter 12, an effective cure is available for tuberculosis, which involves taking a combination of antituberculosis drugs for a minimum of 6 months. The patient is likely to spend the majority of this time being treated on an out-patient basis.

However, this chapter describes the basic elements of nursing care that may be needed by patients with tuberculosis who are in hospital. The range of patient problems and nursing care needs vary according to the patients' duration of hospitalization, the severity of their illness, their response to treatment and the presence of complicating co-morbidities, such as HIV disease.

Because millions of patients with tuberculosis throughout the world are co-infected with HIV and are therefore more likely to be seriously ill and, consequently, admitted to hospital, this chapter particularly explores their healthcare problems and needs.

The quality and sensitivity of the care that patients receive in hospital can have an impact on their future relationship with the health service for the duration of their treatment and follow-up. Tuberculosis presents many challenges, as it is widely stigmatized through fear of contagion and is strongly associated with poverty, homelessness, alcohol and/or drug dependency, HIV disease and malnutrition. In view of the complexities of the disease, a holistic and individualized needs-based approach is required for the provision of optimal care and support.

Learning outcomes

After studying and reflecting on the material in this chapter, you will be able to:

- describe and use a relevant needs-based, problem-centred approach systematically to assess, plan, implement and evaluate relevant nursing care,
- identify actual and potential problems experienced by patients admitted with suspected or confirmed tuberculosis and relate these to your wider understanding of the disease,
- support colleagues and students in developing confidence and competence in delivering quality nursing care to patients with tuberculosis.

BACKGROUND TO STRATEGIC NURSING CARE

Patients admitted for investigation or treatment of tuberculosis may be in a rapidly changing clinical situation and their nursing care must be assessed, planned and evaluated on a frequent basis. This requires a comprehensive understanding by the nurse of the rationale that underpins strategic nursing care.

Strategic nursing care is that care which is carefully planned and implemented by nurses and which is designed to meet the immediate needs of patients, solve identified actual problems and prevent recognized potential problems from being realized. Because of their training and experience, their comprehensive understanding of the nursing issues involved and their teaching and management skills, nurses are able to assess and plan the individualized nursing care most appropriate for each patient and lead and supervise the nursing team implementing this care. The care delivered must be evaluated frequently (often on a shift-by-shift basis) and modified according to the patient's response to nursing interventions. The nurse is ideally placed to act as the patient's advocate and to liaise effectively between the patient and other members of the healthcare team.

Strategic nursing care embraces the concept of a problem-solving approach to the individualized care of each patient. It is, however, more than a nursing process style of care. It includes the assessment and planning of nursing care on a hospital-wide basis, taking into consideration all the real and possible issues governing the implementation of care, and involves logistical, educational and managerial aspects, which, if not anticipated, may preclude the delivery of individualized, high-quality care.

Needs-based models of nursing, as conceived by Henderson,[4] Roper, Logan and Tierney,[5] and Orem,[6] are valuable tools by which the individualized nursing care of patients with tuberculosis can be planned and implemented efficiently and effectively. These models describe the needs and self-care requisites necessary for normal, healthy living. Their use allows for a systematic nursing assessment that will identify actual problems arising from deficits in self-care abilities. They further facilitate the recognition of potential problems associated with the patient's condition (social, psychological, physical and medical), specific illnesses, hospitalization and medical treatment. Identifying and documenting needs, self-care requisites and both actual and potential problems facilitates the planning of appropriate nursing interventions and allows the effectiveness of these interventions to be evaluated.

Tuberculosis is a communicable disease with serious consequences if treated inadequately, and the patients' responsibility goes beyond achieving their personal recovery to ensuring that the people around them are safe. This can be very difficult without appropriate care and support. The nurse has a responsibility to assess self-care deficits by exploring social, psychological, physical and medical issues in order to plan interventions relevant to the needs of each individual patient. As well as assessing problems and self-care deficits, it is also important to consider what positive factors exist – such as supportive family members, friends and a strong religious faith – which will assist the patient, both in hospital and following discharge.

Because needs-based models used alone can be potentially de-humanizing, the nursing assessment must also include an examination of how this episode of illness is affecting the *person* (as opposed to the body). A simple set of questions that might be used to structure such an assessment could include the following.

- *Who are these people?* What do they, or did they, do for a living? Where do they live? Who do they live with? What family do they have?
- *What health events bring people into hospital?* By getting patients to describe these events, the nurse can ascertain their level of understanding and knowledge about their condition. This can help in identifying knowledge deficits the patients may have and in deciding how to individualize patient education.
- *How are these people feeling?* This question is designed to embrace the physical, emotional, psychological and spiritual aspects of the patients. It allows them to talk about themselves and about any hopes or anxieties they may have, or about anything to do with their current state of mind.
- *How have these events affected patients' usual life-patterns and relationships?* Disruption to health obviously brings with it disruption to normal life. By discussing this, problems as disparate as loss of earnings, loss of ability to engage in leisure activities and loss of intimacy with partners may all be highlighted.
- *What support do these people have?* This question raises the nurse's awareness of who or what the patients use to help them cope during times of stress, such as partners, families, friends, religious or spiritual faith. It can also provide a clearer picture of who the patients are socially and which other people may become involved in their care episodes. The question can also provide information that will be useful when planning discharge.

- *How do these people view their future?* This question raises issues about the meaning of tuberculosis to the patients, as their experience of living with tuberculosis will probably have a strong effect on how they view their future. It should be acknowledged that many will interpret a diagnosis of tuberculosis as a potentially fatal condition that will take their future from them.

This assessment structure is taken from the 'Burford Nursing Development Unit Model'.[7] The idea behind the model is to allow the nurse to 'connect' with patients in a way that conventional nursing models do not always do. In essence, it aims to help the nurse to see people in relation to their illness, as opposed to 'a patient with an illness'. In the acute care setting, gaining information to assist with this may often be neglected in favour of physiological assessment. When one considers the nature of tuberculosis, however, with its impact on the patient physiologically, psychologically and socially, it would seem vital that a *comprehensive* assessment is carried out. To that end, it is suggested that both these assessments are used together, so that information is gained about the person living with tuberculosis (Burford model) in addition to information about the needs that this disease generates for that person (needs-based model).

Additionally, an existing wealth of knowledge will exist and be available to nurses to assist them in planning and delivering appropriate and relevant nursing care. The members of the multi-disciplinary TB team that supports the care of the patient – including specialist nurses such as respiratory or tuberculosis clinical nurse specialists, infection control nurses, physicians, physiotherapists, microbiologists, pharmacists and dieticians – all possess valuable specialist knowledge regarding dimensions of tuberculosis care that the nurse can access and use appropriately when planning, implementing and evaluating a patient's individualized nursing care.

NEEDS-BASED NURSING MODELS

In this chapter, an eclectic needs-based nursing model is used to organize the information provided. Most nurses will already be familiar with this assessment structure, as the list of needs is adapted from Henderson's *Components of basic nursing* and Roper, Logan and Tierney's *Activities of daily living*.[4,5] By meeting these needs, it is hoped that the hospitalized patient may return to health, if not by the time of discharge, then by the completion of treatment.

Fifteen needs are discussed. Each is described as having *potential problems* associated with it. Alongside each of these problems, there is a list of *possible causes*. Neither of these lists is designed to be exhaustive; rather, they are indicative of the problems affecting the patient and their causes that the nurse may most commonly encounter in the ward setting when caring for patients with tuberculosis.

General *objectives of care* are described for each need. This is followed by a description of relevant *nursing interventions*, introduced by identifying important elements of a *nursing assessment*. In the real world of nursing practice, a more comprehensive assessment of each patient (as previously described) is needed to plan appropriate interventions and care most effectively.

As stated previously, nursing care must be regularly *evaluated* and modified according to the response of the patient. A brief description of evaluation (linked to the stated objectives of care) concludes the discussion of each need.

In common with those with other illnesses, patients with tuberculosis have needs that they or others must meet for health to be maintained. The following list itemizes the needs that may be examined during the nursing assessment.

1. The need for adequate respiration.
2. The need for adequate hydration.
3. The need for adequate nutrition.
4. The need for urinary and faecal elimination.
5. The need to control body temperature.
6. The need for movement and mobilization.
7. The need for a safe environment.
8. The need for personal cleansing and dressing.
9. The need for expression and communication.
10. The need for working and playing.
11. The need to maintain psychological equilibrium.
12. The need for adequate rest and sleep.
13. The need for spiritual care.
14. The need to express sexuality.
15. Needs associated with dying.

THE NEED FOR ADEQUATE RESPIRATION

Potential problems	Possible causes
Breathlessness, dyspnoea, hypoxia, tachypnoea, cyanosis	Reduced lung capacity through infiltration and/or tissue damage caused by tuberculosis
	Other lung disease
Chest pain	Excessive coughing and/or pleural effusion
Cough, haemoptysis	Pulmonary tuberculosis, other lung disease

Objectives of care

- To promote optimal respiratory function.
- To keep the patient well oxygenated.
- To alleviate associated symptoms, for example cough, dry mouth, anxiety, and to keep the patient as comfortable as possible.

Assessment

- Assess vital signs (blood pressure, pulse, respiratory rate, body temperature, pulse oximetry). Record as baseline and repeat as appropriate. Pulse oximetry may need to be continuous if respiratory function is poor.
- Assess colour, respiratory effort, chest sounds, sputum production (amount and whether there is blood present) and mental status.
- Assess severity and location of any pain.
- Note history of any other respiratory health problems, e.g. asthma, sarcoidosis, chronic obstructive pulmonary disease (COPD).

- Assess smoking habits and identify potential problems associated with cessation of smoking.
- Obtain sputum specimens for microbiological examination (microscopy for acid-fast bacilli, culture and sensitivity) and be aware of results.
- Be aware of arterial blood gas (ABG) values.

Nursing interventions

Position

The patient should be placed in a position that facilitates good respiratory function. Sitting the patient upright in bed or in a chair, leaning forward and well supported, is useful as it allows the accessory muscles of respiration to assist respiratory effort. Placing pillows on the patient's table and allowing him or her to lean over may facilitate adequate respiration, especially in the patient who is tiring.

Oxygen

Depending on the patient's clinical condition and ABG values (Table 17.1), the physician may prescribe supplemental oxygen (O_2) to be administered or, if pulse oximetry shows the O_2 saturation of a patient to be falling below 95 per cent, the nurse may need to administer O_2 until the physician is consulted. Oxygen saturation should ideally be maintained at above 95 per cent at rest, but *always* above 90 per cent. Oxygen should be considered a drug and, as such, a prescription for its use should be sought as soon as possible. In general, the lowest concentration of O_2 needed to overcome hypoxaemia will be ordered.

TABLE 17.1 Normal range for arterial blood gases

PaO_2	10.6–13.3 kPa (80–100 mmHg)
$PaCO_2$	4.6–6.9 kPa (35–45 mmHg)
pH	7.35–7.45
O_2 saturation	94–100%

Different types of masks will be used, depending on the level of supplemental oxygenation required.

- A standard (Hudson) facemask is suitable for those patients requiring up to 50 per cent O_2 supplementation. These masks cannot, however, guarantee accuracy of administration.
- For patients requiring high levels of supplemental O_2, or when highly accurate administration is needed, a Ventimask or Venturimask is indicated.
- Nasal catheters and cannulae may be used for patients who require low levels of supplemental oxygenation, although the inspired O_2 concentration can be unpredictable (2 L/min of O_2 = approximately 30 per cent O_2 concentration). Patients often prefer these, as they are comfortable and do not interfere with eating, drinking and the wearing of spectacles.

Oxygen therapy should be continuous rather than intermittent, aiming to maintain a constant arterial partial pressure of O_2 (PaO_2) between 10.6 and 13.3 kPa (80 and 100 mmHg). If O_2 is to be administered for more than 12 hours, humidification is required. This prevents excessive drying of the mouth and solidification of secretions.

Patient safety

The patient may be hypoxic and may be confused due to the limited O_2 supply to the brain. This could compromise patient safety. To minimize the potential risks associated with the effects of hypoxia, the nurse should assess patient safety and be prepared to move the confused patient to an area where he or she can be easily observed by the nurse, such as an observation bed on the ward. This may be complicated if there is a need to place a patient in respiratory isolation. In this situation, the patient will need to be regularly observed and the necessary safety precautions will need to be implemented to maximize the patient's safety. There is a potential risk of fire when using O_2 and, accordingly, non-sparking spanners (wrenches) and other equipment should be used when needed. No lighted flames or cigarette smoking are allowed in a room where O_2 is being administered.

It should be remembered that negative-pressure respiratory isolation rooms are a particular risk environment for fire, and every possible precaution needs to be observed to ensure patient safety.

Patient education

Patients should be taught deep breathing, coughing and relaxation exercises. The use of an incentive spirometer (peak flow) is useful for deep-breathing exercises. Advice from a physiotherapist may be useful to supplement the specialist respiratory information nurses give to their patients.

Chest physiotherapy

Chest physiotherapy may be required to help clear the patient's lungs. This should only be carried out in respiratory isolation to reduce the risk of transmission of tubercle bacilli to other patients. The physiotherapist and anyone else present should wear appropriate personal respiratory protection. The required infection prevention and control precautions are described in detail in Chapter 20.

Antituberculosis therapy

Antituberculosis drugs can alleviate the symptoms of tuberculosis within a matter of days, depending on the severity of the case. Pain relief may help patients who are coughing excessively and is likely to be necessary for patients with a pleural effusion. Steroids may be used in conjunction with antituberculosis medication to assist respiratory function in cases where tuberculosis has caused severe infiltration in the lungs or where there is a concurrent respiratory condition. It is essential that all medications for tuberculosis are taken under direct supervision (directly observed therapy – DOT) during the patient's stay in hospital. Any problems the patient has with the medication should be recorded and discussed with both the medical and TB teams. The treatment of tuberculosis is discussed in detail in Chapter 12.

Reassurance

Many patients suspected of having tuberculosis or having just been diagnosed are very anxious and need to be reassured that effective treatment is available and that they have an excellent chance of recovery. In countries where resources are scarce, the many problems often associated with accessing consistent antituberculosis treatment and support add to the patients' anxiety.

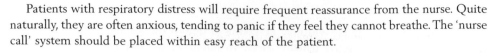

Patients with respiratory distress will require frequent reassurance from the nurse. Quite naturally, they are often anxious, tending to panic if they feel they cannot breathe. The 'nurse call' system should be placed within easy reach of the patient.

Mouth care

Oxygen, even when humidified, may cause dryness of the mucous membranes, and frequent mouth care is required. Patients should rinse their mouth out with water every hour.

Nasal care

If nasal cannulae are used, it is useful if the nostrils are lightly coated with a protective ointment such as Vaseline. With prolonged use, oxygen facemasks and nasal catheters and cannulae can also cause soreness on the top of the ear. Again, a protective coating of Vaseline is useful.

Evaluation

The patient will be assessed frequently and appropriately to ensure that the objectives of care are being achieved, such as:

- optimal respiratory function is achieved, as evidenced by satisfactory ABG and oximetry values,
- associated symptoms are alleviated,
- side effects of medications have been anticipated, detected and managed promptly.

It is essential that any changes in the patient's respiratory status are reported to the physician immediately. If improvement is not being made, there may be another underlying infection or other medical condition that has not yet been detected, the patient may not be absorbing the medication as expected, or may have drug-resistant disease. In any case, further investigation is required.

In the rare event that the patient requires artificial ventilation and intensive care, special precautions should be taken in all procedures, especially with regard to maintaining the airway through regular endotracheal suction (as discussed in Chapter 20).

THE NEED FOR ADEQUATE HYDRATION

Potential problems	Possible causes
Dehydration	Fever and sweating
	Inadequate intake of oral fluids due to respiratory distress and/or O_2 administration via facemask
Electrolyte imbalance	Dehydration
Acute renal failure	Nephrotoxicity of some antituberculosis drugs, existing renal disease

Objectives of care

- To maintain optimal hydration and electrolyte balance.
- To prevent or correct dehydration and electrolyte imbalance.
- To maintain optimal renal function.

Assessment

- Assess the patient's ability to maintain his or her own hydration.
- Identify oropharyngeal disease.
- Assess level of sweating.
- Assess level of consciousness and cognitive ability.
- Assess drug chart for medications that alter renal function.
- Assess the patient for signs of systemic hypovolaemia.
- Assess skin turgor daily.
- Initiate fluid balance chart for ongoing assessment.
- Be aware of current blood chemistry results.
- Weigh the patient on a regular basis.

Nursing interventions

Fluid balance chart

Where possible, encourage patients to keep their own record of fluid intake. They will need education and supervised practice in measuring input and output. Toilets (or bedside commodes, bedpans, urinals) and measuring jugs need to be easily accessible to patients to aid compliance with output measurement. Intake and output information needs to be transferred into the nursing notes at regular intervals.

Oral fluids

Patients should be encouraged to drink frequent, small amounts of fluids as tolerated. Fresh cold water should always be left in an accessible place and alternative drinks should be made available to patients to encourage fluid intake. Patients in respiratory isolation may have difficulty in communicating that they are thirsty and feel uneasy in using their nurse-call system simply to ask for a drink of water.[8] Nurses should always respond sympathetically to all calls for assistance for patients, no matter how trivial their requests may seem. When oral intake is poor even with encouragement, the physician may need to prescribe intravenous fluids.

Intravenous rehydration

The physician may prescribe a regimen of intravenous fluids that must be infused at the correct flow rate. Intravenous insertion sites will need to be inspected regularly by the nurse to ensure they remain patent and free of inflammation and infection. In England, comprehensive national evidence-based guidelines for preventing infections associated with the use of central venous catheters have been published,[9,10] and nurses need to ensure that this guidance is reflected both in local protocols and in routine daily clinical practice (see 'Internet resources' at the end of this chapter).

Electrolyte replacement

The principal electrolyte abnormalities seen in seriously ill patients are decreases in plasma levels of sodium (hyponatraemia) and potassium (hypokalaemia). Excess plasma levels of sodium (hypernatraemia) and potassium (hyperkalaemia) are less frequently encountered. The nurse needs to be aware of the patient's most recent electrolyte values (Table 17.2).

The treatment of hyponatraemia is focused on correcting the underlying cause, restriction of water intake and electrolyte replacement. In general, sodium and potassium

TABLE 17.2 Normal plasma electrolyte parameters

Ion	Normal range in mmol/L (mEq/L)
Potassium (K^+)	3.8–5.0
Sodium (Na^+)	135–145
Chloride (Cl^-)	100–106

depletion is corrected by intravenous infusions of fluids with added electrolytes (potassium, sodium, chloride, bicarbonate). Although potassium and sodium are usually added to intravenous infusions, oral potassium preparations (such as Kloref® or Sando-K®) and/or oral sodium supplementation (such as Slow Sodium®) may be used.

Plasma electrolyte levels need to be carefully monitored and results outside normal parameters reported to the physician immediately.

Mouth care

Patients who are unable to take adequate oral fluids require frequent (2-hourly) mouth care.

Skin care

Dehydrated patients may experience dry skin and may be at increased risk of developing pressure ulcers. They need regular pressure area inspection and care. Emollients (such as Aqueous Cream BP) moisturize the skin and should be applied as appropriate. Emollient bath additives (such as Alpha Keri Bath® or E45® bath oils) may be helpful for some patients.

Patient education

Patients receiving potentially nephrotoxic medications need to be reminded of the importance of drinking sufficient amounts of fluids to help maintain normal renal function. The nurse needs to evaluate the patient's ability to understand any educational input.

Evaluation

The patient will be assessed frequently and appropriately to ensure that the objectives of care are being achieved, such as:

- causes of poor oral intake are addressed and managed,
- fluid loss is adequately replaced by oral and/or intravenous fluids,
- electrolyte imbalance is detected, monitored and reversed,
- risks associated with antituberculosis drugs that alter renal function are managed,
- skin turgor is normal.

THE NEED FOR ADEQUATE NUTRITION

Potential problems	Possible causes
Involuntary weight loss	Fever, wasting associated with tuberculosis and other co-morbidities, e.g. HIV disease
Reduced food intake/malnutrition	Poverty, lethargy, immobility, anorexia, depression
Lack of appetite	Tuberculosis and side effects of some antituberculosis drugs

Objectives of care

- To keep the patient well nourished.
- To prevent further weight loss.
- To increase food intake appropriately in order to enhance weight gain and enable the patient to tolerate antituberculosis drugs better.

Assessment

It is important to obtain an accurate baseline weight on admission and to monitor as appropriate. The nursing assessment will include a history of previous dietary patterns, including likes, dislikes and any known food allergies. Information on the current dietary habit of the patient is recorded, including any special diets he or she may be following and any 'alternative' diets such as macrobiotic diets. A nutritional assessment will include the following.

- Appearance: does the patient look thin or wasted?
- History of recent weight loss: has the patient noticed that clothes have become ill-fitting?
- Normal eating patterns/preferences.
- Lifestyle factors, such as alcohol dependency, chaotic living conditions, homelessness.
- Appetite: any oral/oesophageal conditions that cause difficulties in chewing or swallowing.
- Medications: any dietary restrictions associated with current tuberculosis treatment regimens; any gastrointestinal side effects from any drugs being taken.
- Need for food intake chart.
- Need to liaise with the dietician.

Nursing interventions

Oral nutrition

If patients have lost their appetite as a consequence of having tuberculosis, it can take a while to return. Antituberculosis drugs often contribute to this problem and patients may complain of a bad taste in their mouths and feelings of nausea. It is important to encourage patients to eat little and often according to what they can tolerate. If possible, it is helpful for family and friends to bring in food that the patient enjoys and can have available as and when he or she wants it rather than being restricted to hospital meals provided at certain times.

Antituberculosis drugs are normally prescribed to be taken once daily, usually in the morning 30 minutes before breakfast. All of the drugs in the regimen should be taken at that time, but some patients who experience nausea may tolerate treatment better if they take all their tablets together last thing before they retire for the night. Even then, some patients may only tolerate some antituberculosis drugs if taken with a milk-based drink or food. As their food intake improves, patients are often better able to tolerate the medication.

Splitting the medication into a number of doses to be taken at different times of day can lead to confusion and unintentional partial treatment, especially once patients go home and self-medicate. Nurses should ensure that patients have plenty of fluids to drink so that they can swallow their various tablets.

Referral for social support

If patients are malnourished due simply to not being able to afford sufficient food, it may be helpful to refer them to the hospital social worker to review any benefits they may be entitled to. It is also important to consider this point when planning patients' discharge. There may be food available via hostels and/or day centres, depending on their circumstances. The TB team should be informed of this issue so that they can continue to monitor the situation and support patients once they leave hospital. If patients are unable to afford food, it will be very difficult for them to tolerate the antituberculosis drugs. Support from the tuberculosis service to help patients meet their nutritional needs can therefore help them to adhere to their treatment regimen.

Dietician

Patients who are severely malnourished and/or find it difficult to regain their appetite need to be referred to a dietician for more in-depth assessment and advice. The dietician may recommend appropriate food supplements (such as Ensure®, Enlive® and Complan®) that can be used in addition to meals, although these should not be seen as a replacement for normal meals.

Medication

Anti-emetics, such as metoclopramide hydrochloride (Maxolon®), can help alleviate the symptoms of nausea for patients who are finding it difficult to tolerate antituberculosis drugs; these are generally given at least 30 minutes before meals. They may also help patients who vomit following medication, but alternatives should be explored if the vomiting persists, as it may signal a more serious intolerance of one of the antituberculosis drugs.

Patient education

A healthy diet can often assist patients in making a good recovery, so information should be provided according to the patients' existing dietary habits and access to healthy food.

Evaluation

The patient will be assessed frequently and appropriately to ensure that the objectives of care are being achieved, such as:

- weight gain is appropriate, or at least there is no further weight loss,
- antituberculosis drugs are being tolerated.

THE NEED FOR URINARY AND FAECAL ELIMINATION

Potential problems	Possible causes
Poor access to toilet facilities	Respiratory isolation, lack of en-suite toilet facilities
Diarrhoea	Antituberculosis drugs, gastrointestinal tuberculosis
Constipation	Reduced mobility, poor fibre and fluid intake, treatment related

Objectives of care

- To assist the patient in preventing and/or managing diarrhoea or constipation.
- To ensure good access to toilet facilities if the patient is in isolation without en-suite facilities.
- To prevent or correct dehydration.

Assessment

- Identify the presence of diarrhoea, constipation, and dehydration.
- Review the patient's usual nutrition, hydration, and mobility patterns and usual urinary and defaecation habits.
- Consider the possibility of gastrointestinal tuberculosis and send stool samples for laboratory investigation as necessary.
- Ensure the patient has easy access to toilet facilities while in hospital and in respiratory isolation.

Nursing interventions

Diarrhoea

If the diarrhoea is associated with the antituberculosis drugs, an anti-motility drug such as loperamide hydrochloride may be prescribed by the physician to slow down peristalsis, which will decrease the frequency of bowel movements. If the patient has abdominal pain or cramping, the abdomen should be examined and any rigidity or abdominal guarding reported urgently to the physician.

All patients suffering from diarrhoea need to be advised about correct hand hygiene techniques following bowel movements. **Standard Infection Prevention and Control Principles**[9,10] are used by nurses and other healthcare providers to prevent the nosocomial transmission of any enteric pathogens. Patients in respiratory isolation should have en-suite facilities or, if they do not, should be reassured and made to feel comfortable about calling the nurse when they need to use a bedside commode.

Constipation

A balanced diet with adequate fibre and fluid intake can usually prevent constipation. If patients are constipated, they can be offered a laxative for short-term relief and encouraged to increase their intake of fluid and fibre-rich foods as much as possible. Patients who are in isolation without en-suite facilities may find that waiting for someone to bring them a commode can exacerbate their constipation, and nurses need to be aware of this and develop strategies to ensure that patients have easy and reliable access to toilet facilities.

Evaluation

The patient will be assessed frequently and appropriately to ensure that the objectives of care are being achieved, such as:

- normal patterns of urinary and faecal elimination are resumed,
- hydration is adequate and a balanced diet is being tolerated,
- complications such as dehydration are avoided,
- any risk of the nosocomial transmission of enteric pathogens has been minimized.

THE NEED TO CONTROL BODY TEMPERATURE

Potential problems	Possible causes
Fever and sweating	Tuberculosis, other infections, some antituberculosis drugs

Objectives of care

- Assist in maintaining normal body temperature (36–37.7 °C).
- Alleviate discomfort caused by fever.
- Maintain optimal hydration.

Assessment

- Assess vital signs and body temperature twice a day and, if the patient is febrile, record body temperature every 4 hours.
- Assess for the possibility of a concurrent source of infection in addition to tuberculosis.
- Assess the frequency, duration and timing of sweating experienced by the patient.
- Review the current drug regimen for drugs that may cause fever and/or hepatitis.

Nursing interventions

Fever associated with an infection is a protective response that enhances the body's defence mechanisms. The body's temperature normally fluctuates between 36 and 37.7 °C over a 24-hour period (circadian cycle), being lowest very early in the morning and highest during late afternoon and early evening. Fever occurs when the body temperature is elevated above the normal daily variation or, more precisely, when the temperature, as measured by an oral thermometer, is 37.8 °C (100 °F) or higher or, when measured rectally, is 38.2 °C (100.8 °F) or higher. The hypothalamus in the brain is the control centre for body temperature, and fever results when this centre resets the 'body's thermostat' upwards. Fevers may show particular patterns, such as peaking each day and then returning to normal, or they may be intermittent, with the temperature varying but not returning to normal. Some people, such as young children and the elderly, may actually show a drop in temperature below normal as a response to severe infection.

Patients who have fever associated with tuberculosis often complain of drenching sweats, particularly at night. These can be both alarming and uncomfortable for patients, who may need to have their wet nightclothes and saturated bed linen changed once or more during the night.

Medication

The physician may prescribe antipyretic medication to reduce body temperature, such as paracetamol BP (acetaminophen USP), aspirin or other non-steroidal anti-inflammatory drugs (NSAIDs), for example ibuprofen (Brufen®). Paracetamol is probably the most effective and has the lowest profile of gastrointestinal side effects. Antipyretics should be administered as prescribed, but generally on a regular basis, as intermittent administration may cause unnecessary sweating and thus discomfort. It is useful to record on the temperature chart each time an antipyretic is given so that variations in temperature can be assessed correctly.

Once antituberculosis therapy has been initiated, patients usually become afebrile quite quickly. If a patient remains febrile after 2–3 weeks of antituberculosis treatment, the reasons for this need to be identified. Possible explanations include inadequate antituberculosis therapy or a previously unidentified and often unrelated infection. Ineffective tuberculosis therapy may be linked to a variety of causes, such as primary drug resistance, suboptimal treatment being prescribed, incorrect administration of the prescribed treatment, inadequate absorption of antituberculosis drugs, and non-adherence to the prescribed regimen.

Some antituberculosis drugs, such as rifampicin (rifampin), isoniazid and pyrazinamide, may cause hepatitis or fevers. When the reason for the patient's fever has been established, appropriate nursing and medical interventions need to be implemented and evaluated.

Nutrition and hydration

As prolonged fever increases metabolic processes, catabolism and fluid loss, patients with fever should be encouraged to eat a light, nutritious diet and drink adequate amounts of fluids. Cool drinks must be easily available, and glucose drinks, such as Lucozade® or squash, may be beneficial to some patients, although they may exacerbate diarrhoea in others. Intravenous rehydration may be needed in very ill patients. Those with long-term fevers and associated catabolism, for example fever associated with HIV-related conditions, should be referred to the dietician.

Comfort

The patient's environment should be organized in such a way as to help alleviate as much as possible the discomfort caused by fever. Light, clean and dry bed linen and nightclothes should be readily available and changed frequently. Electric fans are not used in respiratory isolation rooms, as they blow air out of the room each time the door is opened. This results in the liberation of airborne tubercle bacilli into the open ward or corridor and presents a potential risk of nosocomial infection to other patients, visitors and hospital personnel.

Evaluation

The patient will be assessed frequently and appropriately to ensure that the objectives of care are being achieved, such as:

- a normal body temperature is maintained,
- medication is administered as ordered by the physician,
- appropriate action is taken if the fever persists despite antituberculosis therapy,
- the patient remains nourished, well hydrated and comfortable.

THE NEED FOR MOVEMENT AND MOBILIZATION

Potential problems	Possible causes
Pressure ulcers, deep vein thrombosis	Restricted mobility, weakness and bed rest
Weakness and fatigue	Tuberculosis
Painful joints, immobility	Spinal or bone tuberculosis
Peripheral neuropathy	Antituberculosis drugs

Objectives of care

- To alleviate the pain caused by the location of the disease.
- To balance comfort and rest with the need to maintain an adequate level of mobility.
- To be alert to and manage pain associated with antituberculosis medication.

Assessment

- Assess the patient's level of independence and ability to mobilize, as well as any signs of muscle wasting, pressure ulcers or venous thrombosis.
- For patients who are confined to bed, evaluate their ability to move around, sit up and turn on alternate sides.
- Identify any required aids for mobilizing or moving around in bed.
- Determine the level of assistance that is required to ensure safe mobilization/transfer.
- Conduct a risk assessment to identify factors that may contribute to pressure ulcers or deep vein thrombosis.
- Assess the level and location of pain experienced by the patient and explore its possible causes.
- Review current medication regimens and identify any drugs that may contribute to the patient's difficulty in mobilizing.

Nursing interventions

Pain

Some antituberculosis drugs can cause nerve damage (neuropathy) and joint pain (arthralgia), which can impede mobilization. *Isoniazid* causes increased urinary excretion of pyridoxine (vitamin B6), which leads to a pyridoxine deficiency. This manifests itself as a **peripheral sensory neuropathy** with paraesthesia and can progress to overt muscular weakness.[11,12] Early symptoms include tingling, prickling, itching and weakness in the feet, legs and hands. Peripheral neuropathy is treated with pyridoxine and can be prevented by administering pyridoxine to all patients prescribed isoniazid. Elderly and immunocompromised patients and those with a history of chronic alcohol abuse are particularly prone to developing isoniazid-associated peripheral neuropathy. *Pyrazinamide* can cause joint pain, which often responds well to NSAIDs such as ibuprofen. Any symptoms of peripheral neuropathy and/or joint pains need to be reported to the patient's physician.

Extrapulmonary tuberculosis can often result in extreme pain at the site of the disease, for example when it is causing destruction of bones and/or joints or in the case of pleural effusion. It is essential that the level and location of pain are monitored and that attempts are made to alleviate it by the use of analgesic and/or anti-inflammatory medication. Anxiety can often exacerbate the pain, and patients need reassurance and support to help them cope, especially as it can be a few days before pain relief takes effect. While the antituberculosis drugs will treat the disease, pain often persists, especially where damage has been caused to bones and joints. Scar tissue resulting from a healed pulmonary or pleural lesion can also continue to cause pain.

Physiotherapy

Patients who are able to mobilize safely and independently need to be encouraged to do so. If they need assistance, time should be incorporated into daily care plans for this. Those on bed rest or who are chair-bound require regular active and passive lower limb exercises to help prevent deep vein thrombosis and lower limb atrophy. These patients should be assessed by a physiotherapist, who can develop an individualized exercise programme for them and teach them exercises that they can do in bed. Patients with bone, spine and joint tuberculosis may face various degrees of debilitation, with associated reduction in mobility. These patients also need to be referred to physiotherapists so that appropriate mobility aids are provided and individualized exercise programmes are developed.

Patients in respiratory isolation are confined to their rooms. This may not be difficult for very sick patients, but it may be challenging for those who are reasonably well but confined for long periods because they have multidrug-resistant tuberculosis. Physiotherapists may be helpful in suggesting exercises and/or providing exercise equipment that can be used within the isolation room. This can be very helpful for patients who are in long-term isolation.[8]

Pressure area care

Pressure ulcers, previously known as pressure or bed sores or decubitus ulcers, are generally preventable by competent nursing care. Any patient who is experiencing impaired mobility, especially those on bed rest or those spending prolonged periods in a chair, are potentially at risk of developing pressure ulcers. These ulcers frequently occur on the well-recognized pressure points where the weight of the body compresses skin and associated tissues overlying bony prominences (Box 17.1).[5] Several factors contribute to the development of pressure ulcers (Box 17.2) and all patients admitted to hospital should be assessed for their risk of developing such ulcers.

BOX 17.1 Pressure sites[5]

- Elbow
- Heel
- Iliac crest
- Ischial tuberosity
- Knee
- Occiput
- Sacrum
- Scapula
- Shoulder
- Side of foot
- Spinous processes

BOX 17.2 Factors contributing to pressure ulcers

- Pressure:
  - compression of tissue
  - shearing force
  - friction
- Moisture on skin
- Heat
- Poor general nutrition
- Lack of spontaneous body movements
- Age
- Medical diagnosis

There are several well-validated tools in use to identify those patients at risk of developing pressure ulcers. The earliest and still the most widely used is the risk assessment tool developed by Norton and colleagues.[13] This tool uses a scoring scale (as illustrated in Fig. 17.1) where patients with a total score of 14 or less are assessed as prone to develop pressure ulcers, and patients with a total score below 12 are assessed as more likely than not to develop pressure ulcers.

Norton's scoring scale					
Patient's name:			Date:		
Physical condition:			**Mental condition:**		
Good	4		Alert	4	
Fair	3		Apathetic	3	
Poor	2	Score: ______	Confused	2	Score: ______
V.bad	1		Stuporous	1	
Activity:			**Mobility:**		
Ambulant	4		Full	4	
Walk/help	3		Sl.limited	3	
Chairbound	2	Score: ______	V.limited	2	Score: ______
Bedfast	1		Immobile	1	
Incontinent:					
Not	4				
Occasionally	3				
Usually/ur.	2	Score: ______			
Doubly	1				
* * * Total score:					

FIGURE 17.1 *Norton's scoring scale for pressure ulcer risk.*[13]

Another risk assessment method widely used in the UK is the pressure scoring system developed by Waterlow (as shown in Table 17.3).[14,15] Total scores indicate whether patients are 'at risk' (10+), 'high risk' (15+), or 'very high risk' (20+) of developing pressure ulcers.

Both of these tools are easy to use, but their accuracy is dependent upon subjective judgements made by the assessor. Nurses need to assess all patients admitted to hospital or ill in the community for their risk of developing pressure ulcers, using whatever risk assessment tool that has been adopted in their own healthcare facility or service. The risk for the development of pressure ulcers is assessed on admission and weekly thereafter, or whenever there is any significant change in the patient's condition and/or circumstances of care. For those assessed as at risk, a 'relief of pressure' chart (as illustrated in Fig. 17.2) should be commenced.

Preventing pressure ulcers

Patients assessed as at risk of developing pressure ulcers require regular repositioning for pressure area relief. The optimal frequency for regular repositioning has not been established. It is best assessed for each individual patient judged to be at risk in relation to the

TABLE 17.3 Waterlow pressure sore prevention/treatment policy.[14,15]
Ring the scores in the Table, add total, several scores per category can be used

Body weight for height		Skin type visual risk areas		Sex Age		Special risks	
Average	0	Healthy	0	Male	1	Tissue malnutrition e.g.	
Above average	1	Tissue paper	1	Female	2	Terminal cachexia	8
Obese	2	Dry	1	14–49	1	Cardiac failure	5
Below average	3	Oedematous	1	50–64	2	Peripheral vascular disease	5
		Clammy (temperature)	1	65–74	3		
		Discoloured	2	75–80	4	Anaemia	2
		Broken/spot	3	81+	5	Smoking	1
Continence		**Mobility**		**Appetite**		**Neurological deficit**	
Complete/catheterized	0	Fully mobile	0	Average	0	e.g. diabetes, MS, CVA, motor/sensory paraplegia	4–6
Occasional incontinence	1	Restless/fidgety	1	Poor	1		
		Apathetic	2	Nasogastric tube/fluids only	2		
Catheterized/incontinent of faeces	2	Restricted	3				
		Inert/traction	4	Nil by mouth, anorectic	3		
Double incontinence	3	Chairbound	5				
Major surgery/trauma		**Medication**					
Orthopaedic below waist/spinal	5	Cytotoxics, high-dose steroids, Anti-inflammatory	4				
On table >2 hours	5						

Score: 10+, at risk; 15+, at high risk; 20+, at very high risk.
Ring the scores in the table, add total; several scores per category can be used.

Relief of pressure chart

Date	Time	Position of patient	Relief of pressure achieved by	Nurse's signature
12/11	0800	Lying on back	Turned on left side	C. Jones
"	1000	LYING ON LEFT SIDE	TURNED ON RIGHTSIDE	E. KARN
"	1200	Lying on right side	Turned on to back	J. Baird
"	1400	Lying on back	Turned on left side	A. Hilton

FIGURE 17.2 *Relief of pressure chart.*

condition of the skin after 1 hour in a constant position. Consequently, nurses may judge that a particular patient may require repositioning every 2 hours, every hour or even more frequently.[16] Massage of pressure areas with various body lotions and creams is no longer recommended and should not be done because of the risk of damage to the skin.[17] Because it is the weight of the body on pressure points (see Box 17.1) that causes pressure ulcers, the relief of pressure is at the centre of all care strategies designed to prevent them. *Careful repositioning of the patient at regular intervals is the single most effective measure for preventing pressure ulcers*. Using pressure-reducing/relieving aids, such as pressure-reducing cushions, bed cradles and natural sheepskin fleeces (when in chairs), can also help prevent pressure ulcers. In addition, various types of pressure-reducing/relieving beds are now available that are useful for preventing pressure ulcers in those at most risk.[16] Air, rubber or foam rings are no longer recommended.[16,18]

Nurses must be skilful in moving and repositioning patients in order to prevent shearing force to pressure points. The skin needs to be kept clean, and excessive moisture and friction need to be minimized. Dehydration, malnutrition and anaemia are all factors that can lead to the development of pressure ulcers and, when possible, these must be corrected.

Evidence-based guidelines for pressure ulcer risk assessment[19] and prevention[20] and the use of pressure-relieving devices[21] have been developed by the National Institute for Clinical Excellence (NICE) in England and are available online (see 'Internet resources' at the end of this chapter).

Evaluation

The patient will be assessed frequently and appropriately to ensure that the objectives of care are being achieved, such as:

- a level of mobility appropriate to the patient's condition is maintained,
- peripheral sensory neuropathy and arthralgias associated with antituberculosis drugs are identified, reported and managed appropriately,
- pain caused by the location of extrapulmonary tuberculosis is alleviated,
- pressure ulcers, venous thrombosis and excessive muscle wasting are avoided by effective nursing care,
- where pressure ulcers are present, further tissue damage is prevented and healing is promoted by effective wound care.

THE NEED FOR A SAFE ENVIRONMENT

Potential problems	Possible causes
Accidents	Confusion, hospital environment and equipment, visual impairment as a result of drug-related optic neuritis
Fire	Oxygen therapy, negative-pressure respiratory isolation room, cigarette smoking
Healthcare-associated infections	The use of medical devices, e.g. indwelling urethral catheters, peripheral intravenous or central venous catheters
Nosocomial transmission of *Mycobacterium tuberculosis*	Ineffective infection prevention and control practices

Objectives of care

- Provide a safe environment for care and recovery.
- Minimize the risk of confusion due to a change in environment and routine.
- Minimize the risk of accidents and fire.
- Prevent healthcare-associated infections and the nosocomial transmission of *M. tuberculosis* to other patients, visitors, and hospital personnel.

Assessment

- Assess the need for respiratory isolation according to hospital infection control policies.
- Assess the patient's mental status and orientation and determine his or her ability to understand and co-operate with nursing care.
- Review the patient's medication regimen, identifying any drugs that may cause confusion or other side effects that may put the patient at an increased risk for accidents or healthcare-associated infections.
- Assess the patient's normal eyesight, physical condition and ability to mobilize safely and monitor any changes following the commencement of antituberculosis medication.
- Maintain awareness of current microbiological results.
- Review the patient's physical condition, noting any history of visual impairment, vertigo, seizures, syncope, falls, and assess the level of weakness and debilitation, if present.
- Identify any environmental hazards present that may predispose to accidents, such as medical devices, oxygen, hospital equipment, bed height.
- Assess the risks for healthcare-associated infections.
- Assess the patient's ability to understand and co-operate in measures designed to prevent fire.
- Assess the patient's normal habits with regard to smoking and alcohol intake and how these may present a challenge, especially if the patient requires isolation.

Nursing interventions

Preventing nosocomial transmission of M. tuberculosis

The various infection prevention and control measures that are used to reduce the risk of airborne transmission of *M. tuberculosis* are known as **Airborne Precautions**. Unarguably, the most important of these control measures is quickly to identify those patients who are known to have or suspected of having active pulmonary or laryngeal tuberculosis and isolate them in single-bed rooms until it has been determined that they are not infectious. This is known as **respiratory isolation**. Airborne Precautions and other infection prevention strategies for preventing the nosocomial transmission of tuberculosis in healthcare facilities are comprehensively described in Chapter 20, but some important patient management issues associated with respiratory isolation need to be considered here.

Patient education

It is important that a clear explanation is given to patients and their relatives, carers and other appropriate closely involved people in order to reduce their fear and anxiety and encourage patient co-operation with the infection control policy, including keeping the door closed and not leaving the room. Patients also need to know that they can get assistance by using the 'call button'. If the local language is not the patient's first language, arrangements should be made for an interpreter or health advocate to be present as soon as possible in order to ensure that the patient understands and is able to ask any questions (see below). Respiratory isolation can be frightening enough, and patients who do not understand why they are being isolated or what procedures they should follow can become very anxious and agitated, especially if they are 'told off' for not following the 'rules'.

Information

Prompt feedback regarding test results can also help patients who become frustrated if they are frequently being asked for specimens and not being informed of results. Some patients may even refuse to provide samples if they have not received feedback from previous tests – this is simply a way for them to try to maintain some control in a situation in which they feel completely powerless. Maximizing choice can also assist patients in isolation, for example with regard to food, visitors and daily routine.

Privacy

Patients may feel more in control if their privacy is respected. This can be achieved by knocking on the door before entering patients' rooms and asking their permission for a particular person to visit.

Counselling

Patients who are alcohol dependent or are having difficulties coping for any other reason may need to be referred to a counsellor with experience of dealing with people with problems of substance abuse.

Smoking

Heavy smokers will develop withdrawal if deprived of cigarettes and they will find it difficult to co-operate with respiratory isolation requirements. Nicotine replacements may be prescribed for some patients. However, some patients will find not smoking intolerable, and nurses may need to negotiate an agreement and a safety plan that allows them to smoke cigarettes occasionally. This will be entirely dependent on the local setting. Many healthcare facilities are 'smoke-free', and any nurse negotiating permission for a patient to smoke must be aware of the health and safety issues and adhere to the local policy on smoking. The wish to abide by patient choice must be weighed against the risks posed to others through passive smoking and possibly fire.

Preventing infections

All patients are at risk of acquiring new infections when they are admitted to hospital or are receiving clinical care from community or primary care services. These infections are known as **healthcare-associated infections** (HAIs) and, during the last two decades, they occurred in 9 per cent of patients admitted to hospitals in England[22,23] and probably at the same rate in most hospitals in other parts of the UK, in most countries in the European Union and in North America. The risk of acquiring HAIs increases if invasive medical devices are used, especially indwelling urethral catheters and central venous catheters.

There is good evidence from outbreak situations that the contaminated hands of healthcare workers are frequently responsible for transmitting infections to patients. *Effective hand decontamination immediately before each and every episode of direct patient contact/care and after any activity or contact that potentially results in the hands becoming contaminated* is the single most important measure that nurses and other healthcare professionals can take to reduce the incidence of HAIs. National evidence-based guidelines in England describe Standard Principles for preventing HAIs and define key points for effective hand hygiene that all nurses and other healthcare professionals need to observe (Box 17.3).[9,10] It is not always necessary to *wash* hands to achieve effective decontamination, and alcohol-based hand rubs offer a practical and acceptable alternative to handwashing when hands are not grossly soiled.

BOX 17.3 Key points for hand hygiene[9,10]

- Hands must be decontaminated immediately before each and every episode of direct patient contact
- Hands must be washed if they are visibly or potentially contaminated with dirt or organic material
- Alcohol-based hand rub may be used to decontaminate hands between caring for different patients and different caring activities for the same patient
- Effective technique ensures thorough hand decontamination and protects skin integrity

Disposable gloves are worn whenever there is a potential for exposure to blood, body fluids, secretions and excretions and for all contact with instruments contaminated with blood or other body fluids, and non-intact skin or mucous membranes during general care and invasive procedures. Because gloves can leak, hands need to be decontaminated after they have been removed.

A clean hospital environment is also important in preventing HAIs, and national guidelines clearly require that both the environment and the equipment used within the environment are clean, that statutory regulations are met and that staff involved in hospital hygiene are aware of their important role in helping to prevent HAIs.[9,10]

Preventing accidents

When admitted to hospital, many patients have some degree of confusion and disorientation due to a new and foreign environment. Stress, difficulties in mobilization, weakness and any intellectual impairment all compound the risk for accidents.

Equipment must be put away after use and not left to obstruct the patient's pathway, especially the path between the bed and the toilet. The nurse-call system should be checked regularly to ensure that it is working and that it is within easy reach for the patient, especially if he or she is in isolation.

Patients receiving the antituberculosis drug *ethambutol* require regular assessments of their vision, as this drug is occasionally associated with optic neuritis. Decreasing visual acuity increases the risk of accidents, as does isoniazid-associated peripheral neuropathy, which can interfere with stability. If either condition is suspected, the patient's physician must be notified.

Patients with a history of syncope (fainting), falling or seizures are assessed as being particularly vulnerable to having an accident. If a nursing assessment indicates that seizures may occur, special care is required, including ensuring that equipment for airway maintenance and suction are available at the bedside and that the bed is kept in the low position.

A careful (and ongoing) *nursing assessment* will identify those most at risk of accidents and an *environmental risk assessment* will help nurses and other healthcare professionals to modify the care setting to minimize this risk. The following aspects must be taken into account when care is planned in order to maintain a safe environment and prevent accidents.

Oxygen

When O_2 is in use, cigarette smoking is not allowed (and is generally not allowed in hospitals unless there is a designated smoking area) and 'Hazard' notices are prominently displayed in the patient's room or by the bedside. If spanners (wrenches) are needed for O_2 tanks, 'non-sparking' wrenches must be used.

Equipment

All equipment must be carefully put away after use so that it does not present a hazard to patients who are ambulatory. It is essential that a clear pathway is maintained between the patient's bed and the toilet.

Bedrails

If patients are confused or sedated, bedside rails are kept in the upright position when they are in bed, the bed is kept in the low position and they are closely observed. It is likely that there are more accidents caused by patients trying to get out of bed when the bedrails have been raised than there are due to patients falling out of bed when there are no bedrails in place, so it is important to remain vigilant if the bedrails have been raised. This is especially so for those patients with diarrhoea or frequency and urgency of urination, who may suddenly need to get out of bed to use the toilet and who are reluctant to use the nurse-call system.

Fire

In addition to the risk of fire associated with the use of medical gases such as O_2, fires can occur from a variety of sources in all healthcare facilities. Nurses need to know about and have frequent drills in how to respond appropriately to different types of fires, how to locate and activate fire alarms, appropriately use available fire-fighting equipment, and safely and efficiently evacuate patients from an area where they are in danger from fire. During evacuations, it is important not to forget to evacuate patients in single rooms, *especially those in negative-pressure rooms, where smoke and fire will quickly be drawn into the room because it has a lower atmospheric pressure then the outside corridor*.

Noise

Hospital activities are frequently noisy and patients need protection from this, as noise can cause irritation, difficulty in concentrating and thinking, discomfort, stress and lack of rest and sleep. Although noise may not directly cause accidents, it is detrimental to care and recovery, and every effort needs to be made by nurses to identify potential sources of noise and develop strategies to decrease noise as an environmental pollutant.

Miscellaneous

Floors need to be kept clean and dry and corridors need to be well lit and free of clutter. The nurse-call system should be checked to ensure that it is working properly and positioned within easy reach of the patient.

Evaluation

The patient will be assessed frequently and appropriately to ensure that the objectives of care are being achieved, such as:

- respiratory isolation is implemented as appropriate and the risk of transmission of tubercle bacilli to other patients, visitors and hospital staff is minimized,
- the frustration and loneliness of respiratory isolation are alleviated by negotiated care,
- patient factors that may predispose to accidents or infections and potential environmental safety hazards are identified and documented by a comprehensive nursing and environmental risk assessment and, where possible, rectified,
- the risk of acquiring HAIs is reduced by good standards of infection prevention and control practices.

THE NEED FOR PERSONAL CLEANSING AND DRESSING

Potential problems	Possible causes
Poor oral hygiene	Dehydration, malnutrition, infections
Inadequate body hygiene	Immobility, lack of privacy, lethargy and/or isolation without en-suite facilities
Discomfort	Excessive sweating

Objectives of care

- Maintain good oral and body hygiene.
- Maintain the patient's comfort.

Assessment

- Assess the need for mouth care, identifying the current state of oral health, usual mouth care routine (tooth brushing, dental flossing), fluid and dietary intake, and underlying physical and mental conditions that may interfere with maintaining good oral health.
- Determine the patient's level of independence/dependence and assess the need for personal care assistance to help the patient maintain body hygiene.
- Assess the care environment for anything that may hinder the patient in maintaining good levels of personal hygiene.

Nursing interventions

Mouth care

Mobile patients should be encouraged to brush their teeth with a soft toothbrush after each meal (or at least twice daily) and taught how to use dental floss or dental tape to keep the teeth clean. Some patients complain that the antituberculosis drugs leave them with an unpleasant taste in their mouth, and regular tooth brushing may help alleviate this. Ensure that cool, fresh water is constantly available and within reach and encourage the patient to drink small amounts frequently. The patient's physician needs to be notified if oral infection is suspected, such as oropharyngeal candidiasis (thrush).

Body hygiene

Cleansing and grooming are both individual and personal. While patients with fever or incontinence, and those who are seriously ill and/or weak, may require specific interventions to maintain cleanliness, the regularity and timing of personal cleansing should be left to the discretion of each individual patient whenever possible. Those confined to bed should be offered a daily bed bath and the opportunity to wash their hair once or twice per week. If a patient declines, or asks to be helped later, this should be respected whenever possible. Patients must also be given the opportunity to wash their hands before eating and after using the toilet.

Those with fever and/or night sweats may need assistance in washing and drying and a change of nightclothes and bed linen after an episode of diaphoresis (sweating) will be needed. This will be particularly important for patients in respiratory isolation, who may become more frustrated and depressed if they also feel uncomfortable.

In the industrially developed countries, most patients in respiratory isolation will have en-suite facilities. Elsewhere this is usually not the case, and before the patient leaves the room to have a bath or shower, a clinical risk assessment needs to be undertaken, particularly if the patient is being treated for suspected or confirmed multidrug-resistant tuberculosis (see Chapter 12).

Patients should be encouraged or helped to keep the skin well moisturized, and the use of a simple moisturizer, such as aqueous cream, is ideal.

Preventing pressure ulcers

Regular assessment and preventive measures, as described previously, for preventing pressure ulcers are needed for all patients except those who are fully ambulatory.[17,19–21]

Evaluation

The patient will be assessed frequently and appropriately to ensure that the objectives of care are being achieved, such as:

- cleaning and grooming are carried out according to the patient's wishes,
- any impediments to good oral and body hygiene are identified and a plan of care that ensures mouth care and assistance with body hygiene is implemented,
- the mouth and skin remain clean, intact and free of secondary infections,
- the patient remains as comfortable as possible.

THE NEED FOR EXPRESSION AND COMMUNICATION

Potential problems	Possible causes
Anxiety	Potential or actual diagnosis of tuberculosis
Feelings of fear, powerlessness and loneliness	Respiratory isolation and associated infection control precautions, such as mask wearing
Disorientation and/or distress	Respiratory isolation, language barriers, pre-existing neurological condition, anxiety, substance abuse, e.g. alcohol

Objectives of care

- Promote effective communication and supportive relationships with healthcare professionals.
- Encourage the maintenance of social contacts with people important to the patient.
- Prevent the deleterious effects often associated with isolation.

Assessment

- Establish the patient's usual communication patterns and first language.
- Assess the patient's orientation to time, place and events, including his or her understanding of the reason for admission and, if relevant, respiratory isolation.
- Assess the patient's reaction to the suspected or confirmed diagnosis of tuberculosis.
- Confirm and document visitors the patient wishes to see (and any he or she does not wish to see).
- Document carefully and clearly who is aware of the patient's diagnosis.

Nursing interventions

Reality orientation

All patients need to be orientated to the ward and the daily ward routine. Basic information needs to be given, such as where the toilets and shower/bathing facilities are, meal times, visitor regulations, fire precautions and evacuation procedures, and, importantly, when patients can expect to see their doctor. Patients who are confused need to be gently reminded of their environment, day and date, and reassured that they are safe.

During the initial assessment, it is important to find out how the patient wishes to be addressed. It is generally useful if first names are used when speaking to patients unless they have objected to this. There is nothing wrong in nurses using their own first names when talking to patients, and this will generally help build a better relationship between them. Patients should be introduced to other patients and healthcare professionals and to the nurse in charge and the nurse principally responsible for their care (the 'named nurse' or primary nurse). All healthcare staff should wear photo identification passes and/or name badges that state their name and role.

Communication aids

Patients should have easy access to a telephone, stamps and stationery. If in a single room, it may be possible for them to have a television set. They should have a bedside radio (with earphones), newspapers and magazines and there should be a clock and a calendar in the room. The nurse-call system should be within easy reach.

If a patient has difficulty communicating in the local language, interpreters should be utilized. This will help prevent feelings of fear and social isolation, which are both distressing to the patient and may prevent him or her from co-operating with care (especially if in respiratory isolation). Visitors should be encouraged to provide newspapers and magazines in the patient's first language.

The use of technical language and jargon should be kept to a minimum and, when used, should be carefully explained to the patient.

Time for talking/listening/touching

Consideration should be given to how patients communicated with their partners, friends and families before their admission to hospital and how best to facilitate the continuation of these communications while they are in hospital. Whether or not they are in isolation, patients are likely to be very anxious about an actual or possible diagnosis of tuberculosis. Nursing care plans must take into account the fact that patients need to talk to their nurses. Listening, holding patients' hands and just quietly being with them are necessary aspects of nursing art. Complex social or psychological concerns may be appropriately referred to a counsellor or mental health nurse consultant.

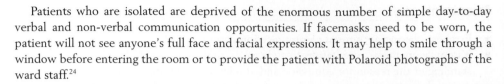

Patients who are isolated are deprived of the enormous number of simple day-to-day verbal and non-verbal communication opportunities. If facemasks need to be worn, the patient will not see anyone's full face and facial expressions. It may help to smile through a window before entering the room or to provide the patient with Polaroid photographs of the ward staff.[24]

Visitors

Caring for a patient's visitors is often a delicate task, especially if they do not know the patient's diagnosis. This is particularly challenging with regard to an isolated patient, as the visitors will have to conform to the infection control precautions. *No information on any aspect of the patient's condition may be given to any visitors, no matter who they are, without the patient's express consent*. As always, all visitors to the hospital must be treated with respect and consistent courtesy. An officious or abrupt manner displayed by healthcare workers to visitors can do immeasurable damage to their willingness to visit and is demoralizing to the patient. If possible, friends and family should be encouraged to visit throughout the day and early evening.

Due to the stigma associated with tuberculosis, some patients may have been abandoned by both friends and family. With the patient's permission, it is possible to contact voluntary support groups who can arrange for members from their organization to visit the patient. The hospital's voluntary services may also be able to provide this service.

Infection prevention

While it is necessary to prevent transmission of disease by isolating known or suspected cases of pulmonary tuberculosis, excessive infection prevention precautions (such as inappropriate isolation or protective clothing) are barriers between the patient and other human beings and must be avoided. If a patient is under investigation for tuberculosis, it is essential to feed back results as soon as possible so the need for isolation can be confirmed or cancelled without delay. This will also alleviate anxiety for patients, who are often eagerly awaiting their results. Patients who are fully ambulatory should be encouraged to use communal ward facilities, such as sitting rooms and television rooms, and to mix with other patients.

Evaluation

The patient will be assessed frequently and appropriately to ensure that the objectives of care are being achieved, such as:

- the patient remains orientated to his or her condition and environment,
- time and space are made available for the patient to communicate with family, friends and hospital staff,
- feelings of anxiety, loneliness and powerlessness are addressed, particularly those associated with the experience of respiratory isolation.

THE NEED FOR WORKING AND PLAYING

Potential problems	Possible causes
Economic hardship	Loss of employment
Boredom and loneliness	Respiratory isolation

Objectives of care

- Provide access to appropriate financial resources.
- Minimize effects of boredom and loneliness.

Assessment

- Assess the effects of absence from usual employment and lifestyle. The nursing history should include information relating to any dependants the patient may have and how loss of earnings will affect the patient and his or her dependants.
- Sensitively assess immigration status and any likelihood of pending repatriation or change in accommodation that may interrupt treatment.
- Document the patient's past leisure-time activities, hobbies and interests.
- Assess the patient's neurological status and the presence of any sensory deficits or physical disablement.
- Indicate if the patient expects and would welcome visits from partner, friends and family.

Nursing interventions

Financial problems

It is possible that patients with tuberculosis will need to claim any available state benefits to which they are entitled. As the social security systems in many countries – if, indeed, they exist at all – are confusing and complex, such patients should be interviewed by a social worker as soon as possible following admission.

The prompt issue of medical and sickness certificates while patients are in hospital is important and should not be left until they ask for them. Another real issue for some patients who are having financial difficulties is their ability to maintain rent or mortgage payments. The need for stable housing is very important to the patient's ability to continue treatment with the necessary support from the TB team following discharge. If there are likely to be problems with housing, the TB team should be informed before the patient's discharge. The hospital social worker will be able to advise patients about their housing situation and may also be able to assist those who have been dismissed by their employers as a result of illness.

Leisure-time activities

In settings in which such luxuries are available, it is important that patients have access to a telephone, television viewing and a radio. Any available hospital library services should be explained and arrangements made for patients to purchase newspapers and magazines. Boredom can be a serious problem for isolated patients. 'Home from home' comforts that can be brought in will help to maintain their psychological well-being during their confinement and make their rooms less like hospital wards.[8]

For those who are not isolated, a comfortable area for sitting and socializing can provide patients with a change of scenery and promote social interaction. This room needs to be accessible at all times and patients should be made aware of its location.

Visitors

Visiting times must be flexible and visitors encouraged. Where appropriate, visitors can be encouraged to take patients off the ward, as this can provide a very welcome break from the monotony of ward life. It is also necessary to respect patients' privacy when partners are visiting and allow them the time and space to be with one another without interruption.

With their permission, the hospital's volunteer services or a voluntary organization may be able to arrange visitors for patients who do not have any. It is also important for patients to have visits from healthcare workers, especially if they are being nursed in single rooms. Time must be made available to visit and talk to patients, rather than only entering the room to 'do' something.

Substance abuse

It is recommended that alcohol is avoided when taking antituberculosis medication, due to the potential hepatotoxic effects of most of the antituberculosis drugs. This may present a challenge to people who enjoy social drinking and may find it difficult to explain their change in drinking habits to their friends if they have not told them about their diagnosis. It is important that this is discussed with patients before their discharge. Patients who have drug or alcohol dependency may benefit from being referred to appropriate specialist agencies and should either be referred directly (with their permission) or be given the relevant information in order that they may refer themselves. If these patients are likely to have difficulties adhering to their treatment regimen, especially following discharge, the tuberculosis specialist nurse should arrange for them to receive directly observed therapy (DOT). In any case, it is important that the specialist nurse is informed as soon as possible of any patients with drug or alcohol dependency.

Evaluation

The patient will be assessed frequently and appropriately to ensure that the objectives of care are being achieved, such as:

- an opportunity is given for the patient to address any financial issues related to maintaining his or her standard of living while in hospital and on discharge,
- leisure-time activities and visiting arrangements are organized as much as possible according to the preference of the patient,
- drug or alcohol dependency is managed effectively.

THE NEED TO MAINTAIN PSYCHOLOGICAL EQUILIBRIUM

Potential problems	Possible causes
Depression	Rejection, powerlessness, isolation
Anxiety and stress	Fear of long-term illness, stigma, death
Loss of self-esteem	Stigma, infectiousness, unemployment
Exacerbation of concurrent psychiatric illness	Rifampicin reducing efficacy of some anti-psychotic drugs

Assessment

- Assess any indications of psychological distress, such as anxiety, depression, ineffective coping, feelings of isolation and low self-esteem.
- Assess pre-existing psychiatric conditions.
- Ascertain the patient's level and source of emotional and social support.

Nursing interventions

Anxiety

Anxiety is neither inappropriate nor uncommon in people with serious illness, including those with tuberculosis, especially during periods of hospitalization. Manifestations of anxiety occur on several levels, ranging from mild tension to sympathetic nervous system overflow and panic (Table 17.4). Many patients will require assistance in coping with excessive anxiety.

TABLE 17.4 Levels of anxiety

Level of anxiety	Characteristics
Level 1 (mild)	The patient is alert, enquiring and relatively relaxed and defence mechanisms are working well. In this level, patients are receptive to information.
Level 2 (moderate)	Increased alertness and heightened emotional state. The patient is more receptive to sensory information than factual information and is able to learn relaxation techniques. In this level, patients are able to solve most problems on their own.
Level 3 (severe)	Sympathetic nervous system overflow is present, with typical fight-or-flight responses. With severe anxiety, patients are no longer able to solve problems on their own, needing the advocacy skills of the nurse. Physical signs and symptoms of anxiety are often present, such as tachycardia, restlessness, irritability and a feeling of 'butterflies in the stomach'. The patient is frightened.
Level 4 (panic)	The patient is overwhelmed by fear and is unable to concentrate, having more pronounced physical signs of sympathetic over-activity, such as insomnia, tachycardia, profuse perspiration (especially on the palms and forehead), frequency of micturition and defaecation, rapid breathing and vertigo.

Patients do not progress from level 1 through to level 4, but fluctuate from one level to another. Stressful events (Box 17.4) occurring during illness may precipitate progression to more severe levels of anxiety. Interventions designed to alleviate excessive anxiety include discussing patients' fears with them, rationally highlighting their identifiable strengths to cope with stressors, and encouraging socialization and leisure-time activities. In some coun-

BOX 17.4 Some stressors for patients with tuberculosis

- Fear and loneliness due to respiratory isolation
- Stigmatization related to having tuberculosis (see Chapter 15)
- Rejection from family, partner, friends, employer, faith community, school
- Unemployment, financial worries, poverty
- Homelessness
- Difficulties adhering to prescribed antituberculosis chemotherapy
- Development of resistance to antituberculosis chemotherapy
- Progressive changes in body image
- Inappropriate infection control precautions while in hospital or clinic
- Prejudice and discrimination
- Disclosing diagnosis of tuberculosis to spouse or partner, family, friends, neighbours, employers
- Threatened (or actual) loss of confidentiality

tries, many hospitals have qualified counsellors and clinical psychologists on their staff who can offer more skilled assistance to patients in alleviating anxiety and teaching relaxation techniques. Severe anxiety or panic generally requires anxiolytic medication (Box 17.5), which is more useful for the short-term management of acute anxiety rather than long-term use.

BOX 17.5 Some anxiolytic, hypnotic and antidepressant drugs[25]

Drugs used for anxiety

Benzodiazepines, including:

- Diazepam
- Chlordiazepoxide
- Lorazepam
- Oxazepam

Hypnotics (drugs used for the relief of insomnia)

Benzodiazepines, including:

- Nitrazepam
- Temazepam
- Loprazolam

Cyclopyrolone

Zopiclone

Antidepressant drugs

Tricyclic and related antidepressant drugs, including:

- Amitriptyline
- Clomipramine
- Imipramine
- Mianserin
- Trazodone

Monoamine oxidase inhibitors (MAOIs),[a] including:

- Phenelzine
- Isocarboxazid

Selective serotonin re-uptake inhibitors (SSRIs), including:

- Fluoxetine
- Citalopram
- Fluvoxamine maleate
- Paroxetine
- Sertraline

[a]See Box 17.6.

Depression

Clinical depression is common in people with chronic illness and its early recognition allows prompt treatment. It is important to assess patients for signs of depression to be able to plan appropriate action and prevent problems that may arise with adherence to medication relating to their depression (see Chapter 14). Patients may despair, complain of sleep disturbances (early-morning wakening, difficulty in falling asleep), lose the ability to concentrate and show a loss of interest and energy and diminished appetite (anorexia). Ideas of self-reproach are associated with feelings of despair, hopelessness and guilt. Mental retardation (as seen in depression) in patients with chronic illness often acts as a brake on suicidal acts, but it cannot be relied upon. In general, antidepressant medication is required for all but the mildest incidents of depression.

Although there are various types of antidepressants (see Box 17.5), the *tricyclic and related group of antidepressants* are the safest and most commonly prescribed. *Selective serotonin re-uptake inhibitors* (SSRIs) are also used and, in addition to their antidepressant properties, many SSRIs also help to alleviate panic attacks. An older group of antidepressants, known as *monoamine oxidase inhibitors* (MAOIs), is less often prescribed but may be used for those refractory to treatment with tricyclic and related drugs or to SSRI antidepressants.

If a patient is prescribed antidepressant medication, it is imperative that the nurse is aware to which group the drug belongs. MAOI antidepressants require specific dietary restrictions, as foods rich in tyramine (Box 17.6) may interact with these drugs and provoke a hypertensive crisis, with the risk of intracranial haemorrhage. MAOI antidepressants also interact with pethidine (meperidine hydrochloride USP), opiates, phenothiazines (e.g. chlorpromazine and haloperidol) and alcohol. If administering MAOIs, nurses will find it useful to seek advice from the pharmacist or consult the latest edition of the *British National Formulary* (BNF),[25] or analogous publications in other countries, for a complete description of side effects and drug and dietary interactions. A new edition of the BNF is published every 6 months and it is also available online (see 'Internet resources' at the end of this chapter).

BOX 17.6 Monoamine oxidase inhibitors (MAOIs) and food interactions[25]

Patients need to be advised to avoid the following foods and drinks while taking MOAI antidepressants.

- Cheese
- Meat or yeast extract or fermented soya bean extract, e.g. Bovril®, Oxo®, Marmite®
- Broad bean pods
- Pickled herring
- Alcoholic drinks (including low-alcohol drinks)

Patients should be advised to eat only fresh foods and avoid food that is suspected of being stale or 'going off'. This is especially important with meat, fish, poultry or offal; game should be avoided.

In the 2–3 weeks before antidepressants become effective, the risk of suicide remains real. Antidepressants are generally very effective; some tend to be sedating, whereas others tend to be stimulating. Treatment may have to continue for several months if a relapse is to be prevented.

Individual counselling and psychotherapy

Patients in long-term isolation, for instance those who have multidrug-resistant tuberculosis, may benefit from referral to a counsellor or psychotherapist.

Family and significant others

It is not only the patient who requires psychological and emotional support. Family (husbands, wives and children), lovers and friends all display various levels of anxiety. Enormous demands are commonly made upon nursing staff, and the highest degree of skill and sensitivity is required in offering appropriate support.

Evaluation

The patient will be assessed frequently and appropriately to ensure that the objectives of care are being achieved, such as:

- any psychological dysfunction is recognized early and nursing interventions and medical treatments are implemented to alleviate or contain the mental distress the patient is suffering,
- psychological equilibrium is maintained through ongoing appropriate management of pre-existing psychiatric disorder,
- in liaison with other healthcare professionals, the patient is taught to use effective coping and relaxation techniques.

THE NEED FOR ADEQUATE REST AND SLEEP

Potential problems	Possible causes
Insomnia	Pain, anxiety, discomfort, depression
Interrupted sleep	Nursing interventions, observations, bouts of sweating during the night

Objectives of care

- Ensure that the patient has uninterrupted periods of sleep.

Assessment

- Ascertain the patient's usual sleeping environment, for example own or shared bed, and habits. This includes noting the time the patient usually goes to bed, periods of wakefulness during the night, frequency of need to urinate during the night, and the usual time of waking.
- Assess the patient for any signs or complaints of pain, discomfort, depression or anxiety, including duration and frequency of night sweats.
- Review the rationale for any nocturnal nursing observations or interventions and determine ways in which disruptions can be minimized.

Nursing interventions

Comfort

Most patients in hospital benefit from an afternoon 'rest period' shortly after lunch. Visitors should be asked not to visit during this time. Noise is a frequent cause of complaint from all patients in hospital. Every effort must be made to eliminate unnecessary noise, especially during the night. This specifically includes loud talking or laughter at the nurses' station. Drinks containing caffeine (tea, coffee, chocolate drinks, colas) should be avoided after the evening meal, and a warm milk drink may be useful in helping to settle the patient. Patients should be assisted to void before retiring, the bed linen should be straightened and they should be asked if they want their bedside light left on or if a nightlight is adequate. Care for seriously ill patients requiring intensive nursing during the night should be planned so that everything necessary is done at one time, allowing them 2-hour periods of uninterrupted sleep.

Medication

The physician may prescribe analgesics, night sedation, anxiolytic or antidepressant medication (see Box 17.5). It is important to remember that night sedation is ineffective if pain is present, and appropriate analgesia is often sufficient to allow patients to fall asleep. If night sedation is required, temazepam or zopiclone is commonly used. Anxiety may have to be treated with short-term anxiolytic medication. Early-morning wakening may be a sign of clinical depression, which usually requires specific treatment with antidepressant medications (see above). When administering these (and any other) drugs, nurses need to be fully aware of their potential side effects and interactions with other drugs, and this information can be found in the current edition of the BNF,[25] and in analogous publications in other countries.

Evaluation

The patient will be assessed frequently and appropriately to ensure that the objectives of care are being achieved, such as:

- the planning of nursing interventions takes account of the patient's need to obtain adequate rest and sleep while in hospital.

THE NEED FOR SPIRITUAL CARE

Potential problems	Possible causes
Religious deprivation	Hospitalization and/or isolation
Spiritual deprivation	Loss of social and/or spiritual support

Objectives of care

- Facilitate patients' access to the hospital chaplain or religious adviser.
- Meet patients' spiritual needs on a wider level.

Assessment

- Ascertain and document the patient's religious faith and any special religious needs.
- Confirm whether patients would like a representative of their religion to visit them.
- Assess patients' level of spiritual support from friends, family, their faith community and religious adviser.

Nursing interventions

Spiritual care

The spirit is what makes human beings human.[26] Spirituality can be seen as a person's beliefs about a higher being and the universe and about such ideas as life, love, hope and forgiveness. Spirituality may be expressed through communal worship and participating in the activities of an organized religion or through more personal and individual means. Spirituality can foster hope, help people cope with the stress of illness and reduce anxiety. Nurses are able to offer spiritual as well as physical support to patients by simple activities such as just listening and talking, especially at times of increased stress and worry, 'being there' for patients when they need support, and creating an environment in hospital in which patients are facilitated to worship, pray and observe religious practices and rites.

Facilitating worship

Chaplains and other religious advisers must, at the patient's wish, have complete access. Patients should not be visited by religious advisers they have not asked to see. It is often possible for patients to be taken to the hospital chapel for religious services or to pray.

It is essential that Christian patients have the opportunity of attending Confession and of receiving holy sacraments. The Sacrament of the Anointing of the Sick (Extreme Unction or Last Rites) is extremely important for many Christian patients, and the wish to be administered this sacrament should be documented in the patient's nursing notes. It should, however, be noted that, to an increasing extent, anointing and the laying-on-of-hands is used in the Ministry of Healing for all patients and not just for those who are terminally ill. Patients should therefore be allowed visits from healers if they so wish. The sacrament of Holy Communion is important to members of all the major Christian churches.

Muslim patients may wish to pray five times a day, and every effort should be made to respect the timing and duration of their prayers and assist in ensuring that an appropriate prayer mat is available. This can often be arranged through visiting family or friends.

Religion is diverse and it is important to respect individual religious beliefs. Every effort should be made by healthcare professionals to recognize and encourage the practices involved within all of the diverse religious beliefs that patients may have. The opportunity to participate in religious worship is a tremendous comfort to many patients who are ill in hospital with tuberculosis. At the patient's request, religious attendants can make sacred texts and other literature available.

Evaluation

The patient will be assessed frequently and appropriately to ensure that the objectives of care are being achieved, such as:

- the patient has opportunities to worship and be comforted by his or her religious beliefs.

THE NEED TO EXPRESS SEXUALITY

Potential problems	Possible causes
Unwanted pregnancy	Interaction of some antituberculosis drugs with oral contraceptives
Loss of libido	Perceptions of infectiousness
Need to modify sexual behaviour	Co-infection with the human immunodeficiency virus

Objectives of care

- Provide patients with information on safer sex and contraception while taking anti-tuberculosis drugs.
- Reassure patients regarding the transmission of tuberculosis to sexual partners.
- Establish patients' HIV status and manage accordingly.

Assessment

- Assess current sexual health, including HIV status.
- Ascertain the patient's attitude to and knowledge of safer sexual practices.
- If the patient is female, ascertain the method of contraception she is using.
- Identify any underlying anxieties or problems that may be interfering with the patient's ability to express his or her sexuality.

Nursing interventions

Sexuality and sexual health

Sexuality is at the core of our personality and it is an essential element of our personhood.[27] It is 'a powerful and purposeful aspect of human nature and it is an important dimension of our humanness'.[28] It is the way we individually and uniquely express and project our identity and inter-relate our physiological and psychosocial processes, which are inherent in the way we sexually develop and sexually respond, both to ourselves and to others.[27,28]

Sexuality is more than just overt sexual behaviour; it spans and underlies the complete range of human experience and contributes to our lives, and to the lives of our family, friends, neighbours, colleagues and clients in many ways.

In positively expressing our sexuality, we are able to build our unique identity, to communicate subtle, gentle or intense feelings, to realize sexual pleasure and physical release, to bond emotionally with others, to achieve a sense of self-worth and, for many, to link with the future through our children.[27] Being able to express our sexuality positively is one of the most joyful and enriching aspects of the human experience, which, for many people in socially and economically deprived communities and countries, helps compensate for many of the less positive aspects of living in our world today. The expression of sexuality is an aspect of life to which all people are entitled and, for many, makes waking up in the morning worthwhile, purposeful and exciting. Being able to express our individual sexuality positively is an essential component of experiencing a healthy sexual life (Box 17.7) and informs the whole of our lives.

Positive sexuality is associated with high self-esteem, respect for self and others, non-exploitive sexual satisfaction, rewarding human relationships and, for many, the joy of desired parenthood.

BOX 17.7 Positive sexuality

Experiencing a healthy sexual life includes:

- having access to sexual information and developing knowledge in relation to sexual and reproductive phenomena
- freedom from unwanted pregnancies and abusive sexual behaviour
- being able to integrate the physical, emotional, intellectual and social aspects of sexual being in ways that are positively enriching and that enhance personality, communication and love[29]
- having an ability to create effective relationships with members of both sexes
- developing a self-awareness and appreciation of our feelings and attitudes towards sexuality and sexual behaviour
- having a positive self-image
- developing a value system that can assist sexual decision making
- having some degree of emotional comfort, interdependence and stability with respect to the sexual activities in which we participate[29]
- a capacity to enjoy and control sexual and reproductive behaviour in accordance with a social and personal ethic
- freedom from fear, shame, guilt, false beliefs and other psychological factors inhibiting sexual response and impairing sexual relationships
- freedom from organic disorders, diseases and deficiencies that interfere with sexual and reproductive functions[30]

Sexuality is socially and culturally constructed, and concepts of sexuality have changed over time and remain dynamic today. There are significant individual, social and cultural variations in sexual values, accepted behaviour and sexual practices in different communities throughout the world, which will impact on the ability of an individual to express their sexuality positively.

Most people would agree, however, that the ability to express our sexuality positively is a major determinant of our sexual and reproductive health, which in turn is an important element of our physical and mental health. Everyone has an inalienable right to health, including sexual health, which is defined by the English Department of Health as follows.

> Sexual health is an important part of physical and mental health. It is a key part of our identity as human beings, together with the fundamental human rights to privacy, a family life and living free from discrimination. Essential elements of good sexual health are equitable relationships and sexual fulfilment with access to information and services to avoid the risk of unintended pregnancy, illness or disease.[31]

In addition, being able to express our sexuality positively is a natural aspiration for most people. Co-infection with HIV can have a significant impact on an individual's ability to achieve or sustain an adequate level of sexual health and may require adjustments to how that person expresses his or her sexuality.

HIV co-infection

Throughout the world, tuberculosis is the most common opportunistic disease seen in HIV-infected people (see Chapter 10). Consequently, everyone diagnosed with active tuberculosis should, within the framework of local legislation and guidelines, be offered and be encouraged to be tested for HIV infection. This allows health education interventions, such as safer sexual practices, to be targeted at infected people to help them minimize the risk of infecting others. Additionally, the detection of HIV infection in people with tuberculosis will allow them to access appropriate treatment, such as antiretroviral therapy, which is increasingly available in many parts of the world. Appropriate and sensitive pre-test discussions are important, and the patient's informed consent is needed before testing.

Sexual health

Everyone, including those living with tuberculosis, can benefit from being able to express their sexuality positively and participate in activities designed to promote and enhance their sexual health. Knowing how to protect oneself from sexually transmitted infections (STIs), including HIV infection, is an important feature of an overall strategy designed to maintain the best possible level of sexual health.

Millions of people with tuberculosis throughout the world are co-infected with HIV. Because these people will have some degree of immunosuppression, newly acquired STIs may be more problematic than they would be in a non-HIV-infected person who is fully immunocompetent. Many STIs, including genital warts, herpes virus infections and various fungi and bacterial infections, may be more aggressive in HIV-infected people, more difficult to treat and more likely to result in recurrent disease. In addition, newly acquired STIs can stimulate HIV replication, increasing the viral load and accelerating HIV disease progression. The presence of ulcerative and/or inflammatory STIs makes it more likely that HIV will be transmitted during sexual intercourse. For those HIV-infected individuals who have not previously been infected with herpes simplex viruses or cytomegalovirus, hepatitis B or hepatitis C viruses, becoming infected with these viruses can immensely complicate HIV disease and worsen clinical outcomes. Finally, having unprotected penetrative sex with another HIV-infected person may result in becoming re-infected with a more pathogenic or drug-resistant strain of HIV, which may increase the rate of disease progression and significantly limit future treatment options.

Although it is everyone's responsibility to protect themselves from STIs, HIV-infected individuals who know their infection status may be more acutely aware of the need to protect their sexual partners from infection. This concern may result in disclosure of their HIV status and negotiation concerning the level of risk that each partner finds acceptable.

Nurses can offer factual advice on reducing the risk of sexual transmission of HIV and the prevention of STIs (Box 17.8) and direct the patient to additional sources of reliable information (Box 17.9).

Patients need to be encouraged to seek prompt diagnosis and treatment if they suspect they may have been exposed to an infectious disease, as untreated STIs increase their risk of becoming infected with a new variant of HIV or transmitting HIV infection to others. Additionally, it is important that HIV-infected people receiving antiretroviral treatment realize that *a low or undetectable plasma HIV viral load does not mean that they are no longer infectious*. They may be less infectious,[32] but they are still potentially infectious, as the level of virus in plasma does not necessarily reflect the level of virus in semen or vaginal secretions, which may be higher due to poor penetration of antiretroviral drugs into these biological compartments. Consequently, all infected people need to take precautions to avoid infecting others, regardless of their plasma viral load measurement.

BOX 17.8 Some sources of reliable information on preventing sexually transmitted infections (including HIV infection) in the UK

- *AIDS reference manual*, regularly published by National AIDS Manual (NAM) Publications, 16a Clapham Common Southside, London SW4 7AB. Telephone: 020 7627 3200; email: <info@nam.org.uk>; website: <www.aidsmap.com>
- Terrence Higgins Trust, 52–54 Grays Inn Road, London WC1X 8JU. Telephone (THT Direct): 0845 1221 200; email: <info@tht.org.uk>; website: <www.tht.org.uk>
- Gay Men Fighting AIDS (GMFA), Unit 43, Eurolink Centre, 49 Effra Road, London SW2 1BZ. Telephone: 020 7738 6872; email: <gmfa@gmfa.demon.co.uk>; website: <http://www.hivsouthlondon.org.uk/gmfa.htm>
- Health Protection Agency (HPA) England. Website: <http://www.hpa.org.uk/>
- National HIV Prevention Information Services (NHPIS) – a free specialist information service on HIV health promotion serving people with a professional interest in HIV prevention across England. Health Development Agency, Trevelyan House, 30 Great Peter Street, London SW1P 2HW. Telephone: 020 7413 2001; email: <nhpis@had-online.org.uk>; website: <http://www.hda-online.org.uk/html/nhpis/>
- The Body – the most comprehensive HIV and AIDS information resource on the Internet at: <http://www.thebody.com/index.shtml>

BOX 17.9 Community-based organizations in the UK that provide information and support for adopting a healthy sexual lifestyle

- Terrence Higgins Trust, 52–54 Grays Inn Road, London WC1X 8JU. Telephone (THT Direct): 0845 1221 200; email: <info@tht.org.uk>; website: <www.tht.org.uk>
- Gay Men Fighting AIDS (GMFA), Unit 43, Eurolink Centre, 49 Effra Road, London SW2 1BZ. Telephone: 020 7738 6872; email: <gmfa@gmfa.demon.co.uk>; website: <http://www.hivsouthlondon.org.uk/gmfa.htm>
- London East AIDS Network (LEAN), 35 Romford Road, Stratford, London E15 4LY. Telephone: 020 8519 9545; email: <info@lean.org.uk>; website: <www.lean.org.uk>
- The Naz Project (support for Black and Asian HIV+ people), Palingswick House, 241 King Street, London W6 9LP. Telephone: 020 8741 1879; email: <npl@naz.org.uk>; website: <http://www.naz.org.uk>
- Blackliners (support for Black and Afro-Caribbean HIV+ people), Unit 46, Eurolink Centre, 49 Effra Road, London SW2 1BZ. Telephone: 020 7738 5274 Best time to telephone: 9.30am – 5.30pm, Monday – Friday.; African Community Health Advisor e-mail: acha@blackliners.org; website: <http://blackliners.mappibiz.com/index.htm>
- Positively Women (support for HIV+ women), 347–349 City Road, London EC1V 1LR. Telephone: 020 7713 0222; email: <poswomen@dircon.co.uk>; website: <http://www.positivelywomen.org.uk/>

Transmission of tuberculosis

It is essential that patients understand how tuberculosis is transmitted and are given a realistic account of the risks to their closest contacts depending on the site of their disease and whether or not they are infectious. They need to be reassured that even if they were infectious to begin with, they will no longer be so after 2 weeks of treatment and they should not become infectious again as long as they adhere to the treatment regimen. As close contacts, their partner(s) may be screened, but there is no reason to abstain from sexual activity during or after treatment. This may be an issue that the patient's partner wishes to discuss, and he or she should feel able to do so.

Contraception

It is important to discuss contraception with female patients of childbearing age, as the administration of rifampicin and related rifamycin antibiotics reduces the effectiveness of oral contraceptives, thereby increasing the risk of unwanted pregnancies. Those women (and their partners) who rely on oral contraceptives need to be educated about alternative methods of contraception, such as condoms or the use of a diaphragm.

Evaluation

The patient will be assessed frequently and appropriately to ensure that the objectives of care are being achieved, such as:

- any underling physical or mental health problem that may be interfering with the patient's ability to express his or her sexuality is identified,
- HIV testing is offered and encouraged, with appropriate pre-test and post-test discussions,
- there is an opportunity for the patient to discuss and explore issues surrounding the development of a healthy sexual lifestyle,
- appropriate referrals are made to the health advisor, counsellor, psychologist and/or relevant community-based organization,
- female patients understand that oral contraception will be ineffective while they are taking a regimen of antituberculosis drugs that includes rifampicin.

NEEDS ASSOCIATED WITH DYING

Potential problems	Possible causes
Fear of death	Belief that tuberculosis is always fatal
Fear, anxiety and loneliness	Impending death, manner of death, loss of power and control
Physical problems associated with dying	Pathophysiology of tuberculosis; HIV disease
Inability to adjust to impending death	Fear, regrets, unfinished business

Objectives of care

- Alleviate anxiety of the majority of patients whose tuberculosis is curable.
- Negotiate and agree with the patient the plan and objectives of care.
- Alleviate or control physical problems associated with end-stage HIV disease.
- Support, comfort and reassure the patient journeying towards death.

Assessment

- Assess (and frequently re-assess) physical symptoms associated with the terminal stages of disease.

- Ascertain and anticipate patients' existential, psychosocial, emotional and spiritual needs as they near the end of their life and identify opportunities for support.
- Ascertain patients' beliefs associated with tuberculosis and their attitude to the information being given.

Nursing interventions

Concerns about death and dying need to be addressed. Many people still believe that tuberculosis is a fatal disease and need reassurance that, with effective treatment that is adhered to correctly, the great majority of patients can be cured. It is important to assess patients in terms of their experience and knowledge of the disease so they can be given the relevant information. Patients who are convinced they are going to die may need repeated reassurance over a number of days.

Patients may be at risk of dying if diagnosis is severely delayed, if they have multidrug-resistant tuberculosis and an adequate second-line regimen is not available, or if they have advanced HIV disease. In these cases it will be necessary to address issues associated with dying.

HIV co-infection

Since the introduction of highly active antiretroviral therapy (HAART) in the early to mid-1990s, the death rate from HIV disease has dramatically fallen in countries in the industrially developed world. It is as yet unknown, however, how long end-stage disease can be postponed with the use of these complex and powerful therapies. If drug resistance is ultimately inevitable, and if unacceptable or severe side effects preclude lifelong drug therapy, health will eventually fail and patients will then require nursing care and support as they near the end of their lives.

In resource-poor countries, most patients with tuberculosis and HIV disease are more likely to progress rapidly to end-stage disease because of their poor nutritional status, other underlying diseases, and a lack of competent and effective medical care, including access to antiretroviral therapy. As discussed in Chapter 10, HIV co-infection worsens tuberculosis and tuberculosis accelerates HIV disease progression.

Death and dying

Death is part of life and dying is simply 'living the end of life.' All those who have thought about the inevitability of death share a common wish to 'live the end of their life' well. Supporting patients during the final phase of their lives requires the best nursing skills and a heightened awareness of the unique needs of the person nearing death. These include the need to be safe and not to be hurt, to be given refuge or sanctuary and to be comforted, and to be accepted, to belong, and to give and receive love. Palliative and terminal nursing care is therefore not about death, but rather about supporting patients to 'live the end of their life' well.

Caring for patients living the end of their life is not just about physical care, but also about nurses and other healthcare professionals meeting a variety of psychosocial, emotional, spiritual and existential needs patients may have. Nurses cannot do this alone, but they can co-ordinate the multi-disciplinary and interdisciplinary support needed from members of the healthcare team.

A variety of physical and psychological problems that may impede patients from living the end of their lives well is typically manifested during the terminal stages of illness (Table

TABLE 17.5 Patient problems and concerns

Physical	
Anorexia/weight loss	Excessive respiratory secretions
Bowel colic	Fatigue/weakness
Constipation	Hiccup
Convulsions	Incontinence
Cough	Nausea and vomiting
Dehydration	Pain
Dyspnoea	Pressure ulcers
Ethical and legal	
Euthanasia	Living Wills/Advanced Directives
Healthcare proxy	
Psychological	
Depression	Stress/anxiety
Restlessness and confusion	

17.5). Almost all of them are generally amenable to skilled medical and nursing interventions and symptom management. In addition, several societal concerns and issues, including legal and ethical dilemmas, frequently need to be confronted and addressed, by both patients and their carers, as the end of life draws near.

Agreeing the plan and objectives of care

Everyone approaches the end of their life differently, with unique needs and aspirations for this important and final stage of living. They will need to make decisions about their treatment and care and, in discussion with their doctors, nurses and other members of the healthcare team, clarify and confirm their wishes. The treatment and care issues that need to be confronted vary greatly according to the disease status of the patient. In the case of HIV-related tuberculosis, commonly occurring issues include the discontinuation of many treatments, including antiretroviral therapy, treatment and/or chemoprophylaxis for various opportunistic infections, the use of corticosteroids and artificial nutrition and hydration, and cardiopulmonary resuscitation. A plan of care needs to be negotiated and agreed and the patient needs to be reassured that the objectives of care can be discussed again at any time. Competent and effective symptom management is what most patients desire during this phase of their life.

Physical problems – symptom control

Nursing and medical interventions focused on the relief of most of the physical problems listed in Table 17.5 are discussed elsewhere,[33] but the management of some of these problems within the context of palliative care deserves further elaboration here. Although only briefly discussed in this chapter, nurses are encouraged to explore symptom management further in the more comprehensive texts on palliative care recommended at the end of this chapter.

Pain

Pain, often severe, is a common patient problem and frequently persists, not because it is refractory to analgesia, but because of various misconceptions patients, their friends and families, and healthcare professionals have about pain and the drugs (especially opioids) that are used to alleviate it. *Analgesics are more effective in preventing pain than in relieving it.* Consequently, the initiation of an opioid analgesic should not be delayed because of concern about tolerance or dependence, because these do not occur in the palliative care setting. The physician will order appropriate analgesia (Table 17.6) according to the type (neuropathic, visceral, somatic, bone), severity and intensity of the pain.

TABLE 17.6 Some analgesics commonly used in palliative care[25]

Non-opioid analgesics	Opioid analgesics
Paracetamol	Codeine
Non-steroidal anti-inflammatory drugs, e.g.	Dihydrocodeine tartrate
aspirin	Morphine
naproxen	Hydromorphone hydrochloride
flurbiprofen	Oxycodone
	Diamorphine hydrochloride
	Fentanyl (transdermal)
	Dextromoramide
	Dipipanone hydrochloride
	Dextropropoxyphene
	Methadone

Morphine is probably the most useful and commonly used analgesic and is best given orally as a solution or immediate-release tablet and, when the patient's 24-hour morphine requirement is established, as a modified-release preparation (12-hour or 24-hour preparations) either once or twice daily. Patients need daily pain assessment and dosage adjustment. If the patient cannot swallow, fentanyl transdermal patches (Durogesic®) can be used in place of morphine. Alternatively, morphine can be given parenterally by subcutaneous injection. In the UK, diamorphine is preferred for subcutaneous injection (and for continuous subcutaneous infusion) because, being more soluble, a larger dose can be given in a smaller volume. Diamorphine is, however, only available in the UK; morphine is used in the rest of the world.

Morphine (or diamorphine) is often administered by a **continuous subcutaneous infusion** via a portable **syringe driver**, which provides good control of pain with little discomfort or inconvenience to the patient.

Nursing staff require adequate training in the correct use of syringe drivers, as they are a common cause of drug errors. Additionally, it is important that the different rate settings on the device are clearly identified and differentiated. Finally, staff caring for patients for whom syringe drivers are being used need to be alert to the potential problems associated with these devices (Box 17.10).

Other drugs, such as haloperidol, hyoscine hydrobromide, levomepromazine (methotrimeprazine) and midazolam, can also be given by continuous subcutaneous infusion via a syringe driver. The general principle that injections should be given into separate sites (and should not be mixed) does *not* apply to the use of syringe drivers in palliative care. As long as there is no known mixing incompatibility, many drugs used in terminal care may be combined with morphine or diamorphine in a syringe driver (Box 17.11).[25] Drugs for injection are usually dissolved in water or in sodium chloride 0.9 per cent (physiological

BOX 17.10 Problems encountered with syringe drivers[25]

The following are problems that may be encountered with syringe drivers and the action that should be taken.

- If the subcutaneous infusion runs too quickly, check the rate setting and the calculation.
- If the subcutaneous infusion runs too slowly, check the start button, the battery, the syringe driver and the cannula, and make sure that the injection site is not inflamed.
- If there is a reaction at the injection site, make sure that the site does not need to be changed – firmness or swelling at the site of injection is not in itself an indication for change, but pain or obvious inflammation is.

N.B. Subcutaneous infusion solution should be monitored regularly, both to check for precipitation (and discolouration) and to ensure that the infusion is being administered at the correct rate. Diazepam, prochlorperazine and chlorpromazine are not administered by continuous subcutaneous infusion via a syringe driver, as they tend to cause skin reactions at the injection site.

BOX 17.11 Drugs that can be safely mixed with diamorphine in a syringe driver for continuous subcutaneous infusion[25]

- Cyclizine[a]
- Dexamethasone[b]
- Haloperidol[c]
- Hyoscine butylbromide
- Hyoscine hydrobromide
- Levomepromazine
- Metoclopramide[d]
- Midazolam

[a]Cyclizine may precipitate at concentrations >10 mg/mL or in the presence of physiological saline or as the concentration of diamorphine relative to cyclizine increases; mixtures of diamorphine and cyclizine are also liable to precipitate after 24 hours.
[b]Special care is needed to avoid precipitation of dexamethasone when preparing. In many palliative care services, dexamethasone is often given by a separate infusion.
[c]Mixtures of haloperidol and diamorphine are liable to precipitate after 24 hours if haloperidol concentration is >2 mg/mL.
[d]Under some conditions, metoclopramide may become discoloured; such solutions should be discarded.

saline solution). Drugs dissolved in water for injection may, however, cause pain at the injection site (perhaps not important if the drug being infused is an analgesic) and drugs dissolved in sodium chloride 0.9 per cent tend to precipitate more often than drugs dissolved in water for injection.

Neuropathic pain, caused by damage to the central or peripheral nervous systems, can be severe and is often described by patients as burning, scalding or stinging and may be experienced as a shooting or lancinating pain. If the pain originates from sympathetic nervous system damage, it is generally described as a burning pain and may be accompanied by other sympathetic nervous system symptoms, such as sweating.[25,34] Neuropathic pain is less responsive to non-opioid and opioid analgesics, but may respond better when these analgesics are given with **analgesic adjuvants** – that is, analgesics enhanced with either a tricyclic antidepressant (amitriptyline, nortriptyline) and/or gabapentin (Neurontin®), an anticonvulsant. Other types of adjuvant analgesia may be used under specialist supervision. Transcutaneous electrical nerve stimulation (TENS) and nerve blocks may also be helpful for some patients.[25,34]

Nurses need to consult the 'Prescribing in palliative care' section of the current issue of the BNF,[25] or analogous texts in other countries, for important information on the route of administration, typical doses and dosing regimens, side effects and drug interactions of these analgesics. Additionally, the 'Palliative care formulary' is an essential resource for nurses and other healthcare professionals,[35] and can be accessed online (see 'Internet resources' at the end of this chapter). As already mentioned, analgesics may be used in combination with anxiolytic and antidepressant drugs (see Box 17.5), or with corticosteroids, muscle relaxants and, occasionally, anticonvulsant drugs.

Cough

Intractable cough is often relieved by the use of moist inhalations or oral morphine. For patients who cannot swallow, chronic intractable cough can be relieved by continuous subcutaneous infusion of morphine or diamorphine via a syringe driver.

Dyspnoea

Regular doses of oral morphine every 4 hours may help the patient breathe easier. Corticosteroids, such as dexamethasone, may also be helpful if there is bronchospasm or partial airway obstruction. Oxygen is often helpful and is administered most comfortably by nasal cannulae. Sedatives, such as diazepam, and diuretics may be prescribed and, if death is imminent, intravenous fluids or nasogastric tube feeds are discontinued, as fluids worsen congestion and increase discomfort. The physician may prescribe anxiolytic medication, such as diazepam, to relieve the anxiety associated with dyspnoea.

Excessive respiratory secretions and bowel colic

Excessive respiratory secretions cause respiratory 'rattling,' a wet, bubbly sound that is distressing to conscious patients and to their visitors. Bowel colic often occurs and is uncomfortable and agitating to patients. Both of these conditions may be relieved by the use of hyoscine hydrobromide, which is generally given by continuous subcutaneous infusion via a syringe driver.

Restlessness and confusion

Patients nearing the end of their lives are often restless and confused. This can be caused by a variety of factors, including remediable causes such as anxiety and fear, unrelieved retention of urine and faecal impaction, side effects of drugs (especially opioid analgesics) and drug withdrawal symptoms following the extended use of drugs such as benzodiazepines, alcohol and nicotine. If restlessness and confusion continue despite the alleviation of any potentially correctable causes, the administration of haloperidol, levomepromazine or midazolam by continuous subcutaneous infusion via a syringe driver may be helpful.

Nausea and vomiting

Haloperidol, levomepromazine, cyclizine or metoclopramide may be prescribed to be given orally, parenterally or by continuous subcutaneous infusion via a syringe driver. Cyclizine is particularly liable to precipitate if mixed with diamorphine or other drugs.

Convulsions

Anticonvulsants will be prescribed and midazolam may be ordered to be given by continuous subcutaneous infusion via a syringe driver.

Pressure ulcers

Regular relief of pressure, as previously described in this chapter, is important because patients in the end-stage disease are generally immobile and at risk of developing pressure ulcers.[17,19–21]

Anorexia

Every opportunity to encourage patients approaching death to eat should be taken and patients are often tempted by (and appreciative of) special foods that they enjoy. Steroids (prednisolone or dexamethasone) may be prescribed for anorexia. In the terminal stages of illness, however, it should be noted that intravenous fluids, total parenteral nutrition and nasogastric tube feedings do not prolong the lives of dying patients, and all are associated with increased discomfort and may, in fact, shorten life. Families and friends need to be comforted and told gently that the patient is dying and that food will not improve his or her strength or substantially delay death. Dehydration and starvation typically occur in dying patients and are associated with an analgesic effect and an absence of any associated discomfort.

Constipation

Constipation is a common and distressing problem for some terminally ill patients and may be due to dehydration, anorexia and (especially) the use of opioid analgesics. It can be prevented by the regular use of a laxative that combines a faecal softener with a peristaltic stimulant, such as docusate sodium (Dioctyl®, Docusol®), or lactulose solution with a senna preparation. A small-volume enema containing docusate sodium, with stool-softening agents (Fletchers' Enemmete®) may also be used.

Dry mouth

A dry mouth may be caused by mouth breathing, oxygen therapy, fungal infections and many of the drugs used for palliative care, such as opioid analgesics, hyoscine, some antidepressants and anti-emetics. Regular and appropriately frequent mouth care is essential and the patient's partner, family members or close friends can be taught how to do this. Measures such as the sucking of ice or pineapple chunks, or the use of artificial saliva, are often useful. Candidiasis should be treated appropriately with antifungal drugs.

Hiccups

Hiccups are often due to gastric distension and can be helped by the use of an antacid with an antiflatulent. Metoclopramide or chlorpromazine may also be prescribed.

Psychological, emotional and social needs

Insight into impending death

It is important to ascertain the extent of the patient's knowledge about his or her own impending death. If the assessment indicates that a terminally ill patient is unaware that he or she is dying, this fact should be made known to the physician who has the primary responsibility of discussing the prognosis with the patient. If (or when) the patient's level of comfort permits, practical aspects of his or her death may be gently discussed. This may include referral to a legal adviser or social worker for patients who have not made a will. Nurses must never become involved in either helping a patient draw up a will or witnessing it. It is extremely important that the nursing notes indicate who is to be informed when the patient dies. This information should come from the patient. It would be tragic simply to inform the family, when the most significant relationship may be the patient's partner or a close friend. Because of the high incidence of cognitive impairment in the terminally ill, this discussion should take place at the earliest appropriate opportunity.

Coming to terms with dying

Dying is as important as being born, only this time, most people have an opportunity to contemplate the final weeks and days of their life. Although it is true that no two individuals react in the same way to impending death, there seem to be commonalities in their reactions. Dr Elisabeth Kübler-Ross has elegantly described these as the 'five stages of dying'[36] (Table 17.7) and this model helps healthcare professionals and the significant people in patients' lives to understand the various reactions many people experience as they attempt to come to terms with the end of their life. In reality, patients go back and forth, from one stage to another, not necessarily in consecutive order. In stage 4, nurses can be helpful in reminding patients of the achievements of their lives, the impact that all human beings have by living a life, however short. Loved ones have time to express their love and respect, reassuring the patient that he or she will be remembered.

TABLE 17.7 Psychological stages of dying[36]

Stage	Characteristic features
1: Denial	'No, not me.' This is a typical reaction when a patient learns that he or she is terminally ill. Denial is important and necessary. It helps cushion the impact of the patient's awareness that death is inevitable.
2: Rage and anger	'Why me?' The patient resents the fact that others will remain healthy and alive while he or she must die. God is a special target for anger, since He is regarded as imposing, arbitrarily, the death sentence. To those who are shocked at her claim that such anger is not only permissible but inevitable, Kübler-Ross replies succinctly, 'God can take it'.
3: Bargaining	'Yes me, but . . .' Patients accept the fact of death but strike bargains for more time. Mostly they bargain with God – even people who never talked with God before. Sometimes they bargain with the physician. They promise to be good or to do something in exchange for another week or month or year of life. Kubler-Ross notes, 'What they promise is totally irrelevant, because they don't keep their promises anyway'.
4: Depression	'Yes me.' First, the person mourns past losses, things not done, wrongs committed. Then he or she enters a state of 'preparatory grief', getting ready for the arrival of death. The patient grows quiet, does not want visitors. Kübler-Ross notes, 'When a dying patient doesn't want to see you any more, this is a sign he has finished his unfinished business with you and it is a blessing. He can now let go peacefully'.
5: Acceptance	'My time is very close now and it is all right.' Kübler-Ross describes this final stage as 'not a happy stage, but neither is it unhappy. It is devoid of feelings but it is not resignation, it is really a victory'.

Living Wills, Advanced Directives and Healthcare Proxies

Some terminally ill patients, including those with end-stage HIV disease, will have made a 'Living Will', also known as an Advanced Directive. For patients who are mentally incapable of making decisions about their treatment and care because they are unconscious or otherwise incapacitated, a Living Will informs doctors about which treatments to extend the end of their life artificially they do not want, such as haemodialysis, endotracheal intubation and respiratory ventilation, nasogastric, enteral or parenteral nutrition and hydration and cardiopulmonary resuscitation. The legal status of Living Wills varies from country to country, and local legislation and guidelines should be consulted. A Living Will is legally enforceable in the UK under common law (that is, law decided by the courts) if it meets certain criteria. The Department of Health (England) advises healthcare professionals that: 'if an incompetent patient has clearly indicated in the past, while competent, that they would refuse treatment in certain circumstances (an 'advance refusal'), and those circumstances arise, healthcare professionals must abide by that refusal'.[37] If patients enquire about making a Living Will, they can be referred to the website of the Terrence Higgins Trust or the Voluntary Euthanasia Society (see 'Internet resources' at the end of this chapter) where they can download forms and obtain comprehensive information free of charge. If a patient has made a Living Will, it is important that healthcare professionals are aware of it, that a copy of it is in the patient's records and, ideally, that an opportunity is found to discuss it before the patient loses the ability to make decisions about his or her care.

Sometimes patients appoint a 'Health Care Proxy,' a relative, partner or friend empowered by them to make decisions about their treatment and care should they lose the ability to do this themselves. In the UK, these appointments are not legally binding on physicians, but may usefully inform any decisions made in regard to continuing treatments at the end of a patient's life.

If patients have a Living Will and/or have appointed a Health Care Proxy, it is essential that they discuss this with their general practitioner and hospital healthcare staff so that everyone is clear about their wishes, and distress and embarrassment are avoided at this sensitive and important time. Nurses can consult the current edition of the *National AIDS manual*[38] for further information on these issues.

Last offices

Usual last offices are carried out. The patient is washed and the room tidied. Family, partners and close friends are allowed to see the body before further procedures are undertaken. The nurse must be accessible during this time to support those grieving for their loss. After the body has been viewed, it is placed in a shroud and then gently placed in a heavy-duty plastic body bag. It is both unnecessary and inappropriate to attach warning labels such as 'infection risk' or 'biohazard' to the body bag. Mortuary staff should assume that all patients are potentially infected with bloodborne viruses and take appropriate precautions to prevent exposure to them. Nurses must wear disposable gloves and a plastic apron when carrying out last offices. Once the body has been placed in the body bag, no further infection prevention precautions are required.

Evaluation

The patient will be assessed frequently and appropriately to ensure that the objectives of care are being achieved, such as:

- problems and symptoms associated with the end of life are controlled or alleviated,
- the patient is free of psychological distress and feels safe, comfortable and well supported by friendly and caring nurses as death approaches,

- grieving family, partner, relatives and friends are supported before and after the patient's death.

Summary

The individualized care of patients with tuberculosis requires skill, competence and confidence. These are based on a factual understanding of the pathophysiology of tuberculosis and a comprehensive knowledge of relevant models of nursing care designed to offer all clients, regardless of race, age, creed, gender, sexual orientation or disease, the highest quality of compassionate, non-judgemental nursing care.

Prologue to next chapter

Although the quality of the general care of patients with tuberculosis contributes greatly to their well-being, the most important aspects of their care are those that lead to the cure of their disease and the prevention of relapse. These require the establishment and efficient implementation of a set of inter-related processes aimed at meeting the needs of the patients fully. These processes are discussed in the next chapter.

REFERENCES

1. Henderson V. *Basic principles of nursing care*. Geneva: International Council of Nurses, 1972.
2. Sherman LF, Fujiwara PI, Cook SV et al. Patient and healthcare system delays in the diagnosis and treatment of tuberculosis. *Int J Tuberc Lung Dis* 1999; **12**: 1088–95.
3. Lemaitre N, Sougakoff W, Coetmeur D et al. Nosocomial transmission of tuberculosis among mentally-handicapped patients in a long-term facility. *Tuber Lung Dis* 1996; **77**: 553–6.
4. Henderson V. The nature of nursing. *Am J Nurs* 1964; **64**: 62–8.
5. Roper N, Logan WW, Tierney AJ. *The elements of nursing*, 4th edn. London: Churchill Livingstone, 1996.
6. Orem DE. *Nursing: concepts of practice*, 2nd edn. New York: McGraw Hill, 1980.
7. John C. *The Burford NDU model; caring in practice*. Oxford: Blackwell Sciences, 1994.
8. Mayho P. Barrier grief. *Nurs Times* 1999; **95**(31): 24–55.
9. Pratt RJ, Pellowe C, Loveday HP et al. and the **epic** Guideline Development Team. The **epic** Project: developing national evidence-based guidelines for preventing healthcare-associated infections. Phase 1: Guidelines for preventing hospital-acquired infections. *J Hosp Infect* 2001; **47**(Suppl.): S1–82. Also available online at <http://www.richardwellsresearch.com>.
10. Pellowe CM, Pratt RJ, Harper P et al. and the Guideline Development Group. Infection control: prevention of healthcare-associated infection in primary and community care. Simultaneously published in *J Hosp Inf* 2003; **55**(Suppl. 2): 1–127; and *Br J Infect Control* December 2003; **4**(Suppl.): 1–120. Also available online at <http://www.richardwellsresearch.com>.
11. Stork CM, Hoffman RS. Toxicology of antituberculosis drugs. In Rom WN, Garay S (eds), *Tuberculosis*. Boston: Little, Brown and Company, 1996, 382–6.

12. Peloquin CA. Clinical pharmacology of the anti-tuberculosis drugs. In Davies PDO (ed.), *Clinical tuberculosis*, 3rd edn. London: Arnold, 2003, 171–90.
13. Norton D, McLaren R, Exton-Smith A. *An investigation of geriatric nursing problems in hospital*. London: National Corporation for the Care of Old People, 1962. (Re-issued by Churchill Livingstone, Edinburgh, 1975.)
14. Waterlow J. Prevention is cheaper than cure. *Nurs Times* 1988; **84**: 69–70.
15. Waterlow J. A policy that protects. *Professional Nurse* 1991; **6**: 258–64.
16. Clark M. Pressure ulcer prevention. In Morrison M (ed.), *The prevention and treatment of pressure ulcers*. London: Harcourt Health Sciences, 2000, 75–98.
17. European Pressure Ulcer Advisory Panel (EPUAP). *Pressure ulcer prevention guidelines*. London: EPUAP, 1998.
18. Torrance C. *Pressure sores: aetiology, treatment and prevention*. London: Croom Helm, 1983.
19. National Institute for Clinical Excellence (NICE). *Pressure ulcer risk assessment and prevention: Clinical Guideline B*. London: NICE, 2001. Also available online at <http://www.nice.org.uk/>.
20. National Institute for Clinical Excellence (NICE). *Pressure ulcer prevention: Clinical Guideline 7*. London: NICE, 2003. Also available online at <http://www.nice.org.uk/>.
21. National Institute for Clinical Excellence (NICE). *The use of pressure relieving devices (bed, mattresses, and overlays) for the prevention of pressure ulcers in primary and secondary care*. London: NICE, 2003. Also available online at <http://www.nice.org.uk/>.
22. Meers PD, Ayliffe GA, Emmerson AM et al. Report on the National Survey of Infection in Hospitals 1980. *J Hosp Infect* (Suppl.) 1981; **2**: 1–11.
23. Emmerson AM, Enstone JE, Griffin M et al. The Second National Prevalence Survey of Infection in Hospitals – an overview of results. *J Hosp Infect* 1996; **32**: 175–90.
24. Mayho P. *The tuberculosis survival handbook*. London: XLR8 Graphics Ltd, 1999.
25. Mehta DK (executive editor). *British National Formulary*, 47th edn. London: British Medical Association and the Royal Pharmaceutical Society of Great Britain, March 2004. (Updated and published every 6 months.) Available from: BMJ Books, PO Box 295, London WC1H 9TE (<www.bmjbookshop.com>). Also available online at <www.BNF.org>.
26. Helminiak DA. *The human core of spirituality: mind as psyche and spirit*. Albany, NY: State University of New York Press, 1996.
27. Fogel CI. Human sexuality and health care. In Fogel CI, Lauver D (eds), *Sexual health promotion*. Philadelphia: WB Saunders, 1990.
28. Fonseca JD. Sexuality – a quality of being human. *Nurs Outlook* 1970; **18**: 25.
29. Langfeldt T, Porter M. *Sexuality and family planning. Report of a consultation and research findings*. Copenhagen: World Health Organization Sexuality and Family Planning Programme, 1986.
30. World Health Organization. *Technical Report Series No. 572*. Geneva: WHO, 1975.
31. Department of Health. *The national strategy for sexual health and HIV*. London: Department of Health (England), 2001. Also available online at <www.dh.gov.uk/>.
32. Quinn TC, Wawer MJ, Sewankambo N et al. Viral load and heterosexual transmission of human immunodeficiency virus type 1. *N Engl J Med* 2000; **342**: 921–9. Also available online at <http://content.nejm.org/cgi/content/abstract/342/13/921>.
33. Pratt RJ. *HIV and AIDS: a foundation for nursing and healthcare practice*, 5th edn. London: Arnold, 2003.
34. Woodruff R. *Palliative medicine – evidence-based symptomatic and supportive care for patients with advanced cancer*, 4th edn. Melbourne: Oxford University Press, 2004.

35. Twycross R, Wilcock A, Thorp S. *Palliative care formulary*, 2nd edn. Oxford: Radcliffe Medical Press, 2002. Also available online at <http://www.palliativedrugs.com>.
36. Kübler-Ross E. *On death and dying*. London: Tavistock Publications, 1969.
37. Department of Health (England). *12 key points on consent: the law in England*. April 2001. Available online at <http://www.dh.gov.uk/>
38. Fieldhouse R (ed.). *AIDS reference manual*, 24th edn. London: National AIDS Manual, October 2001.

FURTHER READING

Alexander MF, Fawcett JN, Runciman PJ. *Nursing practice, hospital & home– the adult*, 2nd edn. London: Churchill Livingstone, 2000.

Cohen FL, Durham, JD (eds). *Tuberculosis: a sourcebook for nursing practice*. New York: Springer Publishing Co. Inc., 1995.

Dickman A, Varga J. *The syringe driver – continuous subcutaneous infusions in palliative care*. Oxford: Oxford University Press, 2002.

Fieldhouse R (ed.). *AIDS reference manual*, 24th edn. London: National AIDS Manual (NAM), October 2001. A new edition is published by NAM each year and is available from: NAM, 16a Clapham Common Southside, London SW4 7AB; telephone: 020 7627 3200; fax.: 020 7627 3101; email: <info@nam.org.uk>; website: <www.aidsmap.com>.

Hinchliff S, Norman S, Schober J. *Nursing practice & health care – a foundation text*, 3rd edn. London: Arnold, 1998.

Kübler-Ross E. *On death and dying*. London: Tavistock Publications, 1969.

Lugton J. *Communicating with dying people and their relatives*. Oxford: Radcliffe Medical Press, 2002.

Mayho P. *The tuberculosis survival handbook*. London: XLR8 Graphics Ltd, 1999, 72.

Morrison M (ed.). *The prevention and treatment of pressure ulcers*. London: Harcourt Health Sciences, 2000.

Neuberger J. *Dying well: a guide to enabling a good death*, 3rd edn. Oxford: Radcliffe Medical Press, 2002.

Neuberger J. *Caring for dying people of different faiths*, 3rd edn. Oxford: Radcliffe Medical Press, 2002.

Pratt RJ. *HIV & AIDS: a foundation for nursing and healthcare practice*, 5th edn. London: Arnold, 2003.

Roper N, Logan WW, Tierney AJ. *The elements of nursing*, 4th edn. London: Churchill Livingstone, 1996.

Sims R, Moss VA. *Palliative care for people with AIDS*, 2nd edn. London: Edward Arnold, 1995.

Twycross R, Wilcock A, Charlesworth S, Dickman A. *Palliative care formulary*, 2nd edn. Oxford: Radcliffe Medical Press, 2002.

Weston A (ed.). *Sexually transmitted infections – a guide to care*. London: Nursing Times Books, 1999.

Woodruff R. *Palliative medicine – evidence-based symptomatic and supportive care for patients with advanced cancer*, 4th edn. Melbourne: Oxford University Press, 2004.

INTERNET RESOURCES

The *British National Formulary* (BNF), published by the British Medical Association and the Royal Pharmaceutical Society of Great Britain, provides up-to-date information in relation to the drugs used in the UK to treat HIV infection and HIV-related diseases; both the hard copy and the online version are updated every 6 months. The online version is available at <http://www.BNF.org/>.

For a comprehensive guide to the drugs used for the prophylaxis and treatment of opportunistic infections and other HIV-related illnesses (including tuberculosis), see the current edition of the *HIV & AIDS treatments directory*, published twice yearly by the National AIDS Manual (email: info@nam.org.uk), and the monthly *AIDS treatment update*, available online at <http://www.aidsmap.com>.

The National AIDS Manual also publishes the excellent and authoritative *AIDS reference manual*, which is updated each year.

A website offering detailed information on the drugs used for palliative care (including comprehensive information on using syringe drivers for the continuous subcutaneous infusion of drugs), based on the *Palliative care formulary* (see Twycross et al. in 'Further reading' above), can be found at <http://www.palliativedrugs.com>.

National evidence-based guidelines for preventing healthcare-associated infections have been developed and published by the Department of Health and the National Institute for Clinical Excellence (NICE) in England and are available online at <http://www.richardwellsresearch.com>.

National evidence-based guidelines for risk assessment and pressure ulcer prevention in primary and secondary care and *Recommendations for the use of pressure-relieving devices* have been developed and published by the National Institute for Clinical Excellence (NICE) in England and are available online at <http://www.nice.org.uk/>.

Living Wills, *Advance Directives* and *Healthcare Proxies*: for detailed information and downloadable forms, direct patients to the London-based website of the Terrence Higgins Trust <http://www.tht.org.uk> or the Voluntary Euthanasia Society (<http://www.ves.org.uk>). Patients and healthcare professionals can consult the website of the Department of Health (England) (<http://www.dh.gov.uk>) for guidance on consent and the requirement to abide by 'advance refusal' (Living Wills).

INTERNET RESOURCES

The British National Formulary (BNF), published [illegible] Royal Pharmaceutical Society [illegible] tion to the drugs used in the UK [illegible] HIV [illegible] HIV-related [illegible] the hard copy and the online version, are updated every 6 months. The online version is available at www.BNF.org

For a comprehensive guide to the drugs used for the prophylaxis and treatment of opportunistic infections and other HIV-related diseases (including [illegible]) [illegible] current edition of the [illegible] published [illegible] Manual [illegible] [illegible]

CHAPTER 18

Nurse-led case management

Introduction

Case management per se is not a new concept or a unique form of practice. It is a familiar method of organizing the delivery of services within health care and many other disciplines. As a nursing activity, case management has evolved relatively recently, only really coming of age over the past 15 years. The opportunity for nursing case management to flourish has occurred largely as a result of changes in the role of nurses and through changes in the profession's relationship to medicine. Increases in the scope of professional practice have to some extent been driven by the need to change the skill mix between doctors and nurses, within multi-disciplinary teams. These reforms have been practice driven, with the consequence that nurses regularly take on greater clinical responsibility. Within some specialist areas this has meant nurses can meaningfully take on, and be made accountable for, the management and co-ordination of patient care. Rather than resulting in a simple and direct transfer of roles from doctors to nurses, this opened the way for care, medicine and its relationship to the patient to be conceived of from a new perspective. *Nurse-led* case management remains substantially medicalized, but it does offer a distinctive and more patient-centred approach to tackling tuberculosis.

Learning outcomes

After studying and reflecting on the material in this chapter, you will be able to:

- outline the principles of case management,
- compare and contrast nurse-led case management and clinical case management,
- describe the components of nurse-led case management,
- discuss possible benefits that may be gained from the adoption or extension of nurse-led case management,
- identify possible practical and disciplinary limits of nurse-led case management.

Within the sphere of tuberculosis, many services already utilize aspects of case management in their co-ordination, planning and implementation of care. This chapter sets out to consolidate existing knowledge of case management and to provide an introduction to those who are less familiar with this method of working. The majority of tuberculosis patients are cared for in the community for most, if not all, of their treatment. The individualized assessment and care planning described in the previous chapter in relation to hospitalized patients can also be used to support effective case management, which is described later in this chapter.

Some readers will be aware that the development of nurse-led case management can enhance the co-ordination and continuity of patient care and thus have a positive effect upon patient outcomes. Others among you may also know that this approach does have certain limitations. The discussion in this chapter explores the benefits and restrictions of this approach in context, focusing on both its theoretical uniqueness and its practical application.

CONTEXT OF CASE MANAGEMENT

After a long and steady decline, rates of tuberculosis levelled out and have begun to increase in many parts of the world. Health services and national governments have been slow to respond to this re-emergence of the disease.[1] While many countries have now established national programmes for the control of tuberculosis, others remain without such control strategies. Even in areas with national control programmes, tuberculosis services on the ground and local networks are often left to their own devices to organize and co-ordinate local and regional tuberculosis control. One of the most pressing problems in this situation is that decentralized services tend to develop in a fragmented and inconsistent fashion if they lack a clear mandate from the centre. Under-investment, fragmentation and inconsistency have all been implicated in loss to follow-up of patients and poor treatment outcomes,[2–4] suggesting that one area that is particularly vulnerable to these service weaknesses is case management. In this context, an attempt is made in this chapter to demonstrate that case management is not only an effective method of organizing care around patient needs, but also provides a framework through which many of the problems presented by decentralization can be circumvented. One of the responses to address these issues has been to develop case management of tuberculosis with a much stronger nursing element.[2,4–6]

WHAT IS CASE MANAGEMENT?

There are many definitions of case management and this is reflected in the number of disciplines that have adopted it as a strategy for meeting particular goals. Within the sphere of social work, for example, there is often an organizational will to increase the autonomy of clients and to maximize their integration within the community.[7] Case management techniques are used to achieve this as an outcome. In medicine and health care, these goals of autonomy and integration are also desirable, but case management in this field is nearly always aimed at achieving the resolution of a specific disease or condition. Despite the differences in goals and perspectives, case management can be distilled down to definitions that are universally applicable. Case management might be described as involving: 'A set of ordered and inter-related processes that seek to identify and co-ordinate quality services efficiently in order that the (full) needs of clients are met'.[7]

Case management in this definition is a system of working that assesses the needs of the client or patient, before organizing the available services around those needs. Although this is quite an ambitious definition in terms of its aspirations, case management may also be applied to more limited goals. For example, the following is a medical definition of case management: 'A system of healthcare delivery in which an individualised treatment plan for the patient is developed by a multi-disciplinary team to achieve established patient care outcomes'.[6]

Despite the differences in orientation of these approaches, the basic principles of the operation of case management remain the same: *the integrated organization of multiple activities to achieve specific outcomes for clients or patients*. In the case of an individual with tuberculosis, these activities are geared towards the successful completion of appropriate drug treatment in order to achieve a cure. The definition quoted above is actually directed towards case management of patients with tuberculosis.[6] The majority of this chapter focuses on case management of tuberculosis from a nursing perspective; however, there may be circumstances in which more comprehensive models of case management, as elaborated in a social work approach, demonstrate greater efficacy. The issue of broadening the concept of case management is discussed more fully towards the end of the chapter.

BACKGROUND: DRIVERS OF NURSE-LED CASE MANAGEMENT

Just as there are a variety of goals to which case management can be applied, there are also many different motives that drive it as a popular current strategy. Case management techniques have been adopted in a variety of contexts to address a number of different issues in the field of tuberculosis, but the motives for doing so are not necessarily uniform or predictable. Featured among these are the drive to develop more patient-centred approaches to care,[8,9] the need to address the fragmentation of service delivery,[10] increased emphasis upon the need for evidence-based practice,[11] demands to respond to the social epidemiology of tuberculosis,[12,13] and the need to ensure that services are cost efficient. The following section briefly explains the context of these issues and how they may be addressed through nurse-led case management.

Patient-centred care

Over the past two decades, an increasing amount of attention has been paid to the needs of patients as individuals. Individualized patient-centred care is partly driven by discourses on choice and consumption within health care; it is also motivated by the will of health services to be more responsive to patient needs. Moreover, patient-centred approaches have demonstrated significant improvements in patient outcomes across a range of medical conditions.[14–16] Patient-centred approaches generally utilize the 'named nurse system', with a strong emphasis on the integrated tailoring of care around patient needs. To this end, the nurse-led case management of patients with tuberculosis entails a more individualized approach. This is an important driving force behind the development of case management within many local and regional programmes for the control of tuberculosis. Improvements in the quality of care and in the management of tuberculosis are implicit in most of the reasons for the adoption of a case management approach.

Fragmentation of service structures

Fragmentation of the process of care and treatment of tuberculosis can occur for a number of reasons and at several different levels of service. For instance, where health care is organized through a mixture of public and private provision, the management of tuberculosis is often disrupted by poor communication, which may be compounded by poor adherence of clinicians to existing guidelines.[2,17] Similarly, fragmentation and clinician non-adherence are also a common outcome in situations in which a proportion of all tuberculosis cases are managed by clinicians that are not specialists in the area of tuberculosis. They are also a feature in areas where there are no clear regional or national strategies for the control of tuberculosis.[10] Thus, in areas where the control of the disease is decentralized, there is a risk that local responses will be confused, inconsistent and poorly co-ordinated. This kind of fragmentation may be particularly acute where members of the TB team are employed by more than one agency, or where there is no process in place for reaching local agreements on priorities, policy or strategy. Fragmentation may also be a product of bureaucratic divisions, where there is poor co-ordination and planning between the organizations that provide for the needs of patients with tuberculosis. These divisions have the effect of producing breaks in the continuity and consistency of care and management.[5]

Through the development of locally agreed service guidelines and standard setting, nurse-led case management can deliver a high quality of care. The structure of a nurse-led case management approach is such that teams can be made accountable for providing a particular level of service. If guidelines and standard setting can be agreed across local or even regional settings, consistency and equality of services can be achieved, even in an environment of decentralized and otherwise fragmented services.

Accountability and effectiveness

There is a tendency within specialist services, such as tuberculosis, for teams or individuals to develop in isolation. This is especially likely to occur in an environment in which services are decentralized and fragmented. In this event, there is a risk that practice within teams can become idiosyncratic, with the result that tuberculosis services are rendered inconsistent with each other and poorly adapted to their objectives. This is notably the case where service management is weak and where practice is not made accountable to any evidence base or to the principles of effective disease control. These problems can, however, be identified and addressed in the process of developing nurse-led case management, as this approach requires a well-defined line of accountability through a strong and unitary management system. To ensure that practice is efficacious, activities should be made accountable to an evidence base, which can be built into this approach through collaborative working and the sharing of good practice. Additionally, team activities can be measured against standards, to ensure that the quality of case management and of the broader service is maintained. The system within which nurse-led case management operates is, therefore, well adapted to address issues of accountability and effectiveness.

Changes in the social epidemiology of tuberculosis

Changes in the profile of people with tuberculosis in the UK have been most marked in urban areas, where caseloads increasingly comprise individuals that are both hard to reach and hard to treat, often resulting in loss to follow-up and treatment failure.[12] As a disease, tuberculosis has the effect of selecting out individuals from populations that are least likely to be detected or served by the majority of social and medical services. In this sense, tuberculosis reflects the 'inverse care law' whereby those most in need of services are least likely to have access to them.[18] Some case management systems have begun to address these issues by broadening their remit in order to explore and effectively address these problems.

Costs

When compared with other methods of care and clinical management, nurse-led case management is initially resource heavy, although research in many other areas of health care demonstrates that case management re-coups these costs.[14] Patient-centred nurse-led case management has produced savings in a number of areas: shorter hospital stays, fewer re-admissions to hospital, reduced loss to follow-up, and earlier identification of poor responses to treatment and of serious side effects from drug treatment.[19] Not all of these benefits are necessarily transferable to the case management of tuberculosis, but it is highly probable that this strategy has the effect of reducing breaks in treatment and loss to follow-up.[2,5] Not only does the patient directly benefit from this, it also has the knock-on effect of reducing the extra costs incurred by the further spread of the disease and the potential development of drug-resistant tuberculosis.

With the exception of the last point on cost, all of the issues described above have a critical impact upon the likelihood of successful treatment outcomes for patients with tuberculosis. Before describing the components of nurse-led case management, a nurse-led case management approach is assessed within the context of medical case management.

MEDICAL CASE MANAGEMENT: BENEFITS AND BURDENS

Traditional regimes of medical management tend to view tuberculosis and other conditions as constituting a set of relatively predictable relationships. In the case of tuberculosis, these relationships occur between the bacterium *Mycobacterium tuberculosis*, the response (and pathophysiology) of the diseased person, and the intervention of medical science. Empirical observation of the diseased body has rendered these relationships predictable, as have controlled trials of various antituberculosis drugs.[20]

The predictability of response to the treatment of tuberculosis means that particular benefits can be accumulated around the processes of treatment and clinical management. Predictable relationships between the course of disease and treatment responses mean that the management of tuberculosis can be systematically approached. In accordance with these observations, guidelines and recommendations for good practice are often made at regional and national levels. If clinical practice actually adheres to such recommendations, the probability of a cure should be maximized. A system of practice based on recommendations is also likely to confer other benefits:

- it provides a *structure* and content that will be consistent and therefore transferable across all areas,
- it has the effect of creating *standards*, which may be measurable,
- it provides a degree of *equity* – of both service and treatment.

Whereas all of these qualities are desirable, and critical to the success of national control programmes, structure, standards and equity can present a two-edged sword where patients are concerned. For example, on the positive side, it means that patients can be informed of the likely course of the disease, its treatment, possible side effects and future management. Providing *knowledge* to patients about the management of the disease and its predictability can give them a greater sense of control and reduces levels of anxiety. On the negative side, there is an expectation and a necessity that patients themselves must *comply* with medical directives so as to maximize the chances of a cure. As a system, clinical management, while securing an effective method of treating the disease, has little appreciation of the wider needs or circumstances of the patient. In this sense it is blind to the contingencies that may be introduced by the patient and therefore fails to differentiate between patients, except in terms of their physiological reactions to drugs or disease. This means that clinical interventions and the accompanying structure of medical services have the effect of *reducing* the patient's degree of control. Even in situations in which healthcare staff are sensitive to the needs of patients, the traditional structure of service and the training and development of staff may often leave little scope for meeting needs that fall outside of the medical model.

Although the 'medical model' of care is often thought of as outmoded and obsolete, the principles driving this model underpin our current practice. The organizing principle of our work is rooted in a disease and the treatment of that disease. For a cure to be attained, the principles reflected in this model would seem to be a necessity. The boundaries of the role of the tuberculosis clinical nurse specialist (CNS) are clearly defined by the well-being of the patient, but only in so far as that patient has tuberculosis. This should not be problematic, but for the fact that the patient's well-being is often influenced by a whole raft of other unmet needs that are no less serious to the patient than the disease itself. These issues can put a great deal of stress on the nurse's role, testing its limits and its limitations, particularly if there is little engagement from other agencies that could assist in supporting the patient. Patient-centred, nurse-led case management sets out to strike a balance between the imperatives driven by clinical management and the more unpredictable needs of the patient, and while nurse-led case management introduces flexibility, responsiveness and continuity to patient care, we must remain aware that it cannot be all things to all patients.

NURSE-LED CASE MANAGEMENT OF TUBERCULOSIS

Components

In a nurse-led case management system, the CNS is the case manager and is responsible for the planning, implementation, evaluation and documentation of care. Each member of the TB nursing team is accountable to either the team leader or a line manager. The tuberculosis specialist physician remains accountable for all clinical decision making. The effective organization of nurse-led case management requires that several components are in place.

Accountability, continuity of care and case management

For nurses to be truly accountable in their scope of professional practice, they must be given the authority and autonomy to make decisions. As some nurse theorists point out, 'Accountability is empty without this process'.[21] To ensure that there is continuity and consistency of care for each patient, it is important that the CNS is provided with the freedom and responsibility to work across all relevant healthcare environments – in acute and community settings, as well as within out-patient departments. With the freedom to work across these settings, the CNS has the flexibility to ensure that the patient receives specialized nursing care from the outset of diagnosis and the commencement of treatment. Flexible working practices also allow the CNS to assess, co-ordinate and monitor care across all necessary spheres. If nurses are to be made accountable for work across these diverse areas, resources must be made available to ensure that the CNS develops the necessary professional competencies.

Communication and case management

Under most nurse-led case management systems, the CNS is placed at the hub of the exchange of information concerning patients identified or suspected of having tuberculosis. Communication policies focused on the newly diagnosed patient need to be clear and to outline precisely the required communication network. One method of achieving this is to make the CNS team responsible for the notification of each new patient (see Chapter 16). This is an effective way to lead the process of communication, as notification of new tuberculosis patients is a legal requirement in many countries. This will give the communication policy the authority that it might otherwise lack. To ensure that the TB team is made aware of all new bacteriologically identified cases, microbiology staff can be requested to inform the TB nursing team of all new positive results – even in the event that a completely separate team may have initiated investigations. So, regardless of the source of the referral, once a positive result is identified, referral to the TB team occurs by default.

Putting the CNS at the centre of local communications is the first step towards ensuring that many of the issues outlined in the introduction to this chapter, such as patient centredness, under-notification, fragmentation of provision and loss to follow-up can all begin to be addressed. Once the TB team has been made aware of a new patient with tuberculosis, they can ensure that, from the point of diagnosis onwards, the patient receives specialist care and clinical management (see Chapters 16 and 17). It also lays the necessary foundation for the continuity of specialist care and management to take place.

Case management and caseloads

Individual case managers may be made responsible for caseloads, to ensure that a single 'named nurse' sees the patient throughout his or her course of treatment. This also sets up clear lines of accountability for action. The 'named nurse' will usually be the member of the team that first met and assessed the patient. This can, however, create problems in the event of sickness or when annual leave is taken. Some services address this issue through sharing patients within individual caseloads, for example a team of two nurses may be responsible for a caseload of 80 or more patients. Where possible the 'named nurse' (who carried out the initial assessment) will continue to see the patient, but, in the event of annual leave or sickness, there is still cover from another member of the team who is familiar with the caseload. For this system to work effectively there must be good documentation and clear communication within the team, facilitated by regular case meetings. One of the team members would be appointed team leader and this nurse would be accountable for the care and management of the caseload.

For role and service accountability to be effective, it is critical that all members of the TB team are made accountable through the same management structure. This will make certain that roles and responsibilities within the team are clear and coherent with each other and ensures that the aims and objectives of the team are unfettered by the agendas of different organizations. If the aims and objectives of the team are clear, this in turn allows the development of more coherent service planning. In the event that members of the same CNS team are managed by different employers, there is the risk that the service will be compromised by incompatible and conflicting priorities.

Skill mix and practice development

The sort of skill mix and practice development that occurs within the TB team will be governed by several overlapping factors. The core skills within a team are likely to be set by local or regional standards or clinical guidelines, but the character of particular teams should be driven by what is appropriate for local populations and local case management.

The potential for practice development will be influenced by the local priority given to tuberculosis, staffing levels, expertise found within the TB team, and the availability of relevant professional development programmes. Regular training and supervision should be integral to the working of the team, and this is especially important in isolated services, where access to research and library materials may be poor.[22] The lead clinician who has overall responsibility for providing tuberculosis services needs to ensure that tuberculosis maintains a significant profile at local and regional levels to attract adequate funding for staffing and for the development of the skills required for local control of tuberculosis. The TB team can play a very active role in the process of defining what kind of skill mix is required. It is, after all, the team that will be most aware of, and most able to identify, the needs and characteristics of local populations. It is these needs and characteristics that should form the bedrock of a dynamic and responsive team with the right skill mix. An example of how this might be pursued is given in Box 18.1.

BOX 18.1 Caseload profiling

Exercises to establish the profile of local caseloads are invaluable for providing information concerning local needs and risk assessment of particular populations, in terms of both vulnerability to disease and likelihood of treatment adherence. If properly designed, profiles also demonstrate the strengths and weaknesses of existing service provision. By providing data on the needs of the local population and the deficits of local services, profiles are an effective tool for establishing the developmental and skill-mix requirements of the local TB team. Critically, caseload profiling provides explicit and measurable justification for resourcing of services. For example, the collection of demographic information may highlight that an increasing number of patients from a particular ethnic group are being seen with tuberculosis. In the course of monitoring, it may also be noted that few of these patients speak English. In the event that language needs are not catered for, these patients are more likely to be lost to follow-up. The risk of treatment failure and the potential for drug resistance provide financial incentive for budget holders to ensure that the advocacy and language needs of patients are catered for. Profiling provides accurate local evidence required for planning and resourcing, and should be made an integral part of the tuberculosis service.

The majority of TB teams are made up of specialist nurses and doctors and this can be the full extent of the 'multi-disciplinary team'. Local demographic information may indicate that the team would be enhanced by skills from other areas of health and social care, such as advocates, social workers or housing advice workers. Although these needs are often highlighted by the social epidemiology of the disease, it is still exceptional to find TB teams that have ready access to these resources. It is of the utmost importance that TB teams remain engaged with research into local conditions to ensure that practice development is responsive to local needs and case management requirements. Tuberculosis teams do, however, have a positive and active part to play in moulding the skill mix around local needs identified by research.

Team leadership

In units where more than one nurse is involved in caring for patients with tuberculosis, motivated team leadership is essential for effective case management. While individual team members are responsible for the case management of patients, the senior nurse within the service takes on the roles of assessment, supervision and development that occur within the team itself. The senior nurse will also ensure that the aims and objectives of the team are met and that they continue to correspond with assessed patient needs in that particular area. It is therefore important that the team leader has the skills and authority to lead on policy formation and role development within the team. He or she will also share responsibility for creating links and working policies established in collaboration with other departments and agencies that are relevant to the care of patients.

Where nurses are working independently, it is important that they are working within a clear local management structure. It may also be useful for them to develop links with other units offering specialist tuberculosis services to ensure that they receive adequate cover and support.

Standard setting

Standard setting per se is not strictly a component of nurse-led case management. However, it has been included here because it is a means of facilitating quality care and it is a process through which each element of case management can be strengthened. Many TB teams set up standards against which a service and individual case management roles may be measured. There is a need for regular monitoring and audit for standard setting to be effective.

A standard can be explicit and direct, for example it may require that every newly diagnosed patient is seen by a CNS within 24 hours, or it may be more generalized, specifying that there should be effective links with relevant local services. What is important when establishing standards is that they are locally agreed as priorities, that they are evidence based or based on accepted principles of good disease control, and that they are accepted as achievable by all the parties concerned.

Standards are also useful on a larger scale, if they can be agreed regionally between local services or through a managed clinical network. This can become a means of ensuring that services are consistent in quality and delivery of care, as well as compatible with each other. If this is achieved, standard setting will become a potent method through which services can become more equitable and quality driven, even in circumstances in which a national strategy is absent.

Equally important is funding. Tuberculosis teams need to be adequately resourced if they are to be accountable for all of the components of tuberculosis control. Agreeing local standards can offer TB teams the opportunity to identify priorities and highlight areas in need of investment.

Practice of case management

Initiation of case management

The case management of tuberculosis may begin within a range of activities, at any given point. If CNSs are involved in processes of screening and the investigation of disease, it is likely that case management may begin before a diagnosis. The processes of case finding and case management are often continuous with one another,[23] for example patient referrals may be made to the TB team for the investigation of symptoms. Typically, such referrals would come from other specialist departments, accident and emergency services or from primary care sources. Equally, patients may first be encountered by the team in the course of the routine screening of 'high-risk' groups, such as the contacts of an index case or the homeless. In these circumstances case management will be initiated before a diagnosis has actually been reached: all screenings and investigations for tuberculosis are potential junctures at which case management may start. Alternatively, it is possible that other specialist departments have already carried out their own investigations into a potential case of tuberculosis. In this event, referrals to the TB team, and thus the initiation of case management, may take place only after a diagnosis has been reached.

Referrals for diagnostic testing may be made to a nominated specialist physician, from whom they are passed on to the CNS for investigation. Alternatively, referrals for screening and investigation may be made directly to the CNS.

In certain circumstances, the nurse's first point of contact with the patient may be from a non-medical referral. Routes from non-medical sources to the TB team can be established where staff work with groups that are highly susceptible to tuberculosis, such as outreach teams for the homeless. These referral arrangements are discussed later in this chapter.

First contact with patient diagnosed with tuberculosis

Once diagnosis has occurred, the CNS's first meeting with the patient should include the following elements: education and information giving; needs assessment; support; collection of contact-tracing data; and issues raised by the patient.

The first time that the patient meets with a member of the TB team is of critical importance. It is during this encounter that the majority of patient assessments that inform the planning of care will take place. During this initial meeting, the foundation of a trusting and therapeutic relationship between the CNS and the patient should take shape. On this point, it is worth remembering that assessment is a two-way process and this is also the occasion when patients will form their first impressions of the CNS and the rest of the team.

As described previously, the nurse's first contact with the patient may occur before, at or after diagnosis. Correspondingly, the site of first contact may vary. The CNS may first encounter the patient on the hospital ward, but is just as likely to meet him or her first in an out-patient clinic or, more rarely, at home. The kind of assessment carried out and the nature of support given will be different according to the site and situation of this first meeting.

The most important elements of the initial encounter with the newly diagnosed patient are education, assessment and support. There is certain information that all patients should be told when they are first seen by the CNS. Some of this information will take the form of facts about the disease process and its relationship to treatment. This will provide a context for instructions about drug treatment and adherence. It is worth developing a checklist of basic information that all patients should receive, as shown in Box 18.2. It is possible, and even likely, that some of this information will already have been communicated by the physician who initiated treatment, but research shows that in clinical environments, patients only absorb and retain a proportion of what they are told, especially at the time of diagnosis. It is therefore worth repeating any information already given.[24]

Providing the patient with appropriate information is critical to the case management process. It is worth bearing in mind that although the TB team is principally responsible for

BOX 18.2 Initial consultation

Communication with all patients on first clinical nurse specialist consultation should include:

- assurance that tuberculosis is a curable disease
- informing the patient of his/her infection status (and, in the event of infectiousness, the length of time he/she is likely to remain in isolation)
- stressing the importance of treatment adherence, including the likely duration of treatment and the reasons why antituberculosis drugs must be taken over such a long period
- explanation of the necessity of taking several drugs simultaneously
- instructions on when and how treatment should be taken
- possible side effects of treatment
- future management of the disease
- process of and rationale for contact tracing

the care and management of patients with tuberculosis, in the majority of cases, it is the patients themselves who have to take the treatment *in the absence* of the TB team.

The news of a diagnosis of tuberculosis and the commencement of a burdensome drug regimen often produce anxiety in the patient. The reasons why a diagnosis of tuberculosis induces stress may be multiple and complex, but some of the issues are predictable and can be partly managed by providing clearly communicated and accurate information. Anxiety is most often generated in patients when they do not understand their situation and when they are unable to anticipate what is likely to happen to them.[25] In the case of tuberculosis, anxiety is likely to be compounded by patients' concern that their disease may be a cause of harm to others. For this reason, the process of contact screening should also be clearly explained.

The goal of clearly communicating the basic information outlined in Box 18.2 should be common to all patients. However, there are circumstances in which this information may need to be given with changes in emphasis or with explanations that are appropriate to specific patient contexts. Consequently, the CNS must be able to assess accurately the patient's existing knowledge. This may be a simple matter of 'filling in the gaps', but it could equally be the case that the patient has an alternative set of health beliefs about tuberculosis. This is not unusual among people from non-Westernized cultures. Research in the USA demonstrates that poor understanding of health beliefs in people from different cultures may negatively impact upon treatment outcomes.[26] The CNS should therefore have a working knowledge of common health beliefs within local populations. With regard to treatment, it is not generally necessary to challenge alternative health beliefs. Within many cultures, indigenous beliefs have co-existed with, and adjusted to, Western drugs and technologies over many years. It is very important, however, to make it clear that antituberculosis drug treatment regimens are the only means of curing the disease and drug treatment must not be stopped or changed in any way without prior medical consultation.

As well as providing factual information, instructions and advice, information giving also functions at a more subtle level by helping to build a trusting relationship between the patient and the CNS case manager. If patients are able to anticipate what is likely to happen to them, they are more likely to experience a greater sense of control and, consequently, to feel less anxious about their predicament.[25] If the CNS case manager is able to give information that accurately predicts the course of events and probable outcomes, then this in turn is likely to foster trust in the knowledge and judgement of the nurse. Research indicates that providing information on the possible side effects of drugs is especially important.[27] In a situation where the patient's care is co-ordinated and often carried out by a specific nurse, the building of this kind of confidence is of critical importance. If patients do not fully trust the nurse responsible for their care, they are unlikely to confide in him or her. In these circumstances it is extremely challenging to assess patient needs accurately and to plan their care. It is therefore important for nurses to monitor their own responses to patient concerns and stated opinions, ensuring that they are always sensitive and constructive.

The giving of patient information and the provision of support and advice are rather like a template for how patient-centred case management should develop. It should not be provided as if 'one size fits all', but should be given in such a way that reflects the specific needs and expectations of each patient. Information giving is an interactive activity, closely bound up with the processes of assessment and planning of individualized patient care.

ASSESSMENT, PLANNING AND IMPLEMENTATION OF CARE

Nurse-led case management is essentially interchangeable with the principles of the nursing process, where a standardized approach is designed to provide a basis for individualized patient-centred care.[23] It is in these terms that assessment, planning and implementation of care take place. These processes are likely to be most intensively pursued at and around the time of diagnosis, but they also constitute a continuous process that occurs throughout treatment in response to patients' changing needs and circumstances.

A range of needs has been considered in the previous chapter, many of which will be relevant to patients being cared for in the community. The interventions may well vary in relation to the patient's environment and living conditions, and the case management approach takes into account the complexities of community-based treatment.

Assessment

Data collection

The success of the initial assessment will be dependent upon comprehensive and accurate data collection. Relevant data can be retrieved from a number of sources, including hospital databases and clinical notes and from members of primary care teams or other specialist departments. Most of the information required for assessment will be collected in the course of direct consultation with patients themselves.

A large amount of the information collected is standardized and generalizable to any clinical data set. This would include, for example, whether patients have other medical conditions, if they suffer from allergies, details of their medical history and of any previous hospital admissions. Demographic details such as age, sex, country of origin, languages spoken and ethnicity are also important. Data that are more specific to tuberculosis should be collected at this time. This would include information such as the nature, duration and severity of signs and symptoms, an assessment of risk for co-infection with the human immunodeficiency virus (HIV), and a family history of tuberculosis. Information concerning the patient's broader social situation should also be collected.

Clinical assessment will also require that the results of certain tests and investigations that may have taken place during diagnosis are available, such as chest radiographs, inflammatory markers and microbiological results. For example, liver function status should be assessed before the commencement of treatment with isoniazid, and vision tests (acuity and colour) undertaken before the commencement of treatment with ethambutol. It is also important to record the weight of the patient at this time. All of these results are used to measure the current condition of the patient and to provide a baseline against which to measure clinical progress.

The collection of data must be accurate and clearly documented. Correct interpretation and appropriate use of acquired data are critical. The interpretation of assessment data is often determined by the context in which the patient is seen. For example, information regarding whether there has been a family history of tuberculosis may be utilized differently depending on the circumstances in which this issue is raised. In the context of screening or investigation, information about the family history of tuberculosis will be used as part of a risk assessment for the likelihood that the patient has been previously exposed to the disease. If, on the other hand, the patient has already been diagnosed, these same data may be used to help assess his or her level of knowledge about the disease. Alternatively, if it is established that there is a recent family history of the disease, and medical data concerning the affected relative have been found to be available, this information may also be used as an interim guide to the patient's likely drug sensitivities.

Assessment

Assessments of newly diagnosed patients focus most heavily upon establishing 'needs'. The patient's needs may be clinical, but they could equally be material or social (see also Chapter 17). Within the context of tuberculosis, assessed needs are apprehended as two distinguishable criteria of risk. First, they may be seen as unmet needs to be addressed in their own right. Second, patient needs are often interpreted as a proxy for the 'risk' of non-adherence to treatment. An obvious example of such a need would be homelessness: research throughout the developed world demonstrates that a large proportion of patients without stable accommodation do not manage to complete their course of antituberculosis drug treatment.[28,29] Homelessness is a major risk to patients' health in general and is associated with non-adherence to antituberculosis drug therapy.

Assessment of needs can be a complex issue. Assessment may identify experiences of the patient that do not demonstrate current needs, but might indicate that the patient is more likely to have problems adhering to treatment (Box 18.3). For example, recent profiling of caseloads in London demonstrated that individuals who have been homeless in the past are less likely to be adherent – even if they are currently in stable accommodation.

BOX 18.3 Common criteria used for risk assessment of likely treatment adherence

- Has the patient previously been treated for tuberculosis?
- Is the patient known to be poorly compliant with treatment?
- Is the patient homeless?
- Has the patient ever been homeless?
- Does the patient have household support (family or close friends)?
- Is the patient affected by drug or alcohol dependency?
- Is the patient affected by mental illness?

Many obstacles to patients' ability to adhere to drug treatment can be identified at this time and addressed before they become a problem. For example, a patient may have problems attending clinic for appointments or the collection of medication, or may simply have problems swallowing tablets. These kinds of obstacles are often easily overcome, provided they are identified *before* they result in an interruption in antituberculosis drug treatment. This kind of information is very important in the planning process, as it will provide an indication of what level of support will be required. Like all criteria, however, it remains only a rough predictor of actual human behaviour.

The use of standardized assessments can assist staff in identifying needs, problems and resources. That said, it is important that the CNS is not solely dependent upon this information. It may not always be possible to establish exactly what sort of problems the patient will face by using structured questions that make up a 'standardized' assessment. Assessments designed by healthcare staff have a tendency to treat people in a 'wholesale' fashion.[30] As a result, there is a risk that we may be missing important issues or concerns that the patient may have. Because of this, it is very important that patients should be given time to speak freely during the assessment.

At initial assessment, patients may not be aware of what obstructions lie ahead of them. These may only become clear when they have been discharged from hospital or have returned home from the clinic. In this sense, the assessment process is continuous. It is always well worth establishing a standard whereby all patients commencing unsupervised antituberculosis drug treatment are promptly visited at home. By adopting this measure, any problems or obstacles that were not identified at initial assessment can be rapidly identified and addressed at the first home visit.

As well as identifying the possible risks and obstacles that the patient may face, assessments should also establish whether the patient has well-developed support networks. The importance of such networks, particularly family, should not be underestimated.[31] Family members or partners should be encouraged to be present at the patient's initial assessment. If the patient is alone for this consultation, the issue of family or other sources of social support should be raised. With the patient's agreement, individuals from his or her support network should be provided with information about the disease, antituberculosis drug therapy and the importance of treatment completion. Relatives and friends are vital in providing encouragement and reassurance to patients. Without any formal agreement or contract, the patient's family and support networks are involved in many of the elements that are central to the processes of case management. Recent research in London demonstrates that one of the most important risk factors for being unable to complete the course of treatment for tuberculosis is that the patient lives alone (Alistair Story, unpublished data). What this suggests is that patients living in these circumstances are likely to require increased support from the TB team. Conversely, this demonstrates how important it is to invest time in working with and teaching family and/or friends about patients' conditions.

While family and other forms of social support are often critical to good treatment adherence and case management, this cannot always be assumed. There are (rare) occasions when those that patients would usually depend upon are either unsupportive or even hostile on hearing news that a close friend or member of the family has tuberculosis. It is important to identify if this is a problem so that it can be addressed promptly. This kind of reaction is often based on misunderstandings about tuberculosis or occurs in circumstances in which the disease is stigmatized within the community (as discussed in Chapter 15). Given the importance of informal support, it is worth investing time to discuss the concerns of patients' families and friends about the disease and to make every effort to address these issues and enlist their support.

Planning and implementation

A large part of the planning process is likely to occur at the first meeting of patient and CNS. Wherever possible, planning should directly involve patients and their families and, if necessary, other members of the TB team. If the patient starts treatment in hospital, ward staff will also be involved (see Chapter 17). The development of care and management will usually be based upon the requirements of clinical case management. So far as it is possible, these 'standardized' requirements should be mediated through other patient needs, as established in the process of assessment. This requires a careful balancing act, as the processes and timing of clinical interventions are not always commensurate with the patient's routines or living situation. Within a nurse-led case management system, it is the CNS who co-ordinates and is made accountable for the care and management of the patient.[4]

There are particular core skills that are necessary for the CNS to conduct effective planning and implementation of care. These include the ability accurately to interpret the data gained from assessment, as well as good communication and co-ordination skills. The CNS will also need to have a working knowledge of the disease process, the treatment of tuberculosis and the routine tests and investigations that take place during clinical management. A comprehensive knowledge of the organization of relevant local services and their referral systems is also a requirement.

Clinical case management and the delegation of responsibilities

The *clinical* management of patients is ultimately the responsibility of their physician. The physician should always be responsible for the decision to commence antituberculosis drug treatment and for any changes in, or cessation of, the treatment regimen. The physician is also responsible for the correct interpretation of the investigations and tests that inform clinical decision making. In many countries, however, the responsibilities for requesting clinical tests and investigations and for dispensing drugs have been extended to registered nurses in general and to CNSs in particular, as nurses' scope of professional practice has broadened. In the area of tuberculosis, this has had a significant impact upon case management.

Extensions in practice have meant that CNSs now share limited responsibilities for clinical management with physicians. Responsibilities for requesting chest radiographs, routine blood tests and the dispensing of repeat prescriptions should be carried out under well-regulated conditions. In the UK, for instance, these activities are managed through protocols agreed with all relevant hospital departments and boards, where the knowledge and competency of specialist nurses are carefully monitored and evaluated.

These extensions in responsibility allow nurses to carry out a large proportion of the routine clinical follow-up of patients, without requiring supervision by physicians. Table 18.1 describes a highly idealized and simplified schedule of routine clinical interventions carried out for a typical case of pulmonary tuberculosis. It shows possible options for clinical responsibility through the course of treatment. It demonstrates that CNSs can see patients in stand-alone clinics and, in the process of carrying out normal nursing activities, they may also supply medication to patients and request routine tests and investigations. CNSs may be charged with checking the results of tests and investigations and with reporting any abnormal results to the patient's physician. There is in this respect a degree of shared clinical accountability between the physician and the CNS. In these circumstances it is essential that

TABLE 18.1 Typical course of treatment and follow-up, with clinical procedures[a]

Time line	Activity	Requested/authorized by
Diagnosis	Baseline liver function test	Physician or CNS
	Baseline vision tests (re ethambutol)	
Day 0	Commencement of treatment	Physician
Week 2	Liver function test	Physician or CNS
Week 4	Review of clinical progress – with relevant tests or investigations, e.g. chest radiograph, inflammatory markers	Review by physician, but tests and investigations may be requested by CNS
Week 8	Review of clinical progress	Reviews to be carried out by physician
	Check drug sensitivities	
	Review of drug regimen	Sensitivity results may be retrieved by CNS or physician
Week 12	Review of clinical progress – with tests and investigations, if required	Physician or CNS
Week 16	Review of clinical progress – with tests and investigations, if required	Physician or CNS
Week 20	Review of clinical progress – with tests and investigations, if required.	Physician or CNS
Week 24	Review of clinical progress – with tests and investigations as required	Physician
	Cessation of treatment, if appropriate	

[a]Some qualification is necessary here: the disease process and treatment course are rarely as straightforward as the table suggests. For example, the table suggests that between week 8 and week 24, the patient *may* only be seen by the clinical nurse specialist (CNS). However, in the event that a patient is seen by nurses in a follow-up clinic and it is identified that he or she is experiencing problems with treatment, or if the patient is not making the expected clinical progress, the CNS should book the patient into the next available physician's clinic. Equally, if other health problems are identified, the nurse should make a referral to the appropriate speciality or to primary care services.

there is agreement as to when patients are referred back to physicians in the event of clinical complications.

Within routine follow-up clinics, nurses should observe for and ask the patient about symptom resolution. Provided that the patient has not presented very late in the disease process, many of the symptoms of tuberculosis should be relieved soon after the start of treatment. Weight gain, cessation of night sweats and reduction of pain or discomfort at the site of disease often occur within a few weeks.

Extended practice and flexibility of service provision

The treatment of tuberculosis can be highly disruptive to the lives of patients.[23] Apart from unwanted drug interactions, side effects and the symptoms of disease, often the most common source of disruption to people's daily lives is clinic appointments. Within many services, the majority of clinical follow-ups would occur in doctors' clinics, often scheduled on a highly limited basis. As a result of other commitments, such as work, childcare or other obstacles, poor attendance of these clinics often results. In order to minimize disruption, clinic appointments should be as flexible as possible, so that they may be more closely integrated into patients' everyday routines. If nurses are able to see patients for routine follow-up, to request tests and investigations, and also to dispense 'repeat prescription' drugs when doctors are not available, the scope for developing more flexible and patient-friendly practices is much enhanced.

Although extensions of practice can improve the flexibility and accessibility of clinical case management, they are not an essential component of nurse-led case management.

Flexibility can be further facilitated by giving patients the choice about whether they wish to be seen in clinic or via home visits for routine check-ups and support. Although more time consuming, home visits are sometimes preferred by nurses, as patients are often more at ease when discussing broader issues that may affect outcomes. For this reason, the home is often a more appropriate environment for assessment and planning. Additionally, the effort of visiting patients at home is often appreciated by patients, and builds on rapport and trust.

Joint clinics

There are circumstances in which children and adults within the same family have tuberculosis. If this is the case, different appointment times can be extremely disruptive. The establishment of joint clinics, such as paediatric and adult tuberculosis clinics run in parallel, can circumvent this problem: with forward planning, all family members can be seen on the same day.

During the assessment and planning process, the needs of the patient may be identified as complex. In this situation, it is advisable for multi-disciplinary case management meetings to be held. There is often a tendency for these meetings to be held only in response to a crisis; however, if they are scheduled on a routine basis, problems are more likely to be anticipated, planned for and pre-empted. Planning that occurs in a multi-disciplinary environment is also a means of providing clarity to the processes of planning and risk assessment and is beneficial to the whole team.[6]

Inter-disciplinary service planning

The processes of planning for the patient are often limited by the availability of, and access to, other services. This is not generally a problem if the patient requires medical attention, since nurse-led case management is already organized from within this sphere. However, many of the challenges faced by patients in adhering to treatment are not medical in nature and they may require interventions that lie outside of healthcare provision.

It is therefore important to establish policy agreements with a range of other services, both statutory and non-statutory. Within the TB team, linking in with other relevant services is a responsibility of the senior nurse. Joined-up multi-agency working is, however, a strategic issue, often requiring input and support from senior levels of the organizations involved. In regions or countries where social and public health services have been amalgamated, as is the case in some areas of Japan, this may be a relatively straightforward enterprise. However, where these sectors are organized separately, it is often useful for a third party to 'broker' the development of multi-agency working. Without the protocols for prioritizing tuberculosis patients or the communication policies to ensure their rapid referral, it is very difficult to plan and implement care in areas such as housing, financial support, immigration and many of the other areas in which patients may have problems. It is often the case that the CNS has some skills and experience in accessing and dealing with agencies that can help with these services. Areas outside of healthcare are, however, highly problematic for TB teams, and this issue is discussed more fully at the end of this chapter.

Adherence and case management

The topic of adherence is complex and challenging and is comprehensively discussed in Chapter 14. There are, however, many areas where the concerns of case management and adherence are synonymous, and some of these overlapping areas are briefly discussed in this section.

The provision of patient education and the processes of assessment, planning and implementation should all be implicitly and explicitly geared toward maximizing patients' chances of successfully completing their course of treatment. Equally, many of the features of a good tuberculosis service, such as the provision of flexible and responsive care, should help to optimize these chances.

Another component that should explicitly feature in a good case management system and help implicitly to improve adherence is the maintenance of dialogue with patients. Systems of clinical and nursing case management normally have a structure through which dialogue with patients is maintained, through follow-up appointments and home visits. These consultations are not only important for monitoring patients' clinical progress, they also provide an opportunity for patients to voice concerns that they may have and for nurses to monitor adherence and re-assess their situation. Continued and regular contact with patients is vital for support and encouragement to be effective.

Patients are particularly vulnerable to poor adherence in the initial phase of treatment. They may have unforeseen problems taking tablets or they may be confused by the drug regimen and anxious about getting the dosage wrong. To avoid this, home visits soon after discharge from hospital or shortly after the commencement of treatment are advisable.

Patients are also vulnerable to poor compliance in the middle and later phases of treatment. During these periods it is often less important for patients to be clinically monitored on a regular basis and, as a consequence, there can be a tendency towards a 'slackening' of regular visits and follow-up appointments. It is during this period that there is least apparent incentive for patients to continue to adhere to treatment, as in most cases the symptoms and ill-effects of the disease are resolved during the initial phase of treatment. It is therefore necessary for the TB team to continue to see patients regularly to remind them that treatment must still be taken for its full course if a cure is to be attained. If patients do not attend their appointments, a protocol for contacting them should be strictly and rapidly applied.

In addition to the 'routine' functioning of tuberculosis services, adherence can be specifically encouraged through a series of measures, including enablers such as travel passes and incentives such as luncheon vouchers or money. Existing research suggests that money is the only incentive proven to have a positive effect on adherence.[32]

There are no conclusive methods of monitoring treatment adherence short of directly observed therapy (DOT). Commonly used methods for checking adherence include tablet counts and urine testing. If a sensitive and non-challenging approach is taken, however, it is often sufficient simply to ask patients whether they have taken their treatment.

There are two strategies for encouraging drug adherence that are particularly compatible with a patient-centred approach: self-administration of medication in hospital and treatment contracts or agreements.

Self-administration of drugs is introduced while patients are still in hospital. It allows them to develop knowledge and confidence regarding their medication in a supportive environment and has been demonstrated to result in patients feeling less anxious and more in control and being more likely to continue the treatment when they return home.[33,34]

With patient contracts, agreement is reached through negotiation between the patient, the CNS and, if available, a third party such as a relative or friend of the patient. The process of negotiation is in itself useful, as it provides an opportunity to identify obstacles that may not have been previously recognized.[6] The third party should ideally be someone that the patient trusts and respects.

Incentives may be useful in the process of negotiating with patients. However, if care is organized on a holistic basis, so that financial, housing or immigration problems can begin to be addressed, the TB team has much more effective bargaining power: rather than simply providing incentives, some of the real obstacles to treatment adherence may be addressed.

There are also various degrees of treatment supervision that can be employed, including DOT.

When patients take their medication, they are in a very real sense assisting us in our work. In conditions in which drug treatment is the most effective form of disease control available, adherent patients form a major element of public health strategy by preventing further transmission of the disease. It is rarely acknowledged that patients are effectively partners, not only in the resolution of their own disease, but also in the reduction of the disease at large.[23] Yet the responsibility for disease control in general is not the patient's, it belongs with public health policy makers and TB teams. Therefore, when a patient is facing challenges in completing his or her treatment, the TB team, and tuberculosis control strategies in general, should ensure that all available support is provided.

Within many discourses on adherence, treatment failures are interpreted as a 'failure' on the part of the patient, with the result that he or she is labelled as 'recidivist' or 'delinquent'.[6] It is unhelpful to see non-adherence as an act of defiance. This transfer of blame has the function of distancing medical and healthcare establishments from any responsibility for failure. It also sets in motion a more insidious process. In a climate in which the patient is reflexively blamed for treatment failure, debates over patient adherence can find an audience that is receptive to the idea of incarcerating the 'offending' patient, without any necessity to ensure that the patient has received adequate support or assistance before such a decision is made. Debates about incentives and incarceration are important, as they have a real and tangible impact upon the practice of case management.

Inter-departmental working

There are certain situations in which patients with tuberculosis benefit from medical expertise that is not available in the TB team. The requirement of input from other departments will depend upon the local epidemiology of the disease. Within populations where rates of the disease are high and continue to rise, it is not unusual to see a high proportion of children with tuberculosis.[35] In areas where there is a substantial immigrant population from countries with high rates of HIV infection, these will be reflected in high rates of co-infection in the host area. In both of these circumstances the patient should receive specialist care and consultation from more than one team.

One response to a caseload that requires expert consultation from more than one source is to set up joint clinics. In these clinics, patients may be seen by a particular specialist physician, for example a paediatric consultant with a special interest in tuberculosis. The institution of joint clinics allows for the paediatrician to liaise with the specialist consultant for tuberculosis within the same clinic. Thus expertise is pooled.

In situations in which joint working is not well established and where more than one form of medical expertise is required, there is a risk that patients may only be seen by one physician who only has limited expertise in the field of tuberculosis. In these circumstances it is very important to ensure that effective referral and communication policies are in place between the TB team and other specialist teams. If such policies are not developed, there is a risk that patients will not receive the services they are entitled to. One possible method of circumventing this problem is through the establishment of posts that effectively bridge the gap between specialist services: a nurse who is skilled and experienced in areas of tuberculosis and HIV, or in tuberculosis and paediatrics.

In the process of establishing joint protocols, it is important that consultations take place between all stakeholders at every stage, to ensure that there is consent among all parties, with clear lines of accountability and responsibility.[4]

CHALLENGES TO AND QUALIFICATIONS OF CURRENT MODELS AND SERVICES

Despite all the advantages that nurse-led case management brings to patient care, there are certain limitations to its application. These can be broadly divided into two categories, those of scale and those of scope.

A nurse-led case management approach is only likely to be sustainable in particular conditions. In areas where there is a low incidence of disease and where TB teams are organized within relatively small localities, it will be difficult to justify service development on the scale required by this type of case management.

Despite this limitation, there are several principles that have been established in the course of building nurse-led teams and patient-centred care that are transferable to, and often already utilized by, services in lower incidence areas. These might include putting the tuberculosis nurse at the hub of the notification process, thus ensuring that the patient is able to benefit from the nurse's input from the time of diagnosis or the development of standard setting to maximize the quality of service.

Nurses in some areas have expressed concerns that nurse-led case management has become heavily medicalized, where extensions to practice have not led to the organization of services around the needs of patients per se so much as filled the clinical gap left by shortfalls in medical manpower. Arguably, this in turn has led to nurses spending more time on the paper work associated with extra clinical duties and less time with the patient. There is no particular need for nurse-led case management to be clinically driven; after the evaluation of service provision in the context of local needs, it may be judged that a less clinically interventionist approach to case management is appropriate. This conclusion may be reached when patient support is considered to be more critical than extensions to nursing practice – in the context of patient outcomes. Yet, while a more clinically driven form of case management may reduce nursing input in one instance, it may produce equally valuable benefits in another. For example, if nurses have more control over clinical functions, they are in a better position to ensure that those aspects of the service are more patient friendly and accessible.

There can be no question that gains have been – and will continue to be – made from the further development of nurse-led case management of tuberculosis. As a strategy, it is a successful means of ensuring that the needs of patients within healthcare settings are met with a consistent and co-ordinated response, and thus the chances of successful treatment completion are maximized. However, as many areas of care and management have been systematically improved within services, other unmet needs of patients with tuberculosis have been brought into relief. Many TB teams are working towards more integrated and collaborative care, but it remains relatively rare for the skill mix within services to be broad or balanced enough to offer truly holistic care that reflects patient needs.

These issues rarely form part of the nurse's professional development, and nurses are not often updated on changes in legislation or other forms of regulation that may occur in nonhealth sectors, such as housing and benefits. Moreover, teams are often left to sort out these wider needs of the patient on a 'case-by-case' basis, which is extremely time consuming, not to say frustrating in the event that the desired results are not attained. When planning care with patients, it is therefore very important to ensure that expectations are not unrealistically raised.

One of the major challenges to TB teams that are led and made up of nurses and other healthcare staff is that the medical needs of patients will be systematically prioritized over virtually all other needs as a result of the case manager's remit and the organizational goals of their employers. This may be stating the obvious, but Paul Farmer gets to the heart of the problem that this presents when he writes that: 'Problems faced by patients may be perceived as being more serious than the disease itself. If these problems are not addressed then they may have a serious impact upon treatment adherence and outcomes'.[13]

Many of these problems faced by patients are non-medical. There is also a great deal of supporting evidence to suggest that marginalized groups that face the most challenges are significantly less likely to adhere to treatment.[31]. Although these challenges are recognized by tuberculosis services, the resources and skills to address them are often lacking within TB teams. Over time, many doctors and CNSs have developed skills and experience in areas such as welfare, housing, immigration and substance abuse. Staff may also apply these skills to improving the situation of patients. Without formal training in these areas, however, or the backing of established policy agreements with the relevant authorities, nurses are often faced with time-consuming challenges that all too frequently end in frustration. Moreover, the bottom line here is that although CNSs identify these problems as critical to case holding and treatment adherence, there is rarely any professional recognition or accountability through which this work is conducted.

There is no reason why the tuberculosis services of the future should not continue to be nurse led. Indeed, the increased input of nursing in the case management of tuberculosis has, in all likelihood, produced a better understanding of why medical models are unable to provide all of the solutions to what are conceived of as medical problems. The extensions of nursing intervention in the case management of tuberculosis have helped shed light on some of the intractable difficulties faced by patients with tuberculosis in urban areas. It has also become clear in many of these areas that the skill mix within TB teams must be extended beyond the scope of nursing if the obstacles to case holding and adherence are to be addressed meaningfully.

Summary

This chapter has identified the principles of case management and related these to the evolution of nurse-led case management approaches in assessing, planning and co-ordinating the range of services needed for the successful management of people with tuberculosis. Case management has been defined and the impetus driving this approach to co-ordinated service delivery outlined. During the discussions in this chapter, the key components of nurse-led case management have been elaborated and the potential benefits and limitations of this concept for co-ordinating care have been noted. Although still evolving as a holistic framework, the authors believe that, within current service structures, nurse-led case management approaches are an important step towards securing comprehensive, organized and appropriate delivery of services, support and care for patients with tuberculosis.

Prologue to the next chapter

Although most patients with tuberculosis will be cared for at home, many will initially require in-patient care in a hospital or other healthcare facility. During this period, there is a potential risk for the transmission of *M. tuberculosis* to other patients, healthcare workers or visitors. The final two chapters in the book focus on assessing the risk of nosocomial transmission and then developing appropriate and relevant evidence-based responses to minimize this risk.

REFERENCES

1. Davies PDO (ed.). Preface to the second edition. *Clinical tuberculosis*, 2nd edn. London: Chapman and Hall, 1998, xv–xvii.
2. Dorsinville MS. Case management of tuberculosis in New York City. *Int J Tuberc Lung Dis* 1998; **2**: 546–52.
3. Frieden TR, Fujiwara PI, Washko RM, Hamburg MA. Tuberculosis in New York City –turning the tide. *N Engl J Med* 1995; **333**: 229–33.
4. Marais F. *Tuberculosis control: a nurse-led model with case management*. London: Foundation of Nursing Studies, 2002.
5. Cohen EL, Cesta TG (eds). *Nursing case management: from essentials to advanced practice application*, 3rd edn. New York: Mosby, 2001.
6. Campbell M, Galanowsky K, Pirog L. *Tuberculosis case management for nurses*. Newark, NJ: National Tuberculosis Center, 2003.
7. Papadopoulos A. *Case management in practice: an introductory guide to developing case management systems for vulnerable people*. Bicester: Winslow Press, 1993.
8. Department of Health. *The NHS Plan: a plan for investment, a plan for reform*. London: Department of Health, 2000.
9. Department of Health. *Getting ahead of the curve: a strategy for combating infectious diseases*. London: Department of Health, 2002.
10. Hayward A. *TB control in London: the need for change*. London: NHS Executive (Department of Health), 1998.
11. National Institute for Clinical Excellence (NICE). Clinical diagnosis and management of tuberculosis, and measures for its prevention and control. London: NICE. Anticipated date of publication September 2005. Will be available online at <www.nice.org.uk>.
12. Craig G, Hall J. The missing link. *Health Serv J* 2003; **11**: 34–5.
13. Farmer P. Social scientists and the new tuberculosis. *Soc Sci Med* 1997; **44**: 347 –58.
14. Suhonen R, Valmaki M, Leino-Kilpi H. Individualised care from patients' relatives' and nurses' perspective – a review of the literature. *Int J Nurs Stud* 2002; **39**: 645–54.
15. Mills PD, Harvey PW. COAG Coordinated Care Trial. Beyond community-based diabetes management and the COAG Coordinated Care Trial. *Aust J Rural Health* 2003; **11**: 131–7.
16. Wilson J. Integrated care management. *Br J Nurs* 1998; **7**: 201–2.
17. Rothe TB, Karrer W. Short course therapy of pulmonary tuberculosis: doctor's compliance. *Tuber Lung Dis* 1996; **77**: 93–7.
18. Tudor Hart J. Commentary: three decades of the inverse care law. *BMJ* 2000; **320**:18–19.

19. Vrijhoef HJ, Diederiks JP, Wesseling GJ, van Schayck CP, Spreeuwenberg C. Undiagnosed patients and patients at risk for COPD in primary health care: early detection with the support of non-physicians. *J Clin Nurs* 2003; **12**: 366–73.
20. Cochrane AL. Effectiveness and efficiency. In Davey B, Gray A, Seale C (eds), *Health and disease: a reader*, 3rd edn. Buckingham: Open University Press, 1995.
21. Cox CL, Reyes-Hughes A. *Clinical effectiveness in practice*. Basingstoke: Palgrave, 2001.
22. Bryar R, Griffiths J. *Practice development in community nursing: principles and processes*. London: Arnold, 2001.
23. Williams V. Patient holding. In Davies PDO (ed.), *Clinical tuberculosis*, 3rd edn. London: Arnold, 2003, 427–35.
24. Comolet TM, Rakotomalala R, Rajaonarioa H. Factors determining compliance with tuberculosis treatment in an urban environment, Tamatave, Madagascar. *Int J Tuberc Lung Dis* 1999; **11**: 1049.
25. Lazarus RS, Averill JR. *Emotion and cognition: trends in theory and research*. New York: Academic Press, 1972. Cited in: Gould D. *Infection and patient care: a guide for nurses*. London: Heinemann, 1987, 186–7.
26. Lester N. Cultural competence: a nursing dialogue. *Am J Nurs* 1998; **98**: 26–41.
27. Crouch D. Sharing medication agreements with patients. *Nurs Times* 2003; **99**: 34–6.
28. Diel R, Niemann S. Outcome of tuberculosis treatment in Hamburg: a survey, 1997–2001. *Int J Tuberc Lung Dis* 2003: **7**: 124–31.
29. Pablos-Mendez A, Knirsch CA, Barr RG, Lerner BH, Frieden TR. Nonadherence in tuberculosis treatment: predictors and consequences in New York City. *Am J Med* 1997; **102**: 164–70.
30. Procter S. The functioning of nursing routines in the management of transient workforce. *J Adv Nurs* 1989; **14**: 180–9.
31. Price B. Mapping the social support networks of patients. Continuing Professional Development Series, CN20. How to construct a social support network map with cancer patients, and understand the importance of lay support. *Cancer Nurs Pract* 2003; **5**: 31–8.
32. Volmink J, Garner P. Systematic review of randomised controlled trials of strategies to promote adherence to tuberculosis treatment. *BMJ* 1997; **315**: 1403–6.
33. Parker R. Self-administration of drugs by older people. *Professional Nurse* 1997; **12**: 328–30.
34. Marland G. Partnership encourages patients to comply with treatment. *Nurs Times* 1998; **94**: 58–9.
35. Rieder HL. *Epidemiologic basis of tuberculosis control*. Paris: IUATLD, 1999.

CHAPTER 19

The tuberculosis infection control plan – risk assessment

Introduction

Tuberculosis is a common infectious disease in many countries throughout the world and exposure to *Mycobacterium tuberculosis* in healthcare settings is a well-recognized hazard. Although the risks associated with this hazard cannot be completely eliminated, they can be controlled and minimized. Hospitals and other healthcare facilities do this by developing and implementing a comprehensive tuberculosis infection control plan that is responsive to the risks that have been identified by means of a structured assessment. This chapter describes the elements of a risk assessment strategy that will assist different healthcare facilities to identify the level of risk in their own institution and will lead to risk management responses that are described in the following chapter.

Learning outcomes

After studying and reflecting on the material in this chapter, you will be able to:

- discuss the evolution of risk management processes in healthcare organizations,
- describe the general elements of a risk assessment for tuberculosis in healthcare facilities,
- participate in an assessment exercise to evaluate the risk for transmission of *M. tuberculosis* in your own area of practice.

HEALTHCARE GOVERNANCE

During the last decade, healthcare systems in many of the industrially developed countries have undergone a transformation as a result of adapting and incorporating the principles of good governance into the management of both clinical and non-clinical services. There is now a major quality improvement and risk management initiative known as **healthcare governance**,[1] which initially involved the introduction of **corporate governance**, a system of financial and risk management based on a code of conduct that incorporates the principles of accountability, probity and openness into non-clinical services. Corporate governance is intended to minimize risk and promote value for money, ensuring that public funds are not wasted.

Corporate governance has continued to evolve in the National Health Service (NHS) in England with the introduction of **controls assurance**, a system for providing evidence to the public and other stakeholders that hospitals and other healthcare organizations are managing risk properly and effectively and protecting patients, staff, visitors and others against risk of all kinds.[2]

As corporate governance continued to be refined, another aspect of governance was introduced – **clinical governance**. This is intended to facilitate quality improvements in all clinical areas and at all levels of healthcare provision, and its key components are a series of quality attributes that include clinical effectiveness and risk management effectiveness.[1]

Clinical effectiveness is concerned with ensuring that clinical care and the delivery of services are based upon the best available evidence of effectiveness, for example *evidence-based infection prevention and control guidelines*. An important component of clinical nursing practice is the protection of patients from new infections during periods when they are receiving nursing care in hospitals, clinics, out-patient departments or in their homes. It is equally important to ensure that nurses and other healthcare practitioners do not acquire an infection from patients as a result of caring for them. Infection control guidelines for preventing healthcare-associated infections (HAIs) are an essential component of the safe delivery of quality care.

GUIDELINES AND POLICIES

Nurses and other healthcare practitioners carrying out clinical procedures should, whenever possible, precisely follow the written infection prevention and control guidelines and *operational policies* issued by their employing authorities. Local infection prevention and control guidelines should incorporate advice and recommendations contained in current evidence-based guidelines developed by government health departments, such as the national evidence-based guidelines for preventing HAIs in England,[3,4] and from a range of other relevant organizations and professional bodies, such as tuberculosis control and prevention guidelines issued by the British Thoracic Society (BTS) in the UK[5] and the Centers for Disease Control and Prevention (CDC) in the USA.[6]

Risk management effectiveness is at the very heart of healthcare governance, and its continuing activity is essential to the provision of a safe environment for nursing care, medical treatment and recovery from illness or trauma. Local infection prevention and control policies need to be based on comprehensive and ongoing assessments of the risks to patients, hospital staff and visitors of exposure to a range of pathogenic microorganisms, including *M. tuberculosis*. This assessment (and periodic re-assessment) conducted in each ward, department, clinic and healthcare facility is essential for developing a proper **risk management strategy**.

RISK ASSESSMENT

The concept of risk management has always been a key feature of proactive infection prevention and control strategies, as a failure to control such risks can have disastrous consequences for healthcare organizations, practitioners and patients. The ongoing cycle of risk management (Fig. 19.1) involves a continual evaluation in order to identify potential risks and assess the methods that are in place to control these.[7] In addition, effective reporting of adverse events, errors and 'near misses' is essential to the ongoing identification of risk and the development of effective risk management responses.

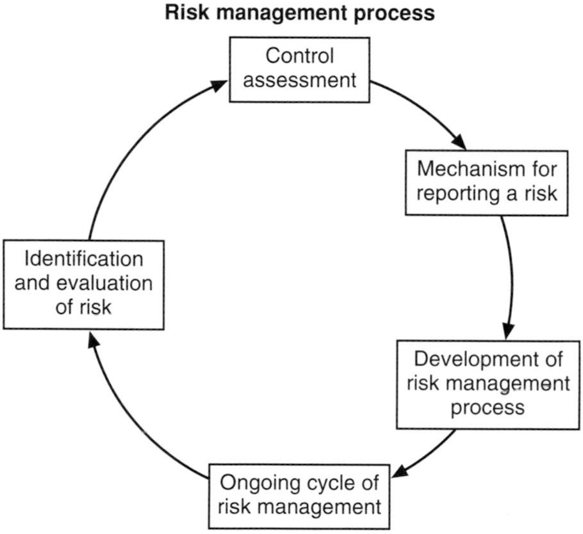

FIGURE 19.1 *Best practice for risk management, defined as the identification, evaluation and control of potential adverse outcomes that threaten the delivery of safe and appropriate care to patients.*

Hospitals in most industrially developed countries are legally required to conduct a formal assessment of the risk of being exposed to 'substances hazardous to health', including the risk of exposure to pathogenic microorganisms such as *M. tuberculosis*.[8] Information from the assessment is used to guide management decisions and policy development focused on efforts to improve patient safety and minimize risk.

Risk assessment exercise – tuberculosis

When conducting a risk assessment exercise for tuberculosis, a variety of data are collected which will enable the precise local nature of the risk from tuberculosis in a given healthcare facility to be assessed (Box 19.1).[6,9] In addition, specific elements of risk, such as environmental, administrative and clinical practice safety deficits, need to be identified.

A *multi-disciplinary assessment team* led by an experienced and qualified member of staff, such as a senior infection control practitioner or risk manager, may usefully include hospital epidemiologists, infectious disease specialists, pulmonary disease specialists, infection control practitioners, hospital managers (administrators), occupational health personnel, engineers

BOX 19.1 Tuberculosis risk assessment exercise[6,9]

The following describes the type of data that can usefully be collected during a risk assessment exercise

1. Review the most recent environmental evaluation and maintenance procedures
2. Establish the local epidemiological profile of tuberculosis
   - Trends in the incidence of new cases of tuberculosis, both pulmonary and extra-pulmonary
   - The number of immunocompromised patients being seen in in-patient and out-patient hospital settings
   - Prevalence of HIV infection and incidence of new infections
   - Incidence of tuberculosis among HIV-infected (and other immunocompromised) individuals
   - Number of patients with infectious tuberculosis admitted to hospital
   - Average length of infectiousness of tuberculosis patients admitted (defined as sputum smear positivity)
   - Number of patients with drug-resistant and multidrug-resistant (MDR) forms of tuberculosis admitted to hospital
   - Length of hospital stay for patients with MDR tuberculosis
3. Review a sample of medical records from tuberculosis patients admitted to hospital to evaluate infection control parameters

   Calculate intervals between:
   - admission until tuberculosis is suspected
   - admission until diagnosis of tuberculosis has been evaluated
   - admission until acid-fast bacilli (AFB) specimens ordered
   - AFB specimens ordered until AFB specimens collected
   - AFB specimens collected until AFB microscopy performed and reported
   - AFB specimens collected until species identification conducted and reported
   - AFB specimens collected until drug-susceptibility tests performed and reported
   - admission until respiratory isolation initiated
   - admission until tuberculosis treatment initiated, and
   - duration of respiratory isolation

   Obtain the following additional information
   - Were appropriate criteria used for discontinuing respiratory isolation?
   - Did the patient have a history of prior admission to the hospital or healthcare facility?
   - Was the antituberculosis drug regimen adequate?
   - Were follow-up sputum specimens collected properly?
   - Was appropriate discharge planning conducted?
4. Conduct a baseline hospital assessment of:
   - current availability of appropriate facilities, personnel, expertise and resources to care for patients with infectious and potentially infectious tuberculosis
   - the infection control strategies in place in relation to caring for patients with infectious and potentially infectious tuberculosis:
     - staff awareness of clinical presentation of patients with pulmonary tuberculosis

- staff familiarity with current infection control guidelines
- provision of continuing tuberculosis in-service education and training

■ quality assurance, audit and policy review mechanisms in place to assure infection control plan is both current, i.e. based on risk assessment data and professional and statutory guidelines, and is being implemented correctly

5. Review occupational health screening data, e.g. tuberculin skin test results of healthcare personnel by area or occupational group

6. Perform an observational review of tuberculosis infection control practices

(with expertise in ventilation and ultraviolet radiation) and local public health personnel. Patient representation on both risk assessment and risk management activities generally enhances the overall quality of the exercise.

Careful and detailed *pre-assessment planning* is needed to ensure that the exercise produces reliable information that can be used to calculate the level of risk and inform risk management responses.

The risk assessment should be conducted for the entire facility and for specific areas, such as medical, tuberculosis, pulmonary and human immunodeficiency virus (HIV) wards; HIV, infectious disease and chest (pulmonary) clinics; accident and emergency departments; mortuary and other areas (both in-patient and out-patient) where patients with tuberculosis might receive care and where cough-inducing procedures are performed.

Following the exercise, a *debriefing* session should be held to discuss the findings and plan the *assessment report*. The report needs to be widely circulated and discussed with staff in order to ensure that appropriate risk management responses are made that will be owned by all members of the hospital community.

A *periodic re-assessment* should be built into the risk management cycle. The frequency of repeat assessments will be determined by the results of the most recent assessment.

The CDC in Atlanta, Georgia, USA, has published a detailed protocol for conducting a tuberculosis risk assessment in a healthcare facility and determining the level of risk in a particular institution.[6] This is available online (see the 'References' at the end of this chapter for the website address) and can be modified and adapted to local circumstances.

Summary

Healthcare practitioners and patients are at potential risk of being exposed to *M. tuberculosis* in hospitals and other healthcare facilities. Before plans can be made to minimize this danger, the level of risk for the transmission of tubercle bacilli in each unit of each healthcare facility needs to be assessed carefully. This chapter gives a description of how the introduction of healthcare governance has placed renewed emphasis on risk management and requires a systematic assessment of the risk to staff and patients of becoming exposed to and infected with *M. tuberculosis* in healthcare settings. Also discussed are the basic structures within which a risk assessment should be conducted and the type of information this exercise is expected to elicit. Although the focus here is on risk assessment in hospitals in countries in the industrially developed world, the principles remain the same wherever assessment of the risk of transmission of *M. tuberculosis* is undertaken.

Prologue to the next chapter

Acquiring a comprehensive understanding of the potential risks for the transmission of tuberculosis currently existing in the different areas of practice in our own hospitals or healthcare facilities is a necessary prelude to developing an effective and relevant tuberculosis infection prevention plan. The majority of risks identified in local assessment exercises will be familiar and will have been previously addressed by others. The next chapter explores how we can use these clinically effective infection control measures, developed and tested by others and shown to be effective, in our own risk management responses to the assessment findings and to develop a locally relevant evidence-based tuberculosis infection control plan.

REFERENCES

1. Pratt R, Morgan S, Hughes J et al. Healthcare governance and the modernisation of the NHS: infection prevention and control. *Br J Infect Control* 2002; **3**: 16–25.
2. Emslie S. Controls assurance in the National Health Service in England – the final piece of the corporate governance jigsaw. *Corporate Governance*, 12 March 2001. London: ABG Professional Information.
3. Pellowe CM, Pratt RJ, Harper P et al. Infection control: prevention of healthcare-associated infection in primary and community care. Simultaneously published in *J Hosp Infect* 2003; **55**(Suppl. 2): 1–127; and *Br J Infect Control* 2003; **4**(6, Suppl.): 1–120. Also available online at <http://www.richardwellsresearch.com>.
4. Pratt RJ, Pellowe C, Loveday HP et al. The Epic project: developing national evidence-based guidelines for preventing healthcare associated infections. Phase 1: Guidelines for preventing hospital-acquired infections. *J Hosp Infect* 2001; **47**(Suppl.): S1–82. Also available online at <http://www.richardwellsresearch.com>.
5. Joint Tuberculosis Committee of the British Thoracic Society. Control and prevention of tuberculosis in the United Kingdom: Code of Practice 2000. *Thorax* 2000; **55**: 887–901. Also available online at <http://www.brit-thoracic.org.uk/index.asp>.
6. Centers for Disease Control and Prevention. Guidelines for preventing the transmission of *Mycobacterium tuberculosis* in health-care facilities, 1994. *MMWR* 1994; **43**(RR-13): 1–133. Also available online at <http://www.cdc.gov/mmwr/PDF/RR/RR4313.pdf>.
7. O'Neill S. Clinical governance in action. Part 2: Effective risk-management strategies. *Professional Nurse* 2000; **15**: 684–5.
8. Control of Substances Hazardous to Health (COSHH). Regulations 2002. London: Stationery Office Ltd. Available online at <http://www.hse.gov.uk/pubns/indg136.pdf>.
9. Interdepartmental Working Group on Tuberculosis. *The Prevention and control of tuberculosis in the United Kingdom: UK guidance on the prevention and control of transmission of (1) HIV-related tuberculosis (2) drug-resistant and multiple drug-resistant tuberculosis.* London: UK Departments of Health, September 1998. Also available by email from the Department of Health (England): <doh@prologistics.co.uk>.

CHAPTER 20

The tuberculosis infection control plan – risk management

Introduction

Nosocomial tuberculosis remains a major concern to healthcare practitioners, patients and the public. Lethal outbreaks of both multidrug-resistant (MDR) and drug-susceptible strains of *Mycobacterium tuberculosis* that occurred in hospitals in New York City,[1] London[2] and other European cities[3] during the last decade have alarmed many and led to questions about the safety of receiving or providing health care.[4]

All healthcare organizations need to have in place a current evidence-based tuberculosis infection control plan that is responsive to the level of risk identified in the baseline risk assessment described in the previous chapter. This plan needs to be integrated into the local tuberculosis policy and the hospital's general policies and procedures for preventing healthcare-associated infections (HAIs). This final chapter explores the dynamics of evolving strategies for preventing HAIs and relates these to developing a plan to minimize the risk of nosocomial tuberculosis.

Learning outcomes

After studying and reflecting on the material in this chapter, you will be able to:

- describe the rationale underpinning current recommendations for preventing HAIs,
- discuss standard and transmission-based infection prevention and control precautions and relate these to your own experience of caring for patients with tuberculosis,
- outline the components of a relevant infection control plan appropriate to different levels of assessed risk for nosocomial tuberculosis,
- explain when a patient with tuberculosis can be considered non-infectious,
- discuss the purpose and characteristics of a respiratory isolation room,
- identify the circumstances when personal respiratory protection should be used.

BACKGROUND

Healthcare strategies designed to protect patients and their carers from becoming infected during periods of hospitalization and community and home care have continued to evolve over many decades. Earlier models for preventing infections in hospitals and in the community consisted of either isolating infectious patients in special 'infectious disease hospitals' or using a cubicle system of isolation (individual rooms or cubicles) with barrier nursing in general hospitals.[5] These models evolved into more sophisticated and detailed category-specific and disease-specific isolation precautions.[6]

NEW CONCEPTS IN ISOLATION PRACTICES

In the early 1980s, a profound change in approaches to infection prevention and control practice occurred with the need to care safely for increasing numbers of patients with the acquired immunodeficiency syndrome (AIDS). *Blood and body fluid precautions* were developed principally to protect healthcare practitioners from becoming infected with the human immunodeficiency virus (HIV) and other bloodborne pathogens, such as hepatitis B virus (HBV). These precautions were used in caring for patients known to be or suspected of being infected with HIV. They focused on preventing injuries from needlesticks and other sharp instruments and on the use of gloves, gowns, masks and eye protection devices to prevent exposure to blood and other body fluids.

As national epidemics escalated and the number of patients with AIDS increased, and as the long asymptomatic incubation period of HIV infection and disease became understood, it was apparent by 1985 that an expanded set of blood and body fluid precautions would need to be 'universally' applied to all patients, regardless of their presumed infection status. This approach became known as *universal precautions* (UP).[7]

A few years later, a new system for preventing infections, known as *body substance isolation* (BSI), was described and rapidly incorporated into clinical nursing practice.[8] This was an elaboration of UP and focused on the isolation of all moist and potentially infectious body substances (blood, faeces, urine, sputum, saliva, wound drainage and other body fluids) from all patients, regardless of their presumed infection status, primarily through the use of gloves. Nurses and other healthcare practitioners wore gloves before any contact with any mucous membranes and non-intact skin from any patient, and before any anticipated contact with moist body substances.

CURRENT ISOLATION PRECAUTIONS

Although there was some evidence to indicate that BSI was effective in reducing the risk of healthcare-associated infections (HAIs),[9,10] infection prevention and control strategies continued to evolve and, in 1996, a new isolation guideline was developed by the Centers for Disease Control and Prevention (CDC) in the USA.[11] This synthesized the major features of UP and BSI into a single set of *standard precautions* to be used in caring for all patients all the time, regardless of their diagnosis or presumed infection status. It also combined and condensed previous category-specific and disease-specific isolation precautions into three sets of precautions based on routes of transmission. These *transmission-based precautions* were designed to reduce the risk of *airborne*, *droplet* and *contact transmission* and are intended to be used when clinically indicated in addition to standard precautions.

STANDARD PRINCIPLES FOR PREVENTING HEALTHCARE-ASSOCIATED INFECTIONS

Evidence-based infection prevention and control guidelines for preventing HAIs in England further elaborate current concepts of standard isolation precautions.[12,13] These *standard principles* provide guidance that should be applied by all healthcare practitioners to the care of all patients all the time regardless of their diagnosis or presumed infection status. They include recommendations for hospital hygiene, hand hygiene, the use of personal protective equipment and the use and disposal of needles and other sharp instruments (Box 20.1). They are not detailed procedural protocols, but are designed to be incorporated into local practice guidelines.

Standard infection prevention and control principles are the first tier of isolation precautions designed to reduce the risk of transmission of infectious microorganisms from both recognized and unrecognized sources of infection in healthcare settings. Their correct and consistent use protects patients and healthcare practitioners from exposure to bloodborne pathogens. Standard infection prevention and control principles apply to:

- blood
- *all* body fluids, secretions and excretions (except sweat)
- non-intact skin, and
- mucous membranes

in all healthcare environments, for all patients, all of the time without exception.

TRANSMISSION-BASED PRECAUTIONS

In addition to consistently using standard principles for preventing HAIs, transmission-based precautions are used for patients who are suspected or known to be infected with highly transmissible or epidemiologically important pathogenic microorganisms. Three types of transmission-based precautions are used: **contact**, **droplet** and **airborne precautions**.[11] These precautions can be combined for diseases that have multiple routes of transmission or for patients who are suffering from multiple infections.

Contact precautions are used to prevent the transmission of infectious microorganisms by direct or indirect contact. Direct contact refers to skin-to-skin transmission. An example of this might be the hands of a nurse becoming contaminated during caring for a patient who is infected or colonized with infectious microorganisms such as *Clostridium difficile* or *Staphylococcus aureus*. Contact precautions are also required for skin infections that are highly contagious, such as skin lesions caused by herpes simplex virus or as a result of reactivation of varicella-zoster virus (shingles) in immunocompromised patients. Indirect contact involves contact with a contaminated intermediate object, such as contaminated medical or surgical instruments, dressings or a contaminated environment.

Droplet precautions are used for patients known or suspected of being infected with microorganisms that are transmitted by large-particle respiratory droplets measuring more than 5 micrometres (μm) in size that are expelled during coughing, sneezing, talking or

BOX 20.1 Standard principles for preventing healthcare-associated infections[12,13]

Hand hygiene

- Hands must be decontaminated immediately before each and every episode of direct patient contact.
- Hands must be washed if they are visibly or potentially contaminated with dirt or organic material.
- Alcohol-based hand rubs may be used to decontaminate hands between caring for different patients and different caring activities for the same patient.
- Effective hand hygiene technique ensures thorough hand decontamination and protects skin integrity.

Gloves

- Gloves must be worn for invasive procedures, contact with sterile sites and non-intact skin, mucous membranes, and all activities that have been assessed as carrying a risk of exposure to blood, body fluids, secretions and excretions, sharp or contaminated instruments.
- Gloves must only be worn once, for one aspect of care and one patient.
- Dispose of gloves as clinical waste and decontaminate your hands following removal of gloves.

Aprons and gowns

- Disposable plastic aprons should be worn when there is a risk that clothing or uniform may become exposed to blood, body fluids, secretions and excretions, with the exception of sweat.
- Full body fluid-repellent gowns should be worn where there is a risk of extensive splashing of blood, body fluids, secretions and excretions, with the exception of sweat, onto the skin of healthcare practitioners.

Facemask and eye protection

- Facemasks and eye protection should be worn where there is a risk of blood, body fluids, secretions and excretions splashing into the face and eyes.

Sharps and needles

- Do not pass sharps from hand to hand and keep handling to a minimum.
- Do not bend or break needles, and do not re-cap/re-sheath or disassemble needles and syringes by hand before disposal.
- Used sharps must be discarded at the point of use into a sharps' container (conforming to UN3291 and BS7320 Standards).

Complete guidelines are available online at <http://www.richardwellsresearch.com>.

during the performance of certain investigations and treatment such as suctioning and bronchoscopy. These large droplets do not remain suspended in air and can only travel short distances, rarely more than 1 metre (approximately 3 feet).[11] Consequently, droplet transmission requires close contact between the source and recipient individuals. Droplet transmission involves contact of the conjunctivae or the mucous membranes of the nose or mouth of a susceptible person with large-particle infectious respiratory droplets. Droplet precautions apply to patients known to or suspected of having invasive disease such as pneumonia, meningitis or sepsis caused by *Haemophilus influenzae* type b, *Neisseria meningitides* disease, and pneumonia and other diseases caused by a variety of other bacteria and viruses.

Airborne precautions are used for patients known or suspected of being infected with microorganisms transmitted by minute *airborne droplet nuclei*, such as those causing measles, varicella, severe acute respiratory syndrome (SARS) and tuberculosis. Droplet nuclei are small-particle residues (5 μm or smaller) of evaporated respiratory droplets containing microorganisms that are suspended in the air and scattered widely by normal air currents within a room, corridor or over long distances.

More detailed information on standard principles for preventing HAIs and transmission-based precautions can be found in the guidelines from CDC,[11] and from the Department of Health and the National Institute for Clinical Excellence (NICE) in England,[12,13] all of which can be accessed online (see 'References' at the end of this chapter for the website addresses).

LOCAL TUBERCULOSIS POLICY

All healthcare authorities, health protection agencies and departments of public health have a comprehensive policy which describes all of the tuberculosis control and prevention measures to be implemented in the local area (Box 20.2).[14] Many of these policy components have been discussed in previous chapters; the remainder of this chapter concentrates on those measures used to prevent the transmission of *M. tuberculosis* in healthcare environments.

All of the recommendations for preventing nosocomial tuberculosis in this chapter are adapted from reliable evidence-based guidelines from the Joint Tuberculosis Committee of the British Thoracic Society (BTS),[14] the CDC (USA),[15] the Francis J. Curry National Tuberculosis Center (USA), [16] and the Department of Health (England).[17] Although these

BOX 20.2 Areas to be covered by the local tuberculosis policy[14]

- Aims and objectives
- Surveillance
- Identification of cases
- Notification
- Treatment
- Case management
- Outcome monitoring
- Hospital infection control
- Screening of vulnerable groups (asylum seekers, refugees, homeless people)
- Contact tracing
- Immunization, including neonatal policy
- Prisons and other institutions
- Education and training
- Continuous quality improvement programme (monitoring and audit)
- Health education
- Provision of adequate resources
- Research and audit
- Contingency arrangements for outbreak investigation

guidelines were developed for healthcare facilities in countries in the industrially developed world, many of the principles, such as administrative controls, are applicable to all countries. All of these guidelines are available online (see 'References' for the website addresses).

TABLE 20.1 Risk categories for nosocomial tuberculosis[15]

Risk	Criteria
Minimal risk	No tuberculosis patients in community or healthcare facility within the preceding year. *Minimal risk category applies only to an entire facility, including many medical and dental offices.
Very low risk	No tuberculosis patients admitted as in-patients to healthcare facility during preceding year and plan to refer patients with confirmed or suspected tuberculosis to a collaborating facility if in-patient care is required. Tuberculosis patients may be seen for triage or diagnostic evaluation in a clinic or emergency department. Those who require in-patient care will be transferred to a collaborating facility. *Very low risk category generally applies only to an entire facility, including many medical and dental offices.
Low risk	Fewer than six tuberculosis patients admitted to area during preceding year, *or* for specific occupational groups, exposure to fewer than six tuberculosis patients for healthcare workers in the particular occupational group during the preceding year. The PPD test conversion rate is not greater than that for healthcare areas or groups in which occupational exposure to *M. tuberculosis* is unlikely or than previous conversion rates for the same area or group. No clusters[a] of PPD test conversions have occurred. Person-to-person transmission of *M. tuberculosis* has not been detected. *Occurrence of drug-resistant tuberculosis in the facility or community, or a relatively high prevalence of HIV infection among patients or healthcare personnel in the area may warrant a higher risk rating.
Intermediate risk	Six or more tuberculosis patients admitted to area during preceding year,[b] *or* for specific occupational groups, exposure to six or more tuberculosis patients for healthcare workers in the particular occupational group during the preceding year. The PPD test conversion rate is not greater than that for healthcare areas or groups in which occupational exposure to *M. tuberculosis* is unlikely or than previous conversion rates for the same area or group. No clusters[a] of PPD test conversions have occurred. Person-to-person transmission of *M. tuberculosis* has not been detected. *Occurrence of drug-resistant tuberculosis in the facility or community, or a relatively high prevalence of HIV infection among patients or healthcare personnel in the area may warrant a higher risk rating.
High risk	The PPD test conversion rate is significantly greater than that for healthcare areas or groups in which occupational exposure to *M. tuberculosis* is unlikely or than previous conversion rates for the same area or group. Epidemiologic evaluation suggests nosocomial transmission, *or* a cluster[a] of PPD test conversions has occurred and epidemiologic evaluation suggests nosocomial transmission of *M. tuberculosis*, or possible person-to-person transmission of *M. tuberculosis* has been detected.

[a]Clusters: two or more PPD skin-test conversions occurring within a 3-month period among healthcare workers in a specific area or occupational group, and epidemiologic evidence suggests occupational (nosocomial) transmission.
[b]Survey data suggest that facilities in which six or more tuberculosis patients are examined or treated each year may have an increased risk for transmission of *M. tuberculosis*.[15]
PPD, Purified Protein Derivative; HIV, human immunodeficiency virus.

PREVENTING NOSOCOMIAL TUBERCULOSIS

A tuberculosis infection control plan incorporates a variety of precautionary measures that are adapted in each healthcare facility depending on the *level of risk* identified during a tuberculosis risk assessment (Table 20.1).[15]

For example, the elements of an infection control programme would be different in a rural hospital or healthcare facility in which the assessment had concluded that there was minimal risk, as opposed to a large, busy urban facility with a high risk of nosocomial tuberculosis. In many countries in the industrially developed world, such as the UK and the USA, most nurses will be working in hospitals or other healthcare facilities that have been assessed as having a minimal or very low risk for the transmission of *M. tuberculosis*. *Minimal-risk* facilities are those that have not admitted tuberculosis patients in the preceding year and are located in a community where tuberculosis has not been reported during the last year. The basic components of a tuberculosis control plan for a minimal-risk facility are listed in Box 20.3. With additional protocols, this will also serve as the basic infection control plan for *very*

BOX 20.3 Tuberculosis control plan: components for minimal-risk and low-risk healthcare facilities[4,15]

- Designated person(s) responsible for tuberculosis infection control plan
- Baseline risk assessment (including community and facility tuberculosis profile) with annual reassessment
- Written tuberculosis infection control plan
- Protocol for identifying patients with active tuberculosis
- Triage system for identifying patients with active tuberculosis in accident and emergency and ambulatory care settings
- Protocol for referring patients who may have active tuberculosis to a collaborating facility (if patients with tuberculosis are admitted, a more comprehensive plan is required)
- Baseline PPD test of healthcare workers[a]
- Educate and train healthcare workers regarding tuberculosis
- Protocol for identifying, evaluating, and managing healthcare workers with positive PPD tests or active tuberculosis
- Protocol for investigating PPD conversions among healthcare workers
- Protocol for investigating possible patient-to-patient transmission
- Protocol for investigating contacts of tuberculosis patients who were not diagnosed or isolated
- Mechanism for reporting patients with tuberculosis to proper public health authority
- Protocols for out-patient areas, such as clinics and accident and emergency departments, that specify how to evaluate and treat patients, how to report laboratory results to appropriate individuals (clinicians, hospital epidemiologist, infection control staff, collaborating referring and receiving facilities, and local public health/health protection departments), and how to protect staff, e.g. a respiratory protection programme[b]

[a]An ongoing PPD skin-testing programme is not needed. However, baseline PPD testing is advisable so that if an unexpected exposure occurs, conversion can be distinguished from positive PPD test results from a previous exposure.
[b]These protocols are only needed for very low-risk facilities.
PPD, Purified Protein Derivative.

low-risk facilities that do not admit patients with tuberculosis and refer those who require in-patient care to a collaborating hospital. *Intermediate-risk* and *high-risk* hospitals and other healthcare facilities that provide in-patient care for patients with active tuberculosis require a more comprehensive plan that outlines and mandates the use of a range of additional infection control measures.

PRIORITIZING CONTROL MEASURES

The infectiousness of patients with tuberculosis is directly related to the number of tubercle bacilli that they expel into the atmosphere. Consequently, a tuberculosis infection control plan should achieve the following goals: early identification of patients with active tuberculosis, prompt respiratory isolation, early diagnostic evaluation, and early effective antituberculosis treatment. These goals are achieved by a variety of control measures that need to be prioritized on the basis of the assessed risk of transmission and their relative effectiveness in reducing that risk. This ranking is referred to as the *hierarchy of controls* and separates these measures into administrative controls, environmental (engineering) controls, and respiratory protection.[4,15]

Administrative controls

Administrative controls are measures intended primarily to reduce the risk of exposing uninfected people to those who have infectious tuberculosis. These controls are the most effective measures that can be taken to reduce the risk of nosocomial transmission and should be implemented first by all healthcare facilities that admit patients with active tuberculosis. Administrative controls include:[15,16]

- developing and implementing effective written evidence-based tuberculosis control policies and procedures based on local-risk assessments,
- in-service education and training,
- screening and counselling employees.

Tuberculosis infection control policies and procedures

Local policies will provide guidance on ensuring the prompt identification, isolation, diagnostic evaluation and treatment of people likely to have infectious tuberculosis. These policies will also detail supervisory responsibility for tuberculosis and outline a series of effective work practices that minimize the risk to healthcare workers, patients and visitors of exposure to *M. tuberculosis*.

Identifying potentially infectious patients

Healthcare personnel with supervisory responsibility for tuberculosis in out-patient (ambulatory care) and in-patient settings need to develop, implement and audit protocols for the prompt identification of potentially infectious tuberculosis patients. During audit, key performance standards should be elicited, for example time from presentation to isolation, to specimen collection, to sputum microscopy result, to initiation of antituberculosis therapy. The criteria used in these protocols will be based on the prevalence and characteristics of tuberculosis in the population served as identified in the risk assessment. A provisional diagnosis of active tuberculosis may be considered for patients who present with the signs and

BOX 20.4 Definition of a suspected infectious tuberculosis patient[15,16]

A diagnosis of infectious tuberculosis may be considered in any patient who has:

- a persistent cough (i.e. a cough lasting for ≥3 weeks) or other signs or symptoms compatible with active tuberculosis, such as bloody sputum, night sweats, weight loss, anorexia or fever (unless the patient's condition has been medically determined to result from a cause other than tuberculosis)
- a positive acid-fast bacilli sputum smear
- been started on antituberculosis therapy for clinical suspicion of active pulmonary or laryngeal tuberculosis but has completed <2 weeks of treatment.

The index of suspicion for tuberculosis will vary in different geographic areas and will depend on the prevalence of tuberculosis and other characteristics of the population served by the hospital or other healthcare facility. Patient characteristics that may increase the index of suspicion include:

- patients from countries with a high prevalence of tuberculosis
- injecting drug users
- alcoholics
- HIV-infected and other immunosuppressed individuals
- homeless people
- current or former prison inmates
- poor nutrition.

HIV, human immunodeficiency virus.

symptoms outlined in Box 20.4. The implementation of these protocols needs to be periodically evaluated and revised appropriately as warranted by new risk assessment data.

Isolation of infectious cases

Patients with suspected infectious tuberculosis need to be cared for in an area away from other patients and certainly away from immunocompromised patients. Ideally, they should be situated in a negative-pressure respiratory isolation room (discussed later), but if this is not possible, they need to be in a single room with the door closed (preferably a room where the air is vented to the outside). Any patient in whom multidrug-resistant tuberculosis (MDR TB) is suspected (Box 20.5) should only be cared for in a negative-pressure respiratory isolation room.[17] All patients with suspected (or proven) infectious tuberculosis being cared for

BOX 20.5 Factors associated with an increased risk for multidrug-resistant tuberculosis (MDR TB)[14]

- Exposed and infected in country with high prevalence of MDR TB
- Previous drug treatment for tuberculosis
- Contact with a case of known MDR TB
- HIV infected
- Failure of clinical response to antituberculosis treatment
- Prolonged sputum smear positive or culture positive while on treatment (sputum smear positive at 4 months or culture positive at 5 months)

HIV, human immunodeficiency virus.

in a ward or unit where there are immunocompromised patients, for example an HIV/AIDS patient care area, must be cared for in a negative-pressure respiratory isolation room.[17] The algorithm developed by the BTS (Fig. 20.1) illustrates appropriate patient placement as determined by a risk assessment.[14] The local tuberculosis infection control policy will outline arrangements for transferring patients with suspected MDR TB or HIV-related tuberculosis to another facility when negative-pressure respiratory isolation rooms are not available.

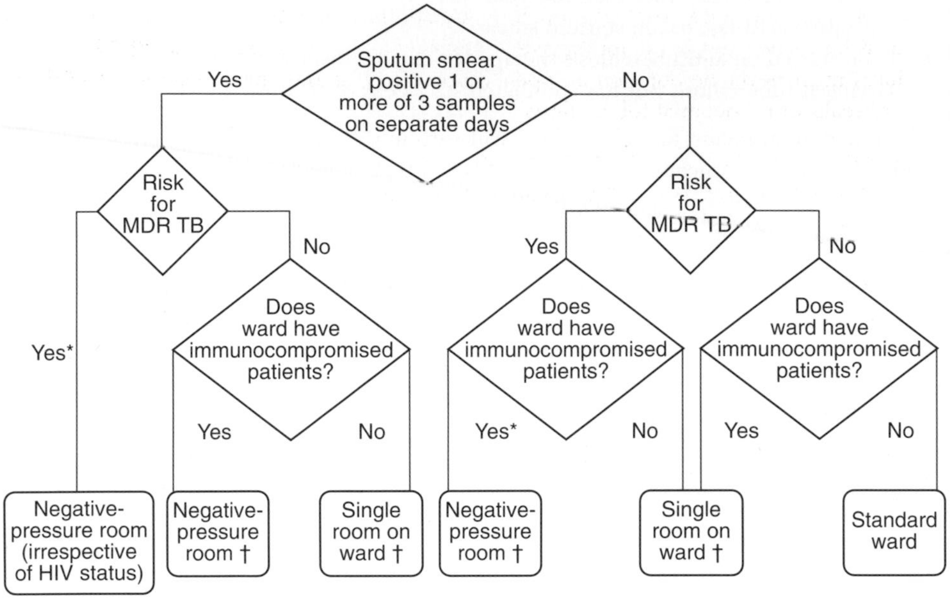

FIGURE 20.1 *Risk assessment of infectivity and other factors. *Molecular tests for identification of* Mycobacterium tuberculosis *and rifampicin resistance strongly recommended. †If previous treatment for tuberculosis or contact with multidrug-resistant tuberculosis (MDR TB), molecular test for rifampicin resistance mandatory; if rifampicin resistance, treat/isolate as MDR TB.[14] Reproduced from the Joint Tuberculosis Committee of the British Thoracic Society guidelines in* Thorax *2000; 55: 890, with permission from the BMJ Publishing Group.*

Additional isolation practices offer added safety and patient benefits.[16]

- *Masking patients* Patients with suspected or known infectious tuberculosis should wear a surgical mask when they are not in a respiratory isolation room or another area where there is exhaust ventilation. The purpose of the mask is to block aerosols produced by the patient when coughing, breathing or talking. A particulate filter respirator (PFR) is not required for this purpose and should not be used. A surgical mask on a co-operative patient provides short-term protection. The mask is changed when damp.
- *Isolating and segregating suspected infectious tuberculosis patients* In order to minimize the risk of transmission further, and to avoid embarrassment and concern to both the patient and others in the department, masked patients should ideally be escorted to a private waiting area or examination room.
- *Fast tracking* Arrangements need to be made in advance for consultations or investigations in other departments so that masked patients can be 'fast tracked' through the procedure. This means they are expected when they arrive and are quickly seen and processed and returned to respiratory isolation. Patients need to be accompanied by a healthcare worker to ensure that they do not remove the mask or get lost.

- *Delay of high-risk procedures* Aerosol-generating and cough-inducing procedures that are not immediately required for diagnosis or treatment should be delayed if at all possible until a suspected or proven infectious tuberculosis patient is no longer infectious.
- *Cough hygiene* Unmasked patients should be instructed to cover their mouth and nose with tissues when they cough. Tissue dispensers should be placed within easy reach of all patients throughout the hospital.
- *Aerosol-generating procedures* For all patients in HIV wards, units and clinics, aerosol-generating procedures, such as bronchoscopy, sputum induction or nebulizer treatment, must be carried out in an appropriately engineered and ventilated area.[14] These procedures must never be done on an open ward or bay, as they have been responsible for outbreaks of nosocomial tuberculosis.[2]

Patients remain in isolation until they are deemed non-infectious by the medical and nursing team caring for them. Patients with sputum smear-positive tuberculosis not known or suspected to have MDR TB usually become non-infectious after 2 weeks of effective antituberculosis treatment (as described in Chapter 12) and remain so if regular adequate treatment is continued, even though tubercle bacilli might still be occasionally seen in sputum smears.[14] In hospitals and other institutional healthcare facilities, segregation for reasons of infectiousness is generally only required for 2 weeks following the commencement of effective antituberculosis therapy.[14] This assumes that patients have had a minimum of 2 weeks of antituberculosis treatment and that their signs and symptoms are regressing, their general condition is improving, they are coughing less and, usually, they have had three negative sputum smears on three consecutive days. However, the criteria for discontinuing respiratory isolation have to be judged individually for each patient. Care must be taken in discontinuing respiratory isolation in a patient being cared for in an HIV ward (Box 20.6),

BOX 20.6 Cessation of respiratory isolation in a human immunodeficiency virus (HIV) setting[14]

A patient with active tuberculosis being cared for on an HIV ward can normally be considered non-infectious if the following criteria are met.

Sputum smear-positive cases

(a) The patient has had a minimum of 2 weeks of appropriate multiple drug therapy, *and*
(b) if being moved to accommodation (in-patient or home) with HIV-infected or immunocompromised patients, has had a *minimum* of three negative sputum microscopic smears on separate occasions over at least a 14-day period, *and*
(c) has shown tolerance to the prescribed treatment and an ability and agreement to adhere to treatment, *and either*
(d) has a complete resolution of cough, *or*
(e) has a definite clinical response to treatment, for example remaining afebrile for 1 week.

Sputum smear-negative cases (three sputum samples on separate days or if no sputum, and bacteriology only from bronchoscopy and lavage):

(a), (c), (d) and (e) above apply.

N.B. The bacteriological response to antituberculosis chemotherapy is equally good in HIV-infected and non-HIV-infected individuals.

as a patient with infectious tuberculosis could present a life-threatening risk to other HIV-infected immunocompromised patients on an open ward.[1–3] Patients with MDR TB will have to remain in respiratory isolation for longer, until they have been judged not to be infectious.

Diagnostic evaluation for active tuberculosis

All patients with a provisional diagnosis of active tuberculosis need to be examined by a physician as soon as possible and appropriate diagnostic procedures conducted (Box 20.7, and as described in Chapter 8). Prompt laboratory results are essential before initiating anti-tuberculosis therapy. Healthcare facilities that do not have their own tuberculosis laboratory need to have arrangements in place for referral to a reference laboratory that uses the most rapid methods for the culture and identification of mycobacteria and for drug-susceptibility testing. The results of sputum microscopy for the detection of acid-fast bacilli (AFB) should be available within 24 hours (or within 1 working day) of specimen collection.[15,17] Serology for HIV infection should be offered and encouraged for all patients with suspected (or proven) tuberculosis.

BOX 20.7 Diagnostic evaluation for active pulmonary tuberculosis[15,17]

Diagnostic measures for identifying active tuberculosis would normally include:

- physical examination and medical history
- microscopic examination and culture of sputum or other appropriate specimens
- tuberculin (PPD) skin test
- other diagnostic procedures, e.g. bronchoscopy or biopsy, as indicated
- chest radiograph (X-ray)

PPD: Purified Protein Derivative.

Early antituberculosis treatment

Patients who have confirmed active tuberculosis or who are considered highly likely to have active tuberculosis should promptly commence appropriate antituberculosis therapy (as described in Chapter 12). Most patients with drug-susceptible tuberculosis are quickly rendered non-infectious within just a few weeks of starting treatment.

In-service education

All healthcare workers, including physicians, should receive training and education regarding tuberculosis that is relevant to their particular occupational group. Ideally, training should be given as part of their orientation/induction programme and repeated on an annual basis. The level and detail of the training given will vary according to the healthcare worker's clinical responsibility and level of risk in the hospital or facility. A suggested educational programme from the CDC is described in Box 20.8.[15] Multi-modal educational methods, such as computer assisted and e-learning, provide opportunities for healthcare workers to update their knowledge and skills without necessarily leaving their wards or departments.

Employee screening, counselling and prevention programme

Occupational health departments need to have effective services in place to screen healthcare workers for tuberculosis. Those who have a positive Purified Protein Derivative (PPD)

BOX 20.8 Tuberculosis in-service education programme for healthcare workers[15]

- The basic concepts of *M. tuberculosis* transmission, pathogenesis and diagnosis, including information concerning the difference between latent tuberculosis infection and active tuberculosis, the signs and symptoms of tuberculosis, and the possibility of re-infection.
- The potential for occupational exposure to people who have infectious tuberculosis in the healthcare facility, including information concerning the prevalence of tuberculosis in the community and healthcare facility, the ability of the facility properly to isolate patients who have active tuberculosis, and situations with increased risk for exposure to *M. tuberculosis*.
- The principles and practices of infection control that reduce the risk for transmission of *M. tuberculosis*, including information concerning the hierarchy of tuberculosis infection control measures and the written policies and procedures of the facility. Site-specific control measures should be provided to HCWs working in areas that require control measures in addition to those of the basic tuberculosis infection control programme.
- The purpose of PPD skin testing, the significance of a positive PPD test result, and the importance of participating in the employee skin-test programme.
- The principles of preventive therapy for latent tuberculosis infection, including the indications, use, effectiveness and potential adverse effects of the drugs.
- The HCW's responsibility to seek prompt medical evaluation if a PPD test conversion occurs or if symptoms develop that could be caused by tuberculosis. Medical evaluation will enable HCWs who have tuberculosis to receive appropriate therapy and will help to prevent transmission of *M. tuberculosis* to patients and other HCWs.
- The principles of drug therapy for active tuberculosis.
- The importance of notifying the facility if the HCW is diagnosed with active tuberculosis so that contact investigation procedures can be initiated.
- The responsibilities of the facility to maintain the confidentiality of the HCW while ensuring that the HCW who has tuberculosis receives appropriate therapy and is non-infectious before returning to duty.
- The higher risks associated with tuberculosis infection in people who have HIV infection or other causes of severely impaired cell-mediated immunity, including (a) the more frequent and rapid development of active tuberculosis after infection with *M. tuberculosis*, (b) the differences in the clinical presentation of disease, and (c) the high mortality rate associated with MDR TB in such people.
- The potential development of cutaneous anergy as immune function (as measured by CD4+ T-lymphocyte cell counts) declines.
- Information regarding the efficacy and safety of BCG vaccination and the principles of PPD screening among BCG recipients.
- The facility's policy on voluntary work re-assignment options for immunocompromised HCWs.

HCW, healthcare worker; PPD, Purified Protein Derivative; MDR TB, multidrug-resistant tuberculosis; BCG, Bacille Calmette–Guérin.

test result, or a PPD test conversion, or symptoms suggestive of tuberculosis should be identified and evaluated in order to rule out a diagnosis of active tuberculosis or commenced on antituberculosis therapy or preventive therapy if indicated.[15] Recommendations for screening healthcare staff in UK hospitals and other healthcare facilities are regularly updated by the Joint Tuberculosis Committee of the BTS and are available online.[14] Other countries have similar recommendations. The UK recommendations include the following measures.

Pre-employment and on-employment measures These are outlined in Figure 20.2 (BTS Guidelines, 2000).[14] A pre-employment personal health questionnaire and on-employment health check should elicit any previous history of tuberculosis or symptoms suggestive of tuberculosis, information of previous Bacille Calmette–Guérin (BCG) vaccination and the presence or absence of a BCG scar and, if indicated, tuberculin (PPD) skin testing and a chest radiograph (X-ray). A tuberculin skin test is only necessary in those new employees who do not have either a definite BCG scar (as recorded by an experienced person) or reliable documentary evidence of previous BCG vaccination. New healthcare employees from a country where the annual incidence of tuberculosis is greater than 40/100 000 of the population and who have not been screened for tuberculosis on entry into the UK or by a previous employer in Britain should routinely have both a chest radiograph and a tuberculin skin test.

Tuberculin-negative employees from countries with a high prevalence of HIV infection should have HIV serological testing before BCG vaccination. As discussed in Chapter 10, HIV-infected people may have a suppressed reaction to tuberculin skin testing and test negative regardless of infection with *M. tuberculosis*, a condition known as anergy.

Healthcare workers in employment Although it is uncommon for healthcare workers to acquire tuberculosis from patients in the UK,[18] it is always a potential risk. In some other countries, the risk to healthcare workers of occupationally acquired tuberculosis may be increased due to the greater prevalence of tuberculosis and lack of adequate resources effectively to diagnose and isolate infectious patients. The in-service education programme described above will increase staff awareness and encourage them to seek medical advice promptly should they experience any signs or symptoms suggestive of active tuberculosis. The risk to patients and other healthcare workers from a member of staff with undiagnosed infectious tuberculosis is severe, especially in those units caring for immunocompromised patients. Routine periodic chest radiography for healthcare workers is not effective in detecting tuberculosis and should not be done.[14,19]

HIV-infected healthcare workers As discussed in Chapter 10, HIV-infected people have an increased susceptibility to develop active tuberculosis following previous infection and/or re-infection. Any protection conferred by previous BCG vaccination will be reduced naturally over time and, more importantly, as a result of a progressive decline in cell-mediated immunity caused by ongoing HIV replication. Consequently, previous BCG vaccination will not protect them following new infection. Additionally, in some countries, a higher than expected incidence of drug and multidrug resistance has been encountered in localized epidemics of HIV-related tuberculosis.

Many HIV-infected healthcare workers choose to care for HIV-infected patients. As tuberculosis is the most common opportunistic infection associated with HIV disease, immunocompromised healthcare workers who work in HIV wards, units and clinics are more frequently exposed to infectious tuberculosis, and probably more frequently exposed in many countries to MDR TB.

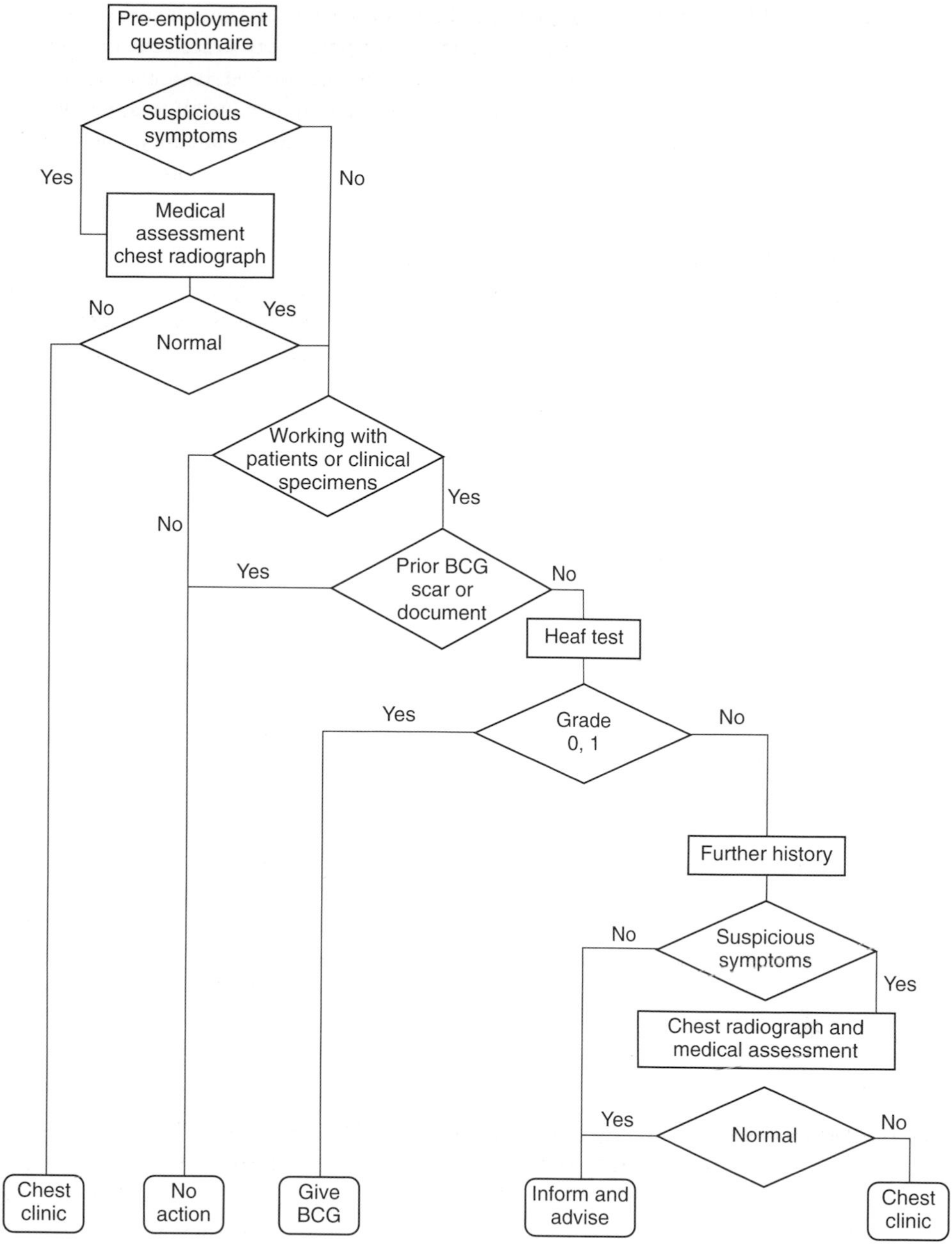

FIGURE 20.2 *Screening of healthcare workers for tuberculosis. Reproduced from the Joint Tuberculosis Committee of the British Thoracic Society guidelines in* Thorax *2000; 55: 891, with permission from the BMJ Publishing Group.*

There is a substantial risk to immunocompromised healthcare workers from HIV-infected patients who have undiagnosed or confirmed active tuberculosis. There is also a serious risk to HIV-infected patients from an immunocompromised healthcare worker who develops active tuberculosis and continues to work before the condition is identified and he or she is isolated and treated.

Consequently, all healthcare workers who believe they may have been exposed to HIV infection under whatever circumstances have an ethical responsibility to seek expert medical advice and serological testing if indicated. If HIV infection is confirmed, they need to inform the occupational health services, which can advise them whether an alternative clinical assignment is necessary to avoid possible exposure to tuberculosis (or any highly infectious disease such as chickenpox or measles).

In no circumstances should immunocompromised healthcare workers care for patients with active tuberculosis. As stated previously, HIV-infected healthcare workers should not receive BCG vaccination, as this is a live vaccine that can cause severe local lesions or even disseminated BCG infection (BCG-osis),[20] as discussed in Chapter 6. All immunocompromised healthcare workers need to remain under the care of specialist medical services and the occupational health service.

Environmental (engineering) controls

Engineering controls are the second level of the tuberculosis control hierarchy and are based primarily on the use of adequate ventilation systems, sometimes supplemented with high-efficiency particulate air (HEPA) filtration and ultraviolet germicidal irradiation (UVGI). These controls are used to minimize further the risk of nosocomial tuberculosis by decreasing the concentration of infectious droplet nuclei in the air, preventing the dissemination of droplet nuclei throughout the hospital or healthcare facility, or rendering droplet nuclei non-infectious by killing the tubercle bacilli they contain.

Ventilation

Ventilation systems for healthcare facilities should meet the needs of the institution risk assessment and be designed and modified when necessary by ventilation engineers in collaboration with infection control and occupational health staff. Hospital ventilation systems are described in detail in CDC guidelines;[15] their diversity and complexity preclude giving specific advice here, except for brief comments on general ventilation and local exhaust ventilation (LEV), and describing the ventilation features of negative-pressure rooms used for airborne infection isolation.

General ventilation

General ventilation systems in healthcare facilities are designed to dilute and remove contaminated air, control airflow patterns within rooms, and control the direction of airflow throughout a hospital or healthcare facility. They are fully described in CDC guidelines.[15,21]

Local exhaust ventilation

Local exhaust ventilation is designed to capture airborne contaminants at or near their source and remove them before they disperse without exposing people in the area to infectious microorganisms.[15] LEV is the preferred source-control technique for enclosing devices used for aerosol-generating procedures, such as laboratory hoods, booths for sputum induction or the administration of aerosolized medications, and hoods and tents made of vinyl or other materials to enclose and isolate patients. Booths, tents and hoods should have sufficient airflow to remove at least 99 per cent of airborne particles during the interval between the departure of one patient and the arrival of the next. The exterior device is usually a hood very near but not enclosing the infectious patient. These devices are more widely used in the USA and are not commonly available in the UK. Further information on their specification and use is available online from the CDC (see reference for website address).[15,21]

Negative-pressure respiratory isolation rooms

Ventilation for respiratory isolation rooms is designed to achieve a negative pressure in the room in relation to adjacent areas, preventing contaminated air from escaping from the room to other areas in the hospital or healthcare facility. Negative-pressure rooms are used for respiratory isolation and this is referred to in the USA as **airborne infection isolation (AII)** – that is, the isolation of patients infected with microorganisms spread via airborne droplet nuclei <5 μm in diameter, such as *M. tuberculosis*. The specification for AII rooms has recently been updated by the CDC (Box 20.9).[21] Isolation rooms need to be monitored on a daily basis when in use to ensure that the negative pressure is maintained. Isolation room exit doors need to be kept closed (preferably having self-closing devices), except when patients or healthcare workers must enter or exit the room, in order to maintain negative pressure. There should be a pressure gauge on the outside of the door, which continuously indicates that the room is under negative pressure.

BOX 20.9 Characteristics of a respiratory isolation room (airborne infection isolation, AII)[21]

- A room used for AII receives numerous air changes per hour (ACH) – preferably ≥12 ACH but not less than 6 ACH.
- AII rooms are under negative pressure, such that the direction of the airflow is from the outside adjacent space, for example the corridor, into the room. A continuous negative air pressure (2.5 Pa [0.01 inch water gauge]) in relation to the air pressure in the corridor is maintained.
- The air in an AII room is preferably exhausted directly outside, away from air intakes and traffic, but may be re-circulated provided that the return air is filtered through a high-efficiency particulate air (HEPA) filter. HEPA filters can be used in ventilation systems to remove droplet nuclei from the air.
- Ultraviolet germicidal irradiation (UVGI) units may also be installed in exhaust air ducts or near the ceiling to irradiate upper room air.
- The use of personal respiratory protection is also indicated for people entering these rooms when caring for patients with tuberculosis (or other airborne transmitted infectious diseases).
- AII rooms are also used for patients with or suspected of having an airborne infection who also require cough-inducing or other aerosol-generating procedures.

High-efficiency particulate air (HEPA) filtration

High-efficiency particulate air filters are sometimes used in ventilation systems to remove droplet nuclei from the air, or are installed in ventilation ducts to filter air for recirculation into the same room or to other areas of a healthcare facility (although air exhaust directly outside is preferable). Portable HEPA filtration units are sometimes used for supplemental air cleaning, but their effectiveness has not yet been adequately evaluated. HEPA filters must be carefully installed and maintained.

Ultraviolet germicidal irradiation

Ultraviolet germicidal irradiation may kill tubercle bacilli contained within drop nuclei. Because exposure to ultraviolet light can be harmful to the skin and eyes, shielded lamps are always installed in the upper part of rooms or corridors where normal air currents circulate contaminated air into an upper room/corridor 'killing zone'. The UVGI may also be installed in ventilation exhaust vents to provide supplemental air cleaning.

Personal respiratory protection

In some healthcare settings in the UK and elsewhere, administrative and engineering controls may not fully protect healthcare workers from infectious droplet nuclei.[22] In these circumstances, special facemasks known as *particulate filter respirators* (PFRs) are used. This is known as *personal respiratory protection* and it is the third level in the hierarchy of controls used to prevent exposure to tubercle bacilli. Personal respiratory protection is not as effective as administrative and engineering controls, but will provide additional protection when appropriately used.

The PFRs are different from surgical masks. Surgical masks are designed to prevent respiratory secretions of the person wearing the mask from entering the air. The PFRs are designed to do the exact opposite, i.e. to filter the air before it is inhaled by the person wearing the respirator. They are capable of filtering out particles with a diameter of 5 μm or smaller.

In many countries in the industrially developed world, approved PFRs are certified by regulatory agencies, such as the National Institute for Occupational Safety and Health (NIOSH) in the USA. In Europe, standards are laid down by the European Union (EU) Parliament.

NIOSH certifies the N-series of PFRs and the EU certifies the EN149 (Personal Protective Equipment) series. NIOSH-certified N-series respirators are required to filter sodium chloride particles to a level of 0.3 μm at a minimum of 95 per cent efficiency. NIOSH certifies the N95 PFR for protection against nosocomial tuberculosis. This PFR is available in the UK as the Kimberly-Clark Tecnol™ PFR95; however, it is not currently certified for use in member nations of the EU for protection against nosocomial tuberculosis.

The EU certifies the EN149 FFP series of PFRs. The FFPS1 PFR is required to filter coal dust at an average of 0.6 μm at 80 per cent efficiency and is recommended for protection against nosocomial tuberculosis. These respirators are available in the UK from 3M™ Health Care. A new respirator manufactured by Kimberly-Clark Tecnol™ (known as the PFR P2) is now certified by the EU for use in the UK and in other European member states when caring for patients with infectious tuberculosis.

The CDC recommends that personal respiratory protection should be used by all people entering rooms where patients with known or suspected infectious tuberculosis are being isolated. The PFRs should also be used by healthcare workers who are present during cough-inducing or aerosol-generating procedures performed on such patients and by people in other settings where administrative and engineering controls are not likely to protect them from inhaling infectious droplet nuclei.[15] In England, the Department of Health recommends that personal respiratory protection be used:

- by all people entering the room of a patient with suspected or confirmed infectious MDR TB,
- by all people during cough-inducing or aerosol-generating procedures on patients with suspected or confirmed pulmonary tuberculosis,

- by healthcare workers caring for any high-dependency patients with known or suspected infectious tuberculosis,
- rarely, in other situations (identified during the risk assessment exercise), for example by people exposed to tuberculosis in settings where ventilation is inadequate, or by healthcare workers who regularly care for patients with infectious tuberculosis, such as on an HIV ward.[17]

Respiratory protection programme

A respiratory protection programme needs to be developed, implemented and periodically re-evaluated in any healthcare facility in which personal respiratory protection is used. All healthcare workers who need to use respirators for protection against *M. tuberculosis* should be included in the programme. The CDC recommends the following programme,[15] which should be used as a template for locally developed programmes.

Assignment of responsibility

Supervisory responsibility for the programme needs to be allocated to designated individuals who have expertise in issues relevant to the programme, including infectious diseases and occupational health. In the UK, infection control nurses and respiratory clinical nurse specialists or nurse consultants are generally assigned this responsibility.

Standard operating procedures

Written standard operating procedures are developed which describe in detail all aspects of the respiratory protection programme.

Medical screening

Healthcare workers need to be screened for pertinent medical conditions when they are first employed (and periodically re-screened) to ensure that they do not have any conditions that would preclude them from using respirators.

Training

Healthcare workers who wear respirators, and the people who supervise them, require education and training focused on the need for personal respiratory protection and the potential risks of failing to use it. Training should also include at a minimum:

- the nature, extent, and specific hazards of *M. tuberculosis* transmission in their respective hospital or other healthcare facility as identified by the most recent risk assessment;
- a description of the natural history of tuberculosis and individual risk factors that increase the likelihood of active tuberculosis following exposure and infection;
- a description of administrative and engineering controls and work practices and the reasons why they do not completely eliminate the need for personal respiratory protection;
- a precise outline of those situations in which personal respiratory protection is required and when it is not;
- instruction and supervised practice in handling the provided respirator, including inspecting it, correctly putting it on, checking for a proper face-seal, and correctly wearing it.

PATIENT NAME: ______________________ Problem No. ☐ PATIENT STICKER

INFECTION CONTROL CARE PLAN FOR A PATIENT WITH (OR SUSPECTED OF HAVING) ACTIVE PULMONARY OR LARYNGEAL TUBERCULOSIS

Tuberculosis should be suspected in any patient, regardless of HIV-infection status, who has a cough without other causes lasting more than 3 weeks, with or without weight loss, anorexia, fever, night sweats or haemoptysis, the presence of cavitating disease or upper lobe disease on chest radiograph (X-ray)

MODE OF TRANSMISSION: From person to person by airborne transmission. The infectious particles are very small respiratory droplets less then 5 micrometres (μm) containing tubercle bacilli expelled during talking, singing or shouting **but especially coughing**.

PRECAUTIONS TO BE LIFTED: When three smear-negative sputa are obtained **and**, if the patient was ever sputum positive, after 14 days' therapy and definite clinical improvement.
NB. Patients who are sputum smear negative but have a positive broncho-alveolar lavage (BAL) will still require isolation precautions.
If after therapy the patient is still smear positive, review risk with consultant microbiologist and/or respiratory/ID physician.

PERSONS MOST AT RISK: Non-immune staff, patients or relatives with prolonged contact. (NB. BCG does not confer full immunity.)
HIV-infected staff or those who are immunocompromised should not care for patients with active tuberculosis.

POTENTIAL PROBLEMS	AIM	INTERVENTION	ASSESSMENT
Unconfirmed diagnosis	Confirm diagnosis	Send three sputum specimens for AFB at three different times – not all on the same day. **Send the specimens to the laboratory urgently and request urgent processing and reporting.**	1 / / Sig. 2 / / Sig. 3 / / Sig.
Possibility of drug-resistant TB	Assess the possibility	Determine if the patient has had or has: *(If yes report to respiratory physician/ICN)* • previous treatment for tuberculosis? • contact with a person with known drug resistant disease? • been resident overseas? • failure of clinical response, e.g. temperature remains elevated after 2 weeks?	/ / / / / / / / / / (day 7 & 14 post therapy)
Cross-infection to patients	Minimize the risk	Nurse the patient in a single room with, if available, negative pressure ventilation. Keep the door closed. Monitor the negative pressure gauge regularly. Encourage the patient to cover the mouth when coughing. Ensure that patient has fresh disposable sputum container and tissues. Discard the sputum container and tissues into clinical waste (yellow) bag. On instruction to end isolation, ensure patient is not nursed next to immunocompromised or HIV-infected patients. Ensure that the patient wears a surgical mask whenever they may need to leave their room.	/ / Sig. / / Sig. Daily Ongoing Daily Ongoing Ongoing / / Sig. Ongoing
Patient understanding of disease process, mode of spread, and need for medication	Educate the patient and provide support	Contact the TB liaison nurse. (TB liaison nurse where possible to do the following.) Explain to the patient how the disease is contracted and how it is spread. Explain the need for infection control precautions. Ask the patient for co-operation & adherence to infection prevention precautions & treatment. Explain the importance of taking the medication as prescribed. Assess the patient's understanding of his/her condition and his/her role in recovery.	/ / Sig. / / Sig. / / Sig. / / Sig. / / Sig. / / Sig.
Failure to comply with therapy	Establish, monitor and promote adherence	Directly Observe Therapy - watch patient swallow tablets. Explain the consequence of non-adherence. Give the patient the opportunity to express fears and anxieties regarding therapy. Explain to the patient side effects of therapy.	Ongoing / / Sig. / / Sig. / / Sig.

PATIENT NAME: ______________________ Problem No. ☐ PATIENT STICKER

POTENTIAL PROBLEM	AIM	INTERVENTION	ASSESSMENT
Cross-infection to visitors	Minimize the risk	Without breaking the confidentiality of the patient, assess the risk for visitors. Advise only visitors who were in close contact with the patient before diagnosis to visit until therapy is established. Advise visitors not to bring children to the ward. Inform relatives of the planned follow-up by TB liaison nurse.	/ / Sig. / / Sig. / / Sig. / / Sig.
Cross-infection to staff	Minimize the risk	Only staff with known immunity should nurse the patient. Wear respiratory protection mask when entering the room for physiotherapy if patient has a productive cough and when **prolonged care** is necessary, or if the patient is dependent. If the patient is smear positive, the nurse-in-charge will give the names of staff who have had close contact with the patient to Occupational Health for follow-up and complete appropriate *pro forma*.	/ / Sig. / / Sig. / / Sig.
Cross-infection to non-ward staff	Reduce the risk	Inform bronchoscopy or other theatre staff of (possible) diagnosis. Inform physiotherapist if referral is necessary. If patient discharged via ambulance whilst still infectious – inform ambulance staff pre-transfer.	/ / Sig. / / Sig. / / Sig
Possible family/close contact outbreak	Inform proper authorities	Ensure notification by medical staff to Department of Public Health/Health Protection Agency. Notify TB liaison nurse – contact via switchboard.	/ / Sig. / / Sig.
Psychological problems as a result of airborne infection isolation	Promote psychological well-being	Ensure patient understands the need for segregation. Ensure the patient has sufficient sensory stimulation, e.g. TV, reading material, access to the phone. Encourage the patient to express fears and anxieties regarding the isolation. Provide the patient with a 'Patients Requiring Isolation Leaflet'. *NB. The door remaining closed will increase the fears and anxieties of the patient.*	/ / Sig. / / Sig. / / Sig. / / Sig.
Continuation of care into the community	Plan discharge	Discuss and agree treatment plan between TB liaison nurse, medical and nursing staff and the patient. Determine: who is going to observe therapy, if required, post-discharge if the patient is still considered infectious clinic follow-up and transport needs prescription: payment, collection requirements that the patient's GP has been informed if support services are necessary the risk of infection, if any, to support staff	/ / Sig.
Cleaning post-discharge	Ensure hygienic standards are achieved	If room is naturally ventilated and not under negative pressure, open the windows with the door closed to disperse air from the room. Undertake normal post-discharge cleaning. Take particular care – as always – with horizontal surfaces. Ensure all waste is discarded from the room as clinical waste.	/ / Sig. / / Sig. / / Sig.

This is a core care-plan and is concerned only with the infection control aspects of the patient's care. Nursing staff using this care plan should endeavour to ensure that it is adapted to meet the individual needs of the patient. Contact the ICN for advice on any aspect of the patient's care.

PATIENT NAME: ______________________ Problem No. ☐ PATIENT STICKER

TUBERCULOSIS RISK ASSESSMENT & NEGATIVE PRESSURE GAUGE MONITORING

Sputum results

Date	Positive or negative smear	Comment NB. 3 consecutive negative smears means non-infectious

Risk assessment for drug-resistant disease	Yes to any means the patient is at higher risk. Contact the ICN if any marked yes
Previous treatment for tuberculosis?	
Close contact with a patient with known drug-resistant disease?	
Likely to have acquired tuberculosis abroad? If so, where?	
HIV-infected?	
Failure to respond to therapy?	

Negative pressure gauge monitoring (Daily)

	Date	Gauge reading		Date	Gauge reading
1			8		
2			9		
3			10		
4			11		
5			12		
6			13		
7			14		

FIGURE 20.3 *Infection control care plan for a patient with (or suspected of having) active pulmonary or laryngeal tuberculosis.*

Face-seal fit testing and fit checking

Healthcare workers need to undergo fit testing to ensure the respirator provided fits them properly. They need to receive full fitting instructions that include demonstrations and practice in how the respiratory should be worn, how it should be adjusted, and how to determine if it fits properly. They also need to be taught to check the fit before each use. Male healthcare workers with facial hair need to be advised that they will be unable to obtain an adequate facial seal when using disposable PFRs.

Periodic evaluation of the programme

The programme needs to be re-evaluated on an annual basis, after which both the written operating procedures and programme administration may need adjusting.

Nursing care plan

Following the assessment of a patient with known or suspected active tuberculosis, an individualized plan of care must be developed, implemented and evaluated on a shift-by-shift basis. It will incorporate a strategy to address the actual and potential problems described in detail in Chapter 17 and the infection control and prevention issues discussed in this chapter. A standardized nursing care plan, such as that developed by the Infection Control Nursing Service at North Glasgow University National Health Service Trust in Scotland (see Fig. 20.3),[23] can be easily adapted to the individual care circumstances and level of risk for patients in any in-patient healthcare facility.

Summary

In this final chapter we have explored the evolution of general infection prevention and the control practices that have resulted in our current strategies to minimize the risks for HAIs in general and nosocomial tuberculosis in particular. These strategies are responsive to specific hazards for exposure to *M. tuberculosis* in each of our healthcare facilities, which we can identify by conducting a risk assessment, as discussed in the previous chapter. The specific *administrative and engineering control measures* and *personal respiratory protection procedures* that we need to incorporate into our local strategies are adapted from a series of evidence-based guidance issued by departments of health and professional organizations such as the CDC in the USA,[11,15,16,21] and the BTS, Department of Health and NICE in the UK.[12–14,17] As tuberculosis continues as a serious threat to human health, and as more and more people develop active disease and seek treatment and care, it also remains a potential hazard to those healthcare practitioners who provide that care. Having well-thought-out evidence-based policies and procedures in place that provide guidance on safe work practices and ensuring that healthcare workers are trained to incorporate this guidance consistently into everyday clinical care are the first steps towards providing a safe environment for health care. In addition, healthcare workers need supervision and support to sustain adherence to policy, and managers of healthcare facilities need to audit practice and re-assess the risks for transmission of *M. tuberculosis* on a regular basis so that any identified risk is minimized and the quality of care is continuously improved.

> New evidence-based guidance for preventing nosocomial tuberculosis will be published by NICE in February 2006 and will be available on their website: <http://www.nice.org.uk/>.

REFERENCES

1. Jarvis WR. Nosocomial transmission of multidrug-resistant *Mycobacterium tuberculosis*. *Am J Infect Control* 1995; **23**: 146–51.
2. Kent RJ, Uttley AHC, Stoker NG, Miller R, Pozniak AL. Transmission of tuberculosis in a British care centre for patients infected with HIV. *BMJ* 1994; **309**: 639–40.
3. Di Perri G, Cruciani M, Danzi MC et al. Nosocomial epidemic of active tuberculosis among HIV-infected patients. *Lancet* 1989; **334**: 1502–4.
4. Pugliese G, Tapper ML. Tuberculosis control in health care. *Inf Control Hosp Epidemiol* 1996; **17**: 819–27.
5. Gage ND, Landon JF, Sider MT. *Communicable disease*. Philadelphia: FA Davis, 1959.
6. Garner JS, Simmons BP. *CDC guideline for isolation precautions in hospitals*. Atlanta, GA: US Department of Health and Human Services, Public Health Service, Centers for Disease Control, 1983. HHS publication No. (CDC) 83–8314; *Infect Control* 1983; **4**: 245–325; and *Am J Infect Control* 1984; **12**: 103–63.
7. Centers for Disease Control. Recommendations for preventing transmission of infection with human T-lymphotropic virus type III/lymphadenopathy-associated virus in the workplace. *MMWR* 1985; **34**: 681–6, 691–5.
8. Lynch P, Jackson MM, Cummings J, Stamm WE. Rethinking the role of isolation practices in the prevention of nosocomial infections. *Ann Intern Med* 1987; **107**: 243–6.
9. Klein BS, Perloff WH, Maki DG. Reduction of nosocomial infection during pediatric intensive care by protective isolation. *N Engl J Med* 1989; **320**: 1714–21.
10. Leclair JM, Freeman J, Sullivan BF, Crowley CM, Goldmann DA. Prevention of nosocomial respiratory syncytial virus infections through compliance with gown and glove isolation precautions. *N Engl J Med* 1987; **317**: 329–34.
11. Garner JS, Hospital Infection Control Practices Advisory Committee. Guideline for isolation precautions in hospitals. *Infect Control Hosp Epidemiol* 1996; **17**: 53–80. Also available online at <http://www.cdc.gov/ncidod/hip/isolat/isolat.htm>.
12. Pratt RJ, Pellowe CM, Loveday HP, Robinson N, Smith GW, and the **epic** Guideline Development Team. The **epic** Project: developing national evidence-based guidelines for preventing healthcare-associated infections. Phase 1: Guidelines for preventing hospital-acquired infections. *J Hosp Infect* 2001; **47**(Suppl.): S1–82. Also available online at <http://www.richardwellsresearch.com>.
13. Pellowe CM, Pratt RJ, Harper P et al. and the Guideline Development Team. Evidence-based guidelines for preventing healthcare-associated infections in primary and community care in England. Simultaneously published in *J Hosp Infect* 2003; **55**(Suppl. 2): 1–127; and *Br J Infect Control* 2003; **4**(6, Suppl.): 1–120. Also available online at <http://www.richardwellsresearch.com>.
14. Joint Tuberculosis Committee of the British Thoracic Society. Control and prevention of tuberculosis in the United Kingdom: Code of Practice 2000. *Thorax* 2000; **55**: 887–901. Also available online at <http://thorax.bmjjournals.com/content/vol55/issue11/index.shtml#BTS%20GUIDELINES>.
15. Centers for Disease Control and Prevention. Guidelines for preventing the transmission of tuberculosis in health-care facilities, 1994. *MMWR* 1994; **43**(RR13): 1–132. Also available online at <http://www.cdc.gov/mmwr/preview/mmwrhtml/00035909.htm>.
16. Francis J. Curry National Tuberculosis Center, Institutional Consultation Services. *Tuberculosis exposure control plan: template for the clinic setting*, 1999: 1–54. Available online at <http://www.nationaltbcenter.edu>.

17. Interdepartmental Working Group on Tuberculosis. *The prevention and control of tuberculosis in the United Kingdom: UK guidance on the prevention and control of transmission of HIV-related tuberculosis and drug-resistant, including multiple drug-resistant, tuberculosis*. London: UK Departments of Health, September 1998.
18. Capewell S, Leaker AR, Leitch AG. Tuberculosis in NHS staff: is it a problem? *Thorax* 1986; **41**: 708.
19. Lunn JA, Mayho V. Incidence of pulmonary tuberculosis by occupation of hospital employees in the National Health Service in England and Wales 1980–84. *J Soc Occup Med* 1989; **39**: 30–2.
20. Grange JM. Complications of bacilli Calmette–Guérin (BCG) vaccination and immunotherapy and their management. *Commun Dis Public Health* 1998; **1**: 84–8.
21. Centers for Disease Control and Prevention. Guidelines for environmental infection control in health-care facilities: recommendations of CDC and the Healthcare Infection Control Practices Advisory Committee (HICPAC). *MMWR* 2003; **52**(RR10): 1–45. Also available online at <http://www.cdc.gov/mmwr/preview/mmwrhtml/rr5210a1.htm>.
22. Curran E, Ahmed S. Do health care workers need to wear masks when caring for patients with pulmonary tuberculosis? *Commun Dis Public Health* 2000: **3**: 240–3.
23. Curran E. *Infection control care plan for a patient with (or suspected of having) active pulmonary or laryngeal tuberculosis*. Glasgow: Infection Control Nursing Service, North Glasgow University NHS Trust, May 2004.

FURTHER READING

Centers for Disease Control and Prevention. Guidelines for preventing the transmission of tuberculosis in health-care facilities, 1994. *MMWR* 1994; **43**(RR13): 1–132. Also available online at <http://www.cdc.gov/mmwr/preview/mmwrhtml/00035909.htm>.

Joint Tuberculosis Committee of the British Thoracic Society. Control and prevention of tuberculosis in the United Kingdom: Code of Practice 2000. *Thorax* 2000; **55**: 887–901. Also available online at <http://thorax.bmjjournals.com/content/vol55/issue11/index.shtml#BTS%20GUIDELINES>.

Glossary

Acid-fast bacilli Bacilli with the property of acid fastness and a term often used synonymously with 'mycobacteria'.
Acid-fastness The ability of the tubercle bacillus and other members of the genus *Mycobacterium* to retain certain dyes after treatment with a dilute mineral acid.
Acquired drug resistance Resistance to antituberculosis drugs developing in a patient due to sub-optimal therapy.
Acquired immunodeficiency syndrome (AIDS) A late symptomatic stage of disease caused by the human immunodeficiency virus (HIV), characterized by a high viral load, a profoundly depressed level of CD4+ T-lymphocytes and certain 'AIDS-defining' opportunist infections (including tuberculosis) and cancers.
Addison's disease Adrenal insufficiency.
Adherence The behaviour of the patient that assures that all medication is taken. The term also refers to the behaviour of healthcare workers and employers that assures that they follow all guidelines pertaining to disease control.
Administrative controls Guidelines for rapidly identifying those patients who may have active tuberculosis, isolating them, prompt diagnostic evaluation, and early initiation of antituberculosis chemotherapy.
Aerobe An organism requiring oxygen for growth and replication.
Aetiology The study or theory of factors that cause disease.
AFB Acronym for **acid-fast bacilli**.
AIDS Acronym for **acquired immunodeficiency syndrome**.
AII Acronym for **airborne infection isolation**, i.e. respiratory isolation.
Airborne infection isolation Isolation of patients infected with microorganisms spread via airborne droplet nuclei <5 μm in diameter.
Allergy A term originally applied to any altered immune response, but now usually restricted to certain hypersensitivity reactions.
Alveoli The small air sacs in the lung in which gaseous exchange occurs.
Anaerobe An organism that grows and replicates in the absence of oxygen.
Anergy The failure of a patient to respond immunologically to an infective challenge. This may be suggested by a negative tuberculin reaction in a patient with active tuberculosis.
Annual incidence (of tuberculosis) The number of new cases of tuberculosis detected over the period of 1 year.
Annual infection rate or **annual risk of infection** The number of people infected with a microbial pathogen in the course of a year. It may be greater than the annual incidence of disease (see **Disease ratio**).
Antibody Also termed **immunoglobulin**. Glycoproteins, produced by plasma cells, that bind to antigen and mediate various immune reactions.
Antigen A molecule that induces an immune response.
Antigen-presenting cell (APC) A broad range of cells, including monocytes, macrophages and dendritic cells, found throughout tissues and able to present antigens to the corresponding antigen-specific T-lymphocytes.
Artificial pneumothorax An operation, commonly done in the days before antituberculosis therapy, to collapse a lung by introducing air into the pleural cavity.

Asymptomatic Without symptoms, but not necessarily without a disease.
Attack rate A special form of **incidence rate** that is used in situations where there is a specific episode of risk.
Attenuation The weakening or loss of virulence of a pathogen, utilized in the development of living vaccines such as BCG.
Autoimmune disease Disease due to the immune system attacking parts of the host body rather than 'foreign' molecules.
Bacille Calmette–Guérin (BCG) The only vaccine currently used to prevent tuberculosis. It was developed by the French scientists Albert Calmette and Camille Guérin at the Institut Pasteur, Lille, between 1907 and 1921. It is a living, attenuated variant of the bovine tubercle bacillus.
Bacillus (pleural **bacilli**) Literally, 'a rod'; this refers to rod-shaped bacteria, in contrast to the circular coccus (pleural, cocci). (The term can be confusing, as one genus of bacteria is called *Bacillus*. This includes the organism causing anthrax – *Bacillus anthracis*.)
Bacteriocidal An antimicrobial agent or an immune mechanism that is able to kill a microorganism.
Bacteriostatic A term applied to antimicrobial agents (and occasionally to immune mechanisms) that prevent the replication of a microorganism but fail to kill it.
Bacterium A large group of single-celled organisms which, together with the blue-green algae, are characterized by having a nucleus that is not confined by a nuclear membrane. Most bacteria are free-living in the environment, but a few cause disease in humans and animals. Bacteria are quite different from viruses.
BCG Acronym for **Bacille Calmette–Guérin**.
BCG-osis Disseminated disease caused by BCG vaccine.
Biopsy Removal of a sample of tissue, by means of a fine needle, bronchoscope or other instrument or through a small incision, for laboratory examination.
B-lymphocytes Also termed B cells; the cells of the immune system that, on activation, mature into **plasma cells** and produce antibody.
Booster effect In tuberculin testing, an enhanced skin reaction seen if the test is repeated after a short time interval.
Bovine tuberculosis Tuberculosis of cattle caused by the bovine tubercle bacillus *Mycobacterium bovis*.
Brawl chancre Tuberculosis of the knuckle acquired by punching a person with open tuberculosis in the teeth. A very rare condition!
Bronchoscopy Examination of the airways by means of a flexible fibreoptic tube (bronchoscope). This procedure enables clinical material to be obtained by washing, brushing or biopsy.
Buruli ulcer A chronic tropical disease characterized by extensive skin ulceration and caused by *Mycobacterium ulcerans*.
Butcher's wart Also called **prosector's wart**; a tuberculous skin lesion acquired by accidental injury while cutting up tuberculous animal carcases or human corpses.
Cachexia The extreme wasting seen in people with advanced tuberculosis, and some other diseases.
Capreomycin A rarely used reserve drug for the treatment of multidrug-resistant tuberculosis. It must be given by injection.
Caseation *See* **Caseous necrosis**.
Case-finding The search for people with tuberculosis, usually by microscopical examination of the sputum of 'suspects' with a cough of more than 3 weeks' duration.

Caseous necrosis The central area of tissue necrosis seen in tuberculous lesions, most evident in post-primary lesions. The term caseous necrosis or caseation is in allusion to the cheese-like nature of this necrotic material.
Cavity, pulmonary A necrotic tuberculous lesion that communicates with the airways, enabling tubercle bacilli to enter the sputum and to be coughed out.
CD Cluster differentiation. A system used to subdivide **T-lymphocytes** into functional subsets – principally CD4+ and CD8+.
Cerebrospinal fluid The fluid surrounding the brain and spinal cord.
Chemoprophylaxis The prescription of antimicrobial agents to prevent those at risk of an infection from developing the disease.
Chemotherapy Treatment of disease (not just cancer) by chemicals. It includes the treatment of tuberculosis by various antibacterial drugs.
Clofazimine Also known as **Lamprene**; an antileprosy drug with some activity against tubercle bacilli and other mycobacteria.
Clonal expansion Following activation by antigen-presenting cells and antigen, the replication of an antigen-specific lymphocyte to produce a sufficient number of such cells to induce an effective immune response.
Cold abscess An abscess without the heat and pain characteristic of acute abscesses.
Combination (drug) preparations Tablets containing several antituberculosis drugs to simplify therapy.
Complement A group of serum and tissue proteins that mediate various immune reactions, including lysis of certain pathogens and enhancement of phagocytosis.
Compliance The behaviour of the patient that assures that all medication is taken. *See* **Adherence**.
Congenital tuberculosis Tuberculosis acquired by a baby while in the uterus. An uncommon but serious form of tuberculosis.
Constrictive pericarditis Scarring of the pericardium following tuberculous pericarditis, leading to constriction of the heart and cardiac failure.
Consumption An old term for tuberculosis, in allusion to the wasting seen in advanced disease.
Contact A person likely to have been infected by a person with open tuberculosis due to close association, e.g. in a household.
Contact tracing The search for people infected by a patient with open or infectious tuberculosis, principally in the patient's household.
Contagion parameter The number of people infected by a single infectious patient.
Corticosteroids Anti-inflammatory hormones prescribed in some cases of tuberculosis (notably tuberculous meningitis and pericarditis) to prevent constrictive scarring.
Crohn's disease A chronic inflammatory disease of the human intestine, suspected by some to be caused by the same mycobacterium (*Mycobacterium avium* var. *paratuberculosis*) that causes Johne's disease in cattle, although confirmation is required.
Cryptic disseminated tuberculosis Widespread tuberculosis occurring in those with suppressed immune function, such as people with AIDS. The tissues contain numerous microscopic lesions teeming with tubercle bacilli. In contrast to the lesions of miliary tuberculosis, these are not easily seen on radiology.
Cultivation The process of growing microorganisms in the laboratory for the purposes of identification, drug susceptibility studies and other investigations.
Culture An imprecise term for **cultivation**. The term is also applied to the bacterial mass obtained by cultivation.

Cycloserine A rather toxic second-line drug for the treatment of multidrug-resistant tuberculosis.
Cytokines From the Greek words meaning 'cell energizers', these are molecules released during immune responses that 'direct' the various cells involved in these responses. Examples include gamma interferon and tumour necrosis factor.
Cytotoxicity The killing of cells. It is applied to cytotoxic drugs as used in chemotherapy for cancer and also certain immune mechanisms that result in the death of an infected or otherwise abnormal cell.
Cytotoxic T-lymphocytes T-lymphocytes, usually of the CD8+ type, that are involved in cell-mediated cytotoxicity.
Delayed type hypersensitivity A rather vague term to encompass cell-mediated immune reactions that are detectable by skin testing. They are termed 'delayed' as they take longer to appear than various antibody-mediated hypersensitivity reactions characteristic of allergic conditions. The positive tuberculin test is a typical example of a delayed hypersensitivity reaction as it takes around 48 hours to develop.
Directly observed therapy (DOT) Administration of antituberculosis drugs under direct supervision. One of the elements of the World Health Organization DOTS strategy.
Disease ratio The ratio of those infected with, for example, the tubercle bacillus and those actually developing the disease.
DNA (deoxyribonucleic acid) The famous 'double helix' forming the basis of the genes and chromosomes. *See also* **Nucleic acid**.
DNA fingerprinting A group of techniques used to divide a species, such as *Mycobacterium tuberculosis*, into many variants by detecting small differences in their DNA structure. This enables the spread of these variants in the community to be studied for epidemiological purposes.
DNA probe A diagnostic reagent used to detect a specific DNA sequence in a clinical specimen or an isolated microorganism.
DOTS The 'brand name' of the World Health Organization strategy for the control of tuberculosis. The components are government commitment, diagnosis principally by sputum microscopy, good-quality drugs supplied free to patients, directly observed therapy and monitoring of the efficacy of the control activities.
DOTS-Plus A modification of the DOTS strategy to manage multidrug-resistant tuberculosis.
Droplet nuclei Minute airborne particles, up to 5 μm in diameter, containing infectious agents produced by evaporation of the fluid in **respiratory droplets**.
Drug interactions The effect of one drug on the absorption, metabolism and activity of another. Several important drug interactions occur between rifampicin and other drugs, especially antiretroviral drugs given to those infected with HIV.
Drug resistance A mutational event in the bacterial cell leading to resistance to an antituberculosis drug. Drug resistance is determined in the laboratory by growing isolated tubercle bacilli on media containing various concentrations of the drug.
Drug susceptibility tests Laboratory procedures for determining whether a microorganism is susceptible or resistant to levels of a drug achievable by therapy.
Ehrlich, Paul The German microbiologist and pathologist, best known for his 'magic bullets' against syphilis, who discovered the characteristic acid-fast staining property of mycobacteria.
Empyema Infection of the pleural cavity leading to the accumulation of pus.
Endemic A disease or condition present in a specific population or geographical region all of the time.

Endobronchial tuberculosis Tuberculous involvement of the bronchial lumen due to erosion of a lymph node or other lesion through the bronchial wall.

Endogenous reactivation (of tuberculosis) Tuberculosis occurring years or even decades after infection due to re-activation of the original infection.

Engineering (environmental) controls Engineering systems used to prevent the transmission of tubercle bacilli in healthcare facilities, including ventilation, high-efficiency particulate air (HEPA) filtration, and ultraviolet germicidal irradiation.

Environmental mycobacteria Species of mycobacteria that usually live freely in the environment. Some of these occasionally cause human disease, notably in those who are immunosuppressed.

Epidemic A sudden and significant increase (outbreak) in the incidence of a previously endemic disease or a new disease within a specified population over a specified period of time.

Epidemiology The study of the causes, distribution, frequency and control of disease in populations.

Epitope Also called an antigenic determinant; a small unit of an antigen that is recognized by a single specific T-lymphocyte.

Epituberculosis Hyper-inflation or collapse of a segment or lobe of the lung secondary to bronchial obstruction by enlarged tuberculous lymph nodes.

Erythema nodosum Firm and painful red patches or nodules, usually on the lower limbs, most often seen in children with primary tuberculosis aged between 5 and 10 years. It may occur in other conditions and as a reaction to certain drugs.

Ethambutol One of the first-line antituberculosis drugs, given during the first 2 months of therapy. Care is required in its use, as it can cause irreversible eye damage. Patients should be instructed to stop taking the drug and seek medical advice if they develop any visual disturbances.

Ethionamide (Etionamide in the USA) A drug used to treat cases of drug-resistant tuberculosis. It is closely related to **prothionamide** (protionamide), a drug used for the same purpose.

Exogenous re-infection (of tuberculosis) Tuberculosis occurring in a person previously infected by tubercle bacilli but due to a new and recent re-infection.

Extrapulmonary tuberculosis Tuberculosis occurring outside the tissues of the lung, but including lesions within the thoracic cage.

Extrathoracic tuberculosis Lesions of tuberculosis occurring outside the thoracic cage.

Facultative pathogen Another term for **opportunist pathogen**.

'Fingerprinting' A term applied to molecular methods for subdividing bacterial strains within a species for epidemiological purposes.

First-line (antituberculosis) drugs The drugs used in the standard short-course regimens for the treatment of tuberculosis: **isoniazid**, **rifampicin**, **ethambutol**, **pyrazinamide** and, under some circumstances, **streptomycin**.

Fish tank granuloma *See* **Swimming pool granuloma**.

Fluorescence microscopy A sensitive way of visualizing acid-fast bacilli as fluorescent rods against a black background.

Fluoroquinolones A class of antibiotics used to treat drug-resistant tuberculosis and some diseases caused by environmental mycobacteria. Examples include **ofloxacin** and **ciprofloxacin**.

Fomites Inanimate objects in close contact with, and in regular use by, patients that may harbour and transmit microorganisms, e.g. clothing and bedding.

Gamma interferon A **cytokine** that is essential for protective immunity in tuberculosis by enabling macrophages to express their full ability to contain the infection.
Gastric aspiration The removal of the gastric contents through a tube passed down the oesophagus. This is used to harvest tubercle bacilli ascending from the lung to the pharynx and being swallowed overnight. It is used in those patients, particularly children, who do not produce sputum.
Genome The complete genetic complement of an organism. In the case of a bacterium, this is a single circular chromosome with, in some strains, small extrachromosomal elements called **plasmids**.
Genus The term used to describe the group of organisms above the level of species. Thus the human tubercle bacillus *Mycobacterium tuberculosis* is just one of 100 or so named species within the genus *Mycobacterium*. (N.B. By convention, the initial letter of a generic name is capitalized and the name itself is printed in italics.)
Ghon focus The initial focus of tuberculous infection in the lung.
Gibbus The angular 'hunchback' deformity characteristic of advanced spinal tuberculosis.
Gram's staining A widely used staining technique based on the ability of bacteria to retain crystal violet dye after treatment with acetone or alcohol. Gram-positive bacteria are violet coloured and Gram-negative bacteria take up the colour of a red counterstain.
Granulocyte White blood cells characterized by distinct granules in their cytoplasm. They are divided into **neutrophils**, **eosinophils** and **basophils** on the basis of the staining characteristics of the granules.
Granuloma Characteristic lesions of chronic infections consisting of a compact aggregate of active macrophages around the infecting agent.
HAART Acronym for **highly active antiretroviral therapy**.
HAI Acronym for **healthcare-associated infection**.
Heaf test The tuberculin test performed by driving six short needles into the skin through a drop of concentrated tuberculin by means of a spring-loaded 'Heaf gun'.
Healthcare-associated infection (HAI) Previously referred to as nosocomial infection and sometimes as hospital-acquired infection.
Helper T-lymphocytes T-lymphocytes, mostly of the CD4+ set, that induce and maintain immune reactions. Two main types, **Th1** and **Th2**, are characterized.
HEPA (high efficiency particulate) filters Special filters that can be used in ventilation systems to help remove droplet nuclei from the air.
Highly active antiretroviral therapy A combination of antiretroviral agents used for the treatment of HIV disease.
HIV Acronym for **human immunodeficiency virus**.
Hong Kong operation A radical operation to prevent and correct deformity in cases of spinal tuberculosis.
Hot tub lung A bizarre and unexplained association between pulmonary disease due to environmental mycobacteria and the practice of bathing in hot tubs.
Human immunodeficiency virus A group of retroviruses – RNA viruses that are reversely transcripted to DNA in the host cell – that are responsible for HIV disease. Two types are recognized – HIV-1 and HIV-2.
Human leucocyte antigens (HLA) A group of molecules on the surface of all cells (except erythrocytes) that are unique to specific individuals and allow the body to distinguish between 'self' and 'non-self'. Also called major histocompatibility complex (MHC) molecules.
Hydrocephalus The accumulation of cerebrospinal fluid in chambers (ventricles) within the

brain. The pressure causes severe damage to the brain and, in infants with pliable skull bones, swelling of the head. It is a serious complication of tuberculous meningitis.

Hypersensitivity reaction An immunological reaction that does more damage to the host than to the causative agent of the reaction.

Hypertrophic enteritis Another name for **Johne's disease**.

Immunoglobulin An antibody molecule. The immunoglobulins are divided into five structural and functional classes – IgA, IgG, IgD, IgE and IgM.

Immunopathology Tissue damage resulting from abnormal, inappropriate or poorly regulated immune reactions including **hypersensitivity reactions**.

Immunosuppression The state in which immune responses fail to function adequately. This may be due to genetic (congenital) factors or later events, such as infection by HIV (acquired).

Immunotherapy The treatment of active disease by vaccines, cytokines, interferons or other immunological reagents.

Inducer T-lymphocytes *See* **Helper T-lymphocytes**.

Induration The disk of firm swelling in a positive tuberculin skin test reaction. It is distinct from non-indurated erythematous reactions, which should not be recorded.

Infection The transmission of an infectious agent from a living host or inanimate object to a human or animal. Sometimes, but inappropriately, used synonymously with 'infectious disease'.

Infectious The potential of humans and animals (and occasionally inanimate objects) to transmit pathogenic microorganisms to other humans and animals.

Infiltrate A collection of fluid and cells in the tissues of the lung; it is visible on a chest X-ray in some people with active pulmonary tuberculosis.

Influenza-like syndrome A side effect of rifampicin. Paradoxically, it is more common when rifampicin is given twice or three times a week than when it is given daily.

Initial drug resistance *See* **Primary drug resistance**.

Insertion sequences Also termed 'jumping genes'; small units of DNA with multiple copies throughout the chromosome, which provide a means of 'fingerprinting' bacteria.

Interferons A group of cytokines produced by T-lymphocytes in response to infection. One of these, gamma interferon (IFN-γ), plays a major role in macrophage activation and granuloma formation in mycobacterial disease.

Interleukins Literally, 'between white cells'; these are **cytokines** that have been well characterized and allocated numbers. Many are involved in immune responses in tuberculosis.

Intermittent (antituberculosis) therapy Therapy administered twice or three times weekly rather than daily. This is acceptable practice provided that all doses are given under direct observation.

Interstitial nephritis, tuberculous A very chronic and non-invasive form of renal tuberculosis that is not easy to diagnose and may proceed to renal failure.

Intracellular pathogens Microorganisms, e.g. the tubercle bacillus, that are resistant to digestion by **phagocytes** and are able to thrive within them.

In vitro Literally, 'in glass'; the occurrence of a biological phenomenon in an inanimate experimental system. In-vitro phenomena do not necessarily reflect what occurs in the living organism.

In vivo Literally, 'in life'; the occurrence of a biological phenomenon in a living organism.

Isoniazid A synthetic agent and one of the first-line antituberculosis drugs. It is particularly effective against actively replicating bacilli in the lung cavities. It is also used for **preventive therapy** in those with latent tuberculosis.

Johne's disease Also called **paratuberculosis** or **hypertrophic enteritis**, this is an intestinal disease of cattle and some other hoofed animals caused by *Mycobacterium avium* var. *paratuberculosis*.

Kanamycin An injectable second-line drug, in the same family (aminoglycoside) as **streptomycin**, used for treating multidrug-resistant tuberculosis.

King's Evil A term used for extrapulmonary tuberculosis, especially cervical lymphadenopathy or **scrofula**. The name refers to the belief that the condition could be healed by the touch of the reigning monarch.

Koch phenomenon A necrotic hypersensitivity reaction induced in the skin of tuberculous guinea-pigs following the injection of tubercle bacilli, leading to destruction of the bacilli and local healing.

Koch postulates Also known as Koch–Henlé postulates; criteria for confirming that a given microorganism is the cause of a specified disease.

Koch, Robert The German microbiologist who discovered the tubercle bacillus in 1882.

Lady Windermere syndrome Pulmonary disease due to environmental mycobacteria in otherwise apparently healthy women; thought to be associated with suppressed coughing.

Lamprene *See* **Clofazimine**.

Langerhans' cells A class of antigen-presenting cells, also termed dendritic cells, found principally in the skin and mucous membranes. Not to be confused with the islets of Langerhans in the pancreas.

Langhans' giant cells Large cells with many nuclei, often in a 'horseshoe' formation. These cells are regularly seen in tuberculous lesions but also occur in granulomas due to other conditions.

Latent tuberculosis A term applied to the status of those infected with the tubercle bacillus but remaining healthy. It is assumed that the tubercle bacilli are in some dormant or resting **persister** state, although the exact nature of this state is hotly debated.

Leprosy A chronic human disease caused by *Mycobacterium leprae* and principally affecting the skin and nerves, leading to disfigurement and deformity.

Löwenstein–Jensen medium The most widely used culture medium for the isolation of tubercle bacilli and other mycobacteria. Basically, it is hard-boiled egg with the addition of glycerol and a few mineral salts.

Lupus vulgaris A very chronic and disfiguring form of skin tuberculosis usually affecting the face. The word *lupus* is possibly a corruption of *lepros* – a term applied in the past to many skin conditions and not just to leprosy.

Lymphadenitis Inflammation of a lymph node. Tuberculous lymphadenitis is one of the commonest forms of extrapulmonary tuberculosis. The lymph nodes of the neck (cervical nodes) are the most commonly affected site.

Lymphadenopathy Any disease of the lymph nodes. The term is often used synonymously with lymphadenitis and usually implies swelling of the nodes.

Lymphocyte Cells of the immune system that are responsible for the recognition of antigen and the mediation of immune reactions. Two main sets are recognized – T and B lymphocytes.

Macrolides A class of antibiotics of which erythromycin is the best-known example. Some newer macrolides – **azithromycin** and **clarithromycin** – are used to treat cases of multidrug-resistant tuberculosis and disease due to certain environmental mycobacteria.

Macrophage One of the classes of phagocytic cells that are particularly involved in chronic infections such as tuberculosis.

MAIS complex A term used in older literature to delineate a group of mycobacteria including *Mycobacterium avium*, *M. intracellulare* and *M. scrofulaceum*.

Mantoux test A method for performing the tuberculin test by injecting a set amount (usually 0.1 mL) of tuberculin into the skin with a hypodermic syringe.
MDR TB Acronym for **multidrug-resistant tuberculosis**.
Memory cells An expanded population of antigen-specific lymphocytes that remain after an infectious disease or vaccination, thereby inducing accelerated immune responses on subsequent challenge by the same antigen(s).
Mesophiles Bacteria that grow over a moderate temperature range.
Meta-analysis The combined analysis of several clinical trials.
Microaerophile A bacterium that grows best in conditions of low oxygen levels, e.g. *Mycobacterium bovis*.
Miliary tuberculosis A form of disseminated tuberculosis occurring in patients with relatively good immune responses. The lesions are millet-seed-sized granulomas (Latin: *milium* – a millet seed) that are easily seen on chest radiographs and, sometimes, on the retina with the use of an ophthalmoscope. Miliary lesions differ from those of **cryptogenic disseminated tuberculosis**.
Monocyte A leucocyte with a round or oval nucleus, to distinguish it from a **polymorphonuclear leucocyte**. Closely related to **macrophages**.
Multidrug-resistant tuberculosis By definition, tuberculosis resistant to rifampicin and isoniazid, with or without resistance to additional drugs.
Mycobacteriophage A virus able to infect and destroy a mycobacterium. These viruses were used in the system of 'phage typing' to subdivide tubercle bacilli for epidemiological purposes before the advent of DNA fingerprinting.
Mycobacteriosis Human or animal disease caused by an **environmental mycobacterium**.
Mycobacterium The name of the genus of bacteria that includes the tubercle and leprosy bacilli and the **environmental mycobacteria**. The name means 'fungus bacteria', in allusion to the mould-like pellicles they form on liquid culture media.
Mycobacterium africanum A member of the *M. tuberculosis* complex, consisting of strains of rather variable properties and mostly found in equatorial Africa.
***Mycobacterium avium* complex (MAC)** A group of closely related mycobacteria containing *M. avium* and *M. intracellulare* which are the commonest **environmental mycobacteria** involved in human disease. (In veterinary usage, the complex also contains *M. paratuberculosis* and *M. lepraemurium*.)
Mycobacterium bovis A member of the *M. tuberculosis* complex and the principal cause of tuberculosis in cattle and an occasional cause of the disease in humans.
Mycobacterium leprae The causative organism of leprosy.
Mycobacterium microti A member of the *M. tuberculosis* complex, also known as the vole tubercle bacillus. It is of low virulence for humans.
Mycobacterium tuberculosis A member of the *M. tuberculosis* complex, also termed the human tubercle bacillus and the predominant cause of human tuberculosis.
***Mycobacterium tuberculosis* complex** A group of very closely related species that cause tuberculosis in humans and other mammals. These are *M. tuberculosis*, *M. bovis*, *M. africanum* and *M. microti* (the vole tubercle bacillus).
Neutrophil A type of granulocyte with faintly staining cytoplasmic granules; it is the principal phagocytic cell in acute bacterial infections.
Nocardia A genus of bacteria, usually weakly acid-fast and branching cells, closely related to the mycobacteria and an occasional cause of human disease, especially in immunocompromised people.
Non-tuberculous mycobacteria Another term for **environmental mycobacteria**, more commonly used in the USA.

Nosocomial disease An adverse occurrence, usually infection, acquired while in hospital or as a result of medical care. *See also* **Healthcare-associated infection**.
Notification The process, required by law in many countries, of informing the appropriate health authority of , for example, a **tuberculosis case**.
Nucleic acid Macromolecules coding for the basic genetic characteristics of an organism. There are two types – deoxyribonucleic acid (DNA) and ribonucleic acid (RNA). DNA is found in the chromosomes within the nucleus and represents the basic genetic 'blueprint' of the cell. RNA consists of three types: messenger RNA (mRNA), which conveys the blueprint for individual proteins to **ribosomes**; ribosomal RNA (rRNA), which is involved in protein synthesis; and transfer RNA (tRNA), which transfers the amino acids required for protein synthesis to the ribosome.
Nucleus In biological terms, the intracellular structure containing the DNA in the form of one or more chromosomes.
Obligate pathogen An organism that can only replicate in a state that causes disease. Obligate pathogens in the genus *Mycobacterium* are the *M. tuberculosis* complex and *M. leprae*.
Old Tuberculin A heat-concentrated filtrate of the medium in which tubercle bacilli have been grown. It was originally produced by Robert Koch in 1891 as a therapeutic agent for tuberculosis, but was subsequently utilized as a skin-testing agent.
Open tuberculosis Infectious tuberculosis with acid-fast bacilli in the sputum.
Opportunist pathogen An organism that does not normally cause disease, but may do so given an 'opportunity', such as immunosuppression or a penetrating injury. Some of the **environmental mycobacteria** are opportunist pathogens.
Opsonization Enhancement of phagocytosis of microorganisms by the binding of antibody and/or complement.
Pandemic A major epidemic that spreads over a very large geographical area or even worldwide.
***Para*-aminosalicylic acid (PAS)** One of the earliest antituberculosis drugs; it is still occasionally used for treating multidrug-resistant tuberculosis.
Paratuberculosis An alternative name for **Johne's disease** or **hypertrophic enteritis**; a chronic intestinal disease of cattle.
Pasteurization Named after Louis Pasteur, a method of killing non-spore-forming pathogens in milk and other fluids by heating to temperatures below boiling.
Pathogen A microorganism able to cause disease. There are two types – obligate and opportunist (or facultative).
Pathogenesis The pathological, physiological and biochemical processes by which a disease develops.
Pericarditis Inflammation or infection of the pericardium – the bag in which the heart lies.
Peripheral neuropathy Damage to the sensory nerves of the hands and feet, causing a tingling sensation or a weakened sense of touch; sometimes caused by the administration of the antituberculosis drug **isoniazid**.
Persister *See* **Latent tuberculosis**.
Phagocyte A cell able to engulf and destroy a microorganism. The two major classes of phagocytes are the **granulocytes** and cells of the **monocyte/macrophage** series.
Phagocytosis The 'eating and digestion' of microorganisms by specialized cells of the immune system. Some pathogens, including the tubercle bacillus, are resistant to digestion and thrive within these phagocytic cells. They are thus referred to as **intracellular pathogens**.

Phlyctenular conjunctivitis Inflammation of the eye with itching or pain, excessive production of tears and sensitivity to light, occasionally occurring in children as a temporary hypersensitivity phenomenon in primary tuberculosis.
Photochromogen A mycobacterium producing pigment (usually yellow) during or after exposure to light.
Phthisis Meaning wasting, an old term for tuberculosis.
Plasma cells Activated B cells that synthesize and secrete antibody.
Plasmids Small additional (extrachromosomal) circular units of DNA that, in some bacterial species, bear functional genes.
Pleura The membranes forming a sac or cavity in which the lungs lie.
Pleural effusion Fluid accumulating in the pleural cavity.
Pleurisy Inflammation of the pleura.
Pneumothorax Air within the pleural cavity restricting the normal expansion of the lung. It may occur as part of the disease process or, in the pre-chemotherapy era, as a therapeutic **artificial pneumothorax**.
Point prevalence The number of cases of a disease in a community at a given point in time.
Polymerase chain reaction (PCR) A technique for amplifying a few specific fragments of DNA in a clinical specimen to millions of fragments that are easily detectable.
Polymorphonuclear leucocytes Also known as polymorphs or polys; white blood cells of the granulocyte series with lobed nuclei. These cells include neutrophils, eosinophils and basophils.
Poncet's disease A form of arthritis, thought to be due to immune reactions, occurring in a small minority of patients with active tuberculosis. It usually resolves when the underlying tuberculosis is successfully treated.
Post-primary tuberculosis Tuberculosis occurring after a period of latency following initial infection (usually appearing 5 or more years after initial infection). The usual site, irrespective of the site of the initial infection, is the apex of the lung, and tissue necrosis leading to cavity formation is evident.
Pott's disease Spinal tuberculosis; named after Sir Percival Pott (1714–1788), a surgeon at St Bartholomew's Hospital, London.
PPD Acronym for **Purified Protein Derivative** of tuberculin.
Prevalence The number of cases of an infectious disease at a given time in a specified population; usually either the number of cases over a year (**annual prevalence**) or at any specified time (**point prevalence**).
Preventive therapy A course of one or more antituberculosis drugs given to those with latent tuberculosis (usually indicated by a positive tuberculin reaction) to prevent the development of active disease.
Primary complex The initial lesion of tuberculosis, consisting of lesions at the site of implantation of the bacilli and in the lymph nodes draining that site.
Primary drug resistance Resistance as a result of infection of a patient by a strain of tubercle bacillus already resistant to one or more drugs.
Primary tuberculosis Active tuberculosis occurring within 5 years of initial infection by the tubercle bacillus.
Progressive primary tuberculosis Direct progression from primary to post-primary lesions without an intervening phase of latency.
Prophylactic therapy A course of antituberculosis drugs given to uninfected people at very high risk of infection to prevent active disease should they become infected.
Prosector's wart *See* **Butcher's wart**.

Pulmonary tuberculosis Tuberculosis of the lung – the most common form of tuberculosis.
Purified Protein Derivative (PPD) A derivative of tuberculin prepared by harvesting precipitated proteins. It is less likely to give non-specific reactions than unpurified tuberculin.
Pyopneumothorax The combination of a **pneumothorax** and **empyema**.
Pyrazinamide One of the first-line antituberculosis drugs.
Pyridoxine Vitamin B6. This is often prescribed with antituberculosis drugs to prevent certain side effects of isoniazid on the nervous system.
Radiometry A rapid automated system for the detection of bacterial growth, based on the liberation of radioactive carbon dioxide from a radiolabelled substrate.
Regimen A prescribed course of therapy or remedial activity. In the case of infectious disease, a course of antimicrobial agents over a specified time.
Resistance, antimicrobial The ability, either natural or acquired by mutation, of a microorganism to resist inhibition or destruction by an antimicrobial agent at a specified concentration or dosage.
Respirator A special type of facemask that is capable of filtering out droplet nuclei and is used for **personal respiratory protection**.
Respiratory droplets Airborne particles of various sizes produced by coughing and sneezing.
Restriction fragment length polymorphism (RFLP) typing The principal technique used for 'fingerprinting' bacteria for epidemiological purposes.
Re-treatment regimens Courses of antituberculosis drugs given to patients who are not cured by standard therapy or who relapse after the completion of treatment.
Ribosomes Small structures (organelles) within cells in which protein is synthesized.
Ribotyping A system for identifying bacteria (and other life forms), usually at the species level, according to structural differences in their ribosomal RNA.
Rifampicin (rifampin in the USA) A member of a class of antibiotics termed the **rifamycins**; the most powerful of the first-line antituberculosis drugs. It has the unique property of killing very slowly replicating bacilli that persist in lesions.
RNA Acronym for **ribonucleic acid**. *See* **Nucleic acid**.
Safe school age The period of life between late infancy and puberty in which children appear relatively immune to tuberculosis.
Scotochromogen A mycobacterium producing pigment (usually yellow) in the dark.
Scrofula An old name for tuberculosis of the cervical (neck) lymph nodes; in previous times often the result of drinking cows' milk containing *Mycobacterium bovis*.
Scrofuloderma Skin tuberculosis spreading from a sinus overlying a tuberculous lymph node or other lesion.
Second-line (antituberculosis) drugs Drugs used to treat patients with drug-resistant tuberculosis or those who develop serious adverse reactions to first-line drugs.
Sensitivity (of a diagnostic test) The measure of the ability of a test to detect a characteristic of a disease (such as microscopical detection of acid-fast bacilli) when it is present.
Short-course chemotherapy (for tuberculosis) A term used for modern antituberculosis regimens, usually lasting 6 months, to distinguish them from the older regimens of 18 months' duration.
Slim disease A wasting condition particularly associated with AIDS. Tuberculosis may be the principal or contributing cause.
Source case A person (or animal) from whom others have acquired an infectious disease.
Specificity (of a diagnostic test) The measure of the ability of the test to distinguish between those with and those without the disease.

Sporotrichoid spread Secondary lesions in the lymphatics proximal to a mycobacterial lesion on a limb, as also occurs in the fungal disease sporotrichosis.
Sputum Phlegm coughed up from the lung; the commonest specimen submitted for bacteriological investigation for tuberculosis. Often but erroneously termed 'spit', it must not be confused with saliva.
Sputum conversion The disappearance of microscopically detectable acid-fast bacilli from sputum smears during the course of therapy. Also applied to the disappearance of viable mycobacteria demonstrable by cultivation.
Sputum induction A process (usually involving the use of bronchodilators, inhaled saline aerosols and physiotherapy) to obtain sputum from patients who cannot produce it spontaneously.
Sputum smear Sputum spread on a microscope slide and stained for acid-fast bacilli. Patients are reported as sputum smear negative or positive.
Steroids *See* **Corticosteroids**.
Stevens–Johnson syndrome A very serious and often fatal skin eruption occasionally caused by antituberculosis drugs, notably **thiacetazone** in HIV-positive individuals.
Streptomycin The first effective antituberculosis drug, discovered by Albert Schatz and Selman Waksman in 1944. It is still used, especially in **re-treatment regimens**, but must be given by injection.
Suppressor T-lymphocytes T-lymphocytes, predominantly of the CD8+ class, that suppress or down-regulate immune responses.
Swimming pool granuloma Also called fish tank granuloma; a chronic warty skin lesion resembling **lupus vulgaris** and caused by *Mycobacterium marinum*. It occurs particularly in those acquiring superficial injuries in swimming pools and in keepers of aquaria.
Symptomatic Having symptoms suggestive of a given disease.
Syndrome A group of symptoms and clinical signs that characterize a disease.
Taxonomy The science of classification of life forms. Bacteria are divided into genera, e.g. *Mycobacterium*, which are then divided into various species, e.g. *Mycobacterium tuberculosis*, *Mycobacterium avium*.
Th1 and Th2 T-lymphocytes Functional T helper cells resulting from different maturation pathways of helper T cells, characterized by the **cytokines** that they secrete.
Thermophiles Bacteria that grow preferentially at high temperatures.
Thiacetazone A weak antituberculosis drug with the dubious advantage of cheapness but the distinct disadvantage of causing serious and sometimes fatal skin reactions, especially in HIV-positive people.
Thoracoplasty A major operation once used to collapse parts of the lung, thereby closing tuberculous cavities, by excision of segments of the chest wall.
Tine test A technique for performing the tuberculin test by means of a single-use device with four prongs (tines) coated with dried tuberculin.
T-lymphocytes Also termed T cells; the cells of the immune system that recognize antigen and initiate various immune reactions. Divided into functional subsets according to their CD (cluster differentiation) antigens.
Transkei heart A term for tuberculous pericarditis, reflecting the unexplained frequency of this condition in the Transkei.
Transmission parameter Another term for **contagion parameter**.
Treatment failure A failure of a patient to respond to treatment of tuberculosis manifesting as a failure to become bacteriologically negative or by worsening of symptoms.
Tubercle Literally, 'a small potato'; the characteristic macroscopic lesions of tuberculosis consisting of a granuloma or cluster of granulomas.

Tuberculides Small necrotic skin lesions, usually multiple, occasionally seen in patients with tuberculosis, especially in the tropics. They are thought to be hypersensitivity reactions to circulating tubercle bacilli, or fragments thereof, which lodge in the skin.
Tuberculin *See* **Old Tuberculin**.
Tuberculin reaction The indurated swelling in the skin induced by injection of tuberculin.
Tuberculin test The skin test that elicits the tuberculin reaction. The methods used today are the **Mantoux**, **Heaf** and **tine** tests.
Tuberculoma A large tuberculous lesion appearing as a tumour-like mass on radiology.
Tuberculosis A chronic infectious disease caused by the closely related species *Mycobacterium tuberculosis*, *M. bovis* and *M. africanum*.
Tuberculosis case An epidemiological term for an instance of diagnosed tuberculosis. The term should only be used to refer to the disease itself, never to the patient with the disease. In some countries there is a legal requirement for **notification** of all cases to the designated health authority.
Tuberculosis orificialis cutis Skin tuberculosis resulting from implantation of bacilli in sputum into minor dermal abrasions, usually around the mouth.
Tumour necrosis factor-alpha (TNFα) A cytokine that, depending on underlying immune regulatory mechanisms, contributes to granuloma formation or gross tissue necrosis as seen in cavitating pulmonary tuberculosis.
Vaccination Derived from the latin *vacca* (a cow), this originally referred to immunization with cowpox to protect against smallpox, but now refers to immunization against any infectious agent.
Virulence A measure of the 'power' of a microorganism to cause disease.
Virus A very small infectious particle containing either RNA or DNA, but never both, and only able to replicate within living cells. Despite the widespread belief of journalists, tuberculosis is *not* caused by a virus, but by a bacterium.
Vole tubercle bacillus The unofficial name for *Mycobacterium microti*.
Ziehl–Neelsen staining The name given to the most widely used technique for acid-fast staining of mycobacteria.
Zoonosis A disease that is normally transmitted between animals but may also be transmitted to humans.

Index

Note: bold numbers indicate glossary references.

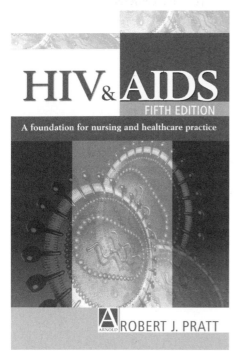

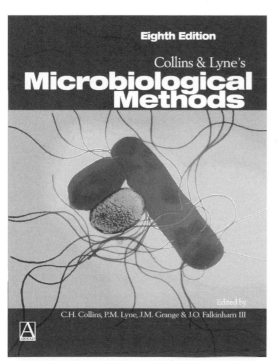